The Pathology of Organ Transplantation

The Pathology of Organ Transplantation

Edited by
George E. Sale, M.D.
Professor of Pathology, University of Washington, Seattle;
Associate Member, Fred Hutchinson Cancer Research Center

With 15 Contributing Authors

Butterworths
Boston London Singapore Sydney Toronto Wellington

Every effort has been made to ensure the drug dosage schedules within this text are accurate and conform to standards accepted at time of publication. However, as treatment recommendations vary in the light of continuing research and clinical experience, the reader is advised to verify drug dosage schedules herein with information found on product information sheets. This is especially true in cases of new or infrequently used drugs.

Library of Congress Cataloging-in-Publication Data

The Pathology of organ transplantation.

Includes bibliographies and index.
1. Transplantation of organs, tissues, etc.—Complications and sequelae. I. Sale, George E.
[DNLM: 1. Postoperative Complications.
2. Transplantation—adverse effects. W0 660 P297]
RD120.7.P37 1990 617.9′5 89-15788
ISBN 0-409-90133-4

British Library Cataloguing in Publication Data
The Pathology of organ transplantation.
1. Man. Organs. Transplantation
I. Sale, George E.
617′.95

ISBN 0-409-90133-4

Butterworth Publishers
80 Montvale Avenue
Stoneham, MA 02180

10 9 8 7 6 5 4 3 2 1

Printed in the United States of America

To the donors

Contents

Contributing Authors

Juhani Ahonen, M.D., Ph.D.
Director, Section of Transplantation, Department of Surgery, Helsinki University Central Hospital, Helsinki, Finland

Margaret E. Billingham, M.D.
Professor of Pathology, Stanford University, Stanford, California

John Chandler, M.D.
Professor and Chairman, Department of Ophthalmology, University of Wisconsin–Madison, Madison, Wisconsin

Wayne W. Hancock, M.D., Ph.D.
Assistant Professor of Pathology, Surgical Research Division, University of Connecticut Hospital, Farmington, Connecticut

Pekka Häyry, M.D., Ph.D.
Professor of Transplantation Surgery and Immunology and Director of Transplantation Laboratory, University of Helsinki, Helsinki, Finland

James L. Madara, M.D.
Associate Professor of Pathology, Harvard Medical School, Brigham and Women's Hospital, Boston, Massachusetts

Wolfgang Muller-Ruchholtz, M.D.
Professor of Immunology, Medical School of the University, Kiel, Federal Republic of Germany

George F. Murphy, M.D.
Professor of Dermatopathology, University of Pennsylvania, Philadelphia, Pennsylvania

George E. Sale, M.D.
Professor of Pathology, University of Washington, Associate Member, Fred Hutchinson Cancer Research Center, Seattle, Washington

Fred Sanfilippo, M.D.
Professor of Pathology, Transplantation and Immunopathology Laboratories, Duke University Medical Center, Durham, North Carolina

Richard K. Sibley, M.D.
Associate Professor of Pathology, Stanford University Medical Center, Stanford, California

Dale C. Snover, M.D.
Professor of Pathology, Department of Laboratory Medicine and Pathology, University of Minnesota–Twin Cities, Minneapolis, Minnesota

Henry D. Tazelaar, M.D.
Assistant Professor of Pathology, Senior Associate Consultant, Mayo Clinic Foundation, Rochester, Minnesota

Eeva von Willebrand, M.D., Ph.D.
Docent in Immunology, Transplantation Laboratory, University of Helsinki, Helsinki, Finland

Samuel A. Yousem, M.D.
Assistant Professor of Pathology, Presbyterian University Hospital of Pittsburgh, Pittsburgh, Pennsylvania

Preface

Organ transplants have assumed a major position in modern medical progress. A National Institutes of Health symposium in 1985 emphasized that for live organ transplantation, seminal advances had occurred in heart, heart-lung, liver, and pancreatic transplants in the preceding three years. When these are added to previous success in renal and marrow transplantation, the field embraces the whole range of diseased human organs. Both the medical economics and the ethics of transplantation have been intensified foci of analytic and policy studies. Econometric studies reviewed by a recent government-sponsored transplantation panel headed by Professor Olga Jonasson of Chicago showed that transplantation is already quite cost effective in persons with chronic renal failure, acute myelogenous leukemia, aplastic anemia, and other hematologic diseases. By now, clinical transplantation has become a major new discipline that crosses conventional interdisciplinary boundaries within the basic and clinical sciences. Departments entirely devoted to transplantation have arisen in Britain, Sweden, Kuwait, Canada, and elsewhere. Here, surgeons, internists, and immunologists team up to cross-fertilize ideas and techniques between fields. Renal and marrow transplants have been used to cure inborn errors of metabolism, to note but two examples. When I was first approached by Butterworth Publishers to edit a book on this subject, the usual anxieties gripped my chest, including doubts about the ripeness of the subject matter. Further inquiries among colleagues outside marrow transplantation convinced me that such a collection would be needed soon. The existence of unified departments of transplantation made it evident that a discipline of transplantation pathology would have to follow in the wake of these new developments. Several of the contributing authors embody that discipline. Our own experience with the expansion of marrow transplantation has clearly indicated the need to disseminate the stern lessons of caring for this fragile patient population. Hence, this book is aimed at pathologists in practice and in referral centers who are already faced with the care of transplant recipients.

Future clinical transplant research will be eclectic and sophisticated. Exciting new currents include adrenal medullary transplants for persons with Parkinson's disease, transfection of methotrexate resistance genes into canine bone marrow [1], and studies of quail-chick chimeras, which demonstrate the ability to transplant behavioral characteristics in embryos [2]. Unresolved ethical issues include the use of human fetal or embryonic tissues.

We are privileged to have assembled a distinguished international group of pathologists, surgeons, internists, and other scientists with experience in clinical transplantation pathology, some with the largest experience in their fields. Dr. Muller-Ruchholtz has broad expertise in the immunopathology of transplantation. Among his major contributions are studies of T-cell depletion in the field of bone marrow transplantation that stimulated a whole wave of clinical trials. Drs. Snover, Sibley, Billingham, Sanfilippo, Madara, Häyry, and the others have worked with major transplant teams in their respective fields and have unique or highly current experience in the experimental and clinical problems in transplanting these organs.

I am grateful for the promptness, enthusiasm, and patience of the contributors and the help I have received from our editors at Butterworth Publishers, Nancy Megley and Susan Warner.

References

1. Lehn PM. Gene therapy using bone marrow transplantation. Bone Marrow Transplant 1987;1:243–58.
2. Balaban E, Teillet M-A, Le Douarin N. Application of the quail-chick chimera system to the study of brain development and behavior. Science 1988;241:1339–45.

Acknowledgments

I would like to thank my colleagues at the Fred Hutchinson Cancer Research Center, particularly Howard Shulman, Robert Hackman, David Myerson, and Betty Gallucci for their support and collaboration of several years and for permission to reproduce some illustrations. In addition, Charles Mahan, Kathleen Schaefers, Lori Richey, Randy Acker, Mary Browne, Clara Bryan, Rudy Lizama, and Clyde Cook have helped with technical work, and Regina Warmoth and Colleen Tuttle have done superb work on the manuscript. A word of thanks for the leadership of the senior faculty in the marrow transplant unit is also appropriate (Reginald Clift, E. Donnall Thomas, Rainer Storb, C. Dean Buckner, and Alex Fefer).

G.E.S.

The Pathology of Organ Transplantation

1

The Immunopathology of Transplantation

WOLFGANG MULLER-RUCHHOLTZ

Transplantation means surmounting the biologic barrier between individuals—one of the dreams of humankind for thousands of years. Interestingly, in Christian history this was considered to be the work not of the devil but of the saints: sculptures and paintings from various places in Europe show the two saints of the medical profession, St. Cosmas and St. Damian, grafting a deceased black man's leg onto a white patient whose own leg had been amputated (Fig. 1.1).

More scientific attention began in the second half of the nineteenth century. Various hypotheses were elaborated to explain the typical results, namely, lack of success. Paul Ehrlich was the first to propose an explanation that was upheld by some scientists until the middle of this century: the primary (!) cause was lack of nutrition in the grafted tissue. Others thought of blood group incompatibilities, i.e., a mechanism similar to that leading to blood transfusion accidents. The pathologist Leo Loeb and his school proposed not group, but individual, specificity; the genetic differences between graft and host were thought to lead to toxic sequences. The origin of the fourth hypothesis, immunologic reactions specific to the individual, dates back to Ehrlich's days and was favored by opponents of Ehrlich, most notably Bashford and Rous. Until the late 1940s, the influential Loeb sharply

Figure 1.1
St. Cosmas and St. Damian, twin brothers coming from Arabia, graft the leg of a deceased black man onto a leprous white patient. They are assisted by three angels. This painting was made in tempera on fir wood at the beginning of the sixteenth century in the Swabian area. It is owned by the Wurttembergische Landesmuseum in Stuttgart, Federal Republic of Germany.

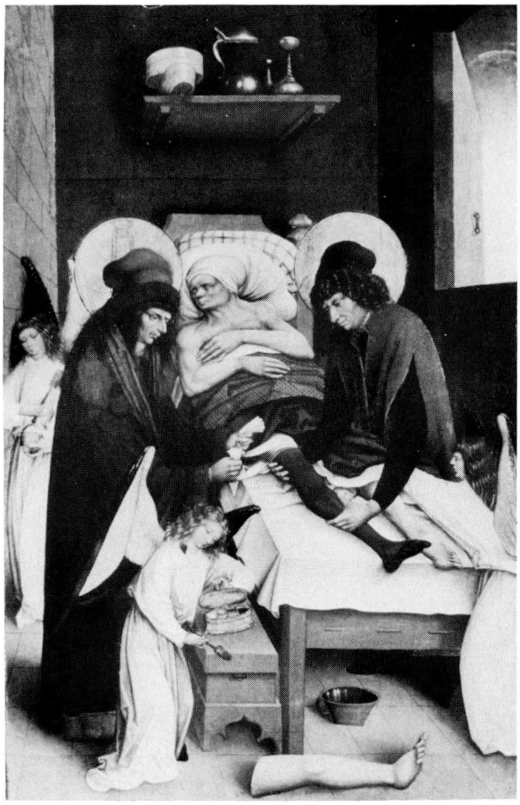

opposed this view and claimed that a second graft would not elicit more intense reactions than the first one did, as would be expected from immunologic reactions. However, Loeb's methods did not ensure that a second graft was derived from the same source.

In 1944 Medawar used an experimental design allowing clear and reproducible observations to present definite evidence for the immunologic nature of foreign graft rejection. Skin grafts were performed between different individuals (originally rabbits); they were rejected faster and with more intense reactions when the second graft came from the same donor.

The concept of immunologic tolerance was advanced by Burnet and Fenner in 1949. They were concerned with explaining how self-components of the vertebrate organism appear to be eliminated without an immune response, and they assumed that all antigens encountered in early developmental stages are recognized as self and therefore do not elicit immune responses. They correctly postulated that self-recognition is acquired early in ontogenesis and would not be inherited. Furthermore, Burnet postulated that foreign antigens presented during the early stages of development will be treated by the body like self-components; i.e., they will induce a state of specific, immunologic unresponsiveness.

First reports on experimentally induced transplantation tolerance were published in 1953 by Billingham, Brent, and Medawar: When mouse embryos of strain CBA were injected with cell suspensions from strain A (this was replaced shortly thereafter by intravenous injections in newborns within 24 hours of birth), these CBA mice specifically tolerated A skin for more than one year, even when it was grafted during adulthood. About the same time, Hasek and coworkers in Prague, Czechoslovakia, joined the chorioallantoic membranes of two different avian embryos. The membranes developed vascular anastomoses, and the embryos exchanged blood; grafts exchanged between the partners in adulthood were specifically accepted.

Today the whole field of immunology may be called "the science of self-nonself discrimination" [1]. Or, in other words, the immune system serves the vital requirement of maintaining an organism's individuality and integrity, especially when it is as advanced evolutionarily as birds and mammals are. Obviously, then, immune reactivity and transplantation after the early stage of ontogeny compete conceptually with each other.

General Graft Terminology

Autograft An *autograft* is a transplant taken from the recipient. If proper surgical procedures are used, an autograft is permanently accepted, since it does not contain any foreign antigens.

Syngeneic Graft A transplant taken from a donor who is (almost) genetically identical is a *syngeneic graft*. Again, no immunogenic foreign antigens are provided, and thus the graft is accepted. Such is the case with identical twins. Also, animals of an inbred strain mutually accept any graft. Each animal of an inbred strain is considered homozygous at all genetic loci; animals have the same alleles at corresponding loci. This genetic state is achieved with high probability after 20 generations of brother-sister mating. Large numbers of genetically well-defined inbred strains exist in the mouse and rat; some exist in guinea pig, hamster, rabbit, and domestic fowl. However, Y chromosome–determined transplantation antigens exist, and in certain strains they may be strong enough to elicit graft rejection between sexes.

Allograft (Formerly Homograft) An *allograft* is a transplant from a genetically different individual of the same species, be it of outbred origin (virtually always in the clinical situation) or from another inbred strain (as should be the case in a well-controlled experiment). An allograft is usually rejected within a few days or weeks, depending on the number and immunogenic strength of the antigens present in the graft but absent in the recipient.

Coisogenic, Congenic, and Recombinant Strain Grafts Two inbred strains have different alleles at at least one of their genetic loci, but never at all of them. A *coisogenic* strain differs at only one locus. This random event can be achieved only by mutation. Grafting to such a strain would allow us to pinpoint the role the alleles at this particular locus play in graft rejection. The immunogenetic researcher cannot wait for these events and compromises by producing a *congenic* strain. It differs at a number of linked genes only and can be obtained by successive backcrossings. *Recombinant* strains are derived by crossing two inbred strains and intercrossing first their F1 progeny and then several of their F2 progeny, followed by continuous brother-sister mating. Such strains are useful for detecting the linkage of newly identified genes and singling out their role in allograft rejection.

Xenograft (Formerly Heterograft) A *xenograft* is a transplant from a donor belonging to a different species than the recipient. The evolutionary relationship between donor and recipient determines the grade of xenogeneity. Because of the pronounced antigenic disparity, a xenograft is usually rejected more quickly than an allograft. Often the presence of cross-reactive "natural" antibodies initiates hyperacute rejection.

Transplantation (Histocompatibility) Antigens

The cytoplasmic membranes of all nucleated cells contain a wide variety of molecules that come into contact with the immunologically competent cells of the allogeneic recipient if the cells are grafted. This is similar to what occurs with genetically determined surface structures of erythrocytes (the so-called blood group substances) in that only some, but by far not all of those substances that are foreign to the recipient elicit an immune response.

Non–Major Histocompatibility Complex Antigens Relevant to Transplantation

In addition to the major histocompatibility complex (MHC, see below), a multitude of distinct histocompatibility antigens have been identified [2,3,23]; each is genetically determined by one allele at a given locus. In the mouse, more than 40 histocompatibility loci at 12 chromosome pairs have been recognized thus far, but the role many of their gene products play in allograft rejection is controversial. The cell surface expression of these gene products varies remarkably among cells; many appear to be restricted to certain cell types (e.g., the Ly series on lymphocytes, Pca on plasma cells, Sk-1 on skin) or to groups of cell types (such as Thy-1 on T lymphocytes and brain). In all other species in which studies on histocompatibility genes have been performed, the existence of a large number of independently segregating loci has been confirmed. The potential of their cell surface gene products to elicit antibody production in a graft recipient does not necessarily imply the initiation of rejection reactions.

Non-MHC antigens have also been termed minor histocompatibility antigens because an individual alloreaction, if triggered, is much weaker than an MHC response. In mice or rats, a non-MHC allogeneic skin graft will be rejected after 20 to 100 days, whereas MHC allogeneic skin is rejected after 7 or 8 days. However, the sum of multiple non-MHC histoincompatibilities may well mount up to a rejection response that is as vigorous as that against MHC. Nevertheless, non-MHC responses can be prevented (rather than overcome following sensitization) more efficiently by immunosuppressive treatment. Furthermore, it is relatively easy to induce tolerance.

Minor lymphocyte stimulating (Mls) antigens are murine alloantigens, which exhibit characteristics quite unlike those of other minor histocompatibility antigens. The Mls-1 locus has two alleles; additional loci are called Mls-2, etc. Mls-1^a activates unprimed T-lymphocytes even at higher frequencies than MHC antigens and, again in contrast to the other minors, T-cell clones recognize this antigen without MHC restriction (see below). But antibodies specific for the Mls-1^a antigen have not yet been isolated. Mls-1^b, on the other hand, is nonstimulating.

In human beings the non-MHC transplantation antigens are less well studied than in other species, but we know of their immunobiologic importance from clinical experience in transplantation between MHC-identical siblings. Most skin grafts are rejected at 15 to 30 days, and no grafted organ is accepted without long-standing immunosuppressive treatment. Still more impressive is the high incidence of lethal graft-vs-host reactions (GVHRs) in MHC-identical bone marrow recipients, despite careful immunosuppressive treatment. Among the known "minors" in humans are ABO blood groups (compatibility is required in most clinical transplantation), the Lewis blood group antigens, the Y (male sex-linked) histocompatibility antigen, and vascular endothelial cell-, monocyte-, and granulocyte-specific antigens.

Major Histocompatibility Complex Antigens

As mentioned, it was early suggested that blood group–like incompatibilities were responsible for allograft rejection. This idea led Gorer (beginning in 1936) to identify a group of antigens in mouse erythrocytes and nucleated cells that were termed histocompatibility antigens H-2 because their identity in donor and recipient markedly improved graft survival. The discovery of a remarkably similar system of antigens in human nucleated cells began in 1954 with Dausset's observation that patients who had received multiple blood transfusions had leukocyte-agglutinating antibodies in their sera. From these studies evolved the description (Dausset, 1958) of the first leukocyte antigen (termed Mac, today HLA-A2) of the so-called human leukocyte system A. It was much later (1968), however, that the term HLA became universally adopted (by the World Health Organization [WHO]) and that HLA was shown to be unequivocally involved in graft rejection. Today it is clear that MHC is the major antigenic determinant of graft rejection. Interestingly, analogous MHC systems have been found in all other mammalian species studied.

Despite the tremendous importance of this complex system in transplantation [1,4], its biologic role is not to complicate humankind's desire to graft tissue. Rather, its molecules appear to regulate cell interactions and are of great biologic importance. Much has been learned about their role in the interaction between immunocompetent cells (see below), but we believe that much more must be learned about their functions. Additionally, MHC is associated with several poorly understood human diseases. The best known is HLA-B27 with ankylosing spondylitis (90% of whites with this disorder

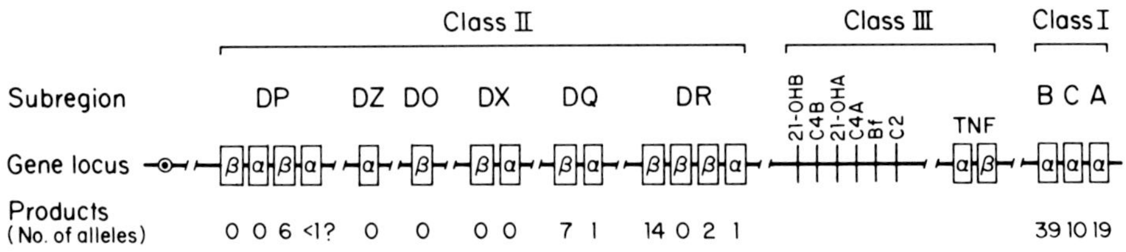

Figure 1.2
MHC region of human chromosome 6. It is located between 6p21.1 and 6p21.3 and includes several gene families clustered in distinct regions. Class I and class II genes encode cell-surface glycoproteins. They are mapped as presently understood. The number and order of the loci remain to be confirmed. Some genes do not appear to be expressed. Some loci demonstrate a genetic polymorphism which is not detectable, as yet, at the cell surface expression level. The total number of allelic products is almost certainly not yet known. So-called class III genes encode the complement factors C2, Bf, C4A, and C4B, and comprise two steroid 21-hydroxylase genes (A and B) and the closely linked tumor necrosis factor (TNF) α and β genes. Not shown are 17 additional class I genes which occur at the telomeric end of the MHC linked to HLA-A. Of these, only HLA-E (the 6.2 gene), the 6.0 gene (HLA-G?), and the 5.4 gene (HLA-F?) are known to be intact.

but only 7% to 9% of the normal population are B27-positive, and a relative risk value of 91 is calculated). Recently MHC molecules have been identified in a number of rodent models as olfactory recognition cues; we have been able to show that a normally restituted MHC fully allogeneic bone marrow graft recipient has not only altered its hemopoietic self but also its odor by superimposing the donor's odor upon its own.

The human MHC is encoded at the shorter arm of chromosome 6 (Fig. 1.2). It comprises a class I and a class II gene family, presumably generated by gene duplication and subsequent diversification events, and, in between, unrelated genes coding for complement components and an enzyme involved in steroid biosynthesis. At present, 17 class I genes and 14 class II genes have been cloned from human DNA. The fascinating polymorphism in MHC alleles and the remarkable variations in gene frequency and linkage disequilibria obviously were established during evolution by selection forces that are still poorly understood and that may be related to the capacity of MHC molecules to present foreign antigens to T lymphocytes (see below).

The gene products on the cell surface are heterodimers consisting of an alpha polypeptide chain noncovalently associated to a beta polypeptide chain (Fig. 1.3). These chains are folded into one or several discrete domains, some of which are stabilized by a disulfide bridge. The class I alpha chain forms highly polymorphic extracellular domains in addition to a transmembrane part and an intracytoplasmic tail. The corresponding beta-2m chain is monomorphic, entirely extracellular, and encoded by a gene on chromosome 15. The class II alpha and beta chains are both membrane anchored and form two extracellular domains; their polymorphism appears to be mainly beta chain–determined (see Fig. 1.2). It is interesting to note that the differences between amino acids that determine specificity are mostly clustered in certain hypervariable regions. Taking into considerations het-

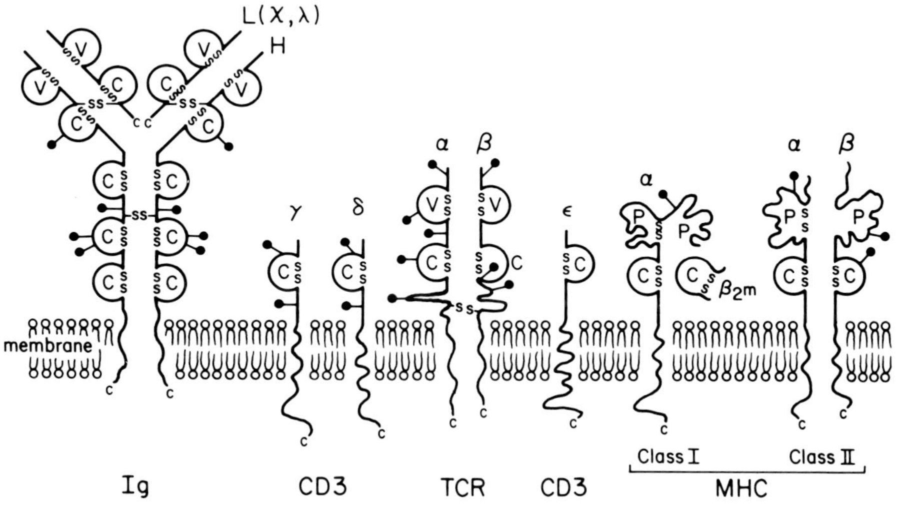

Figure 1.3
Immunoglobulin gene superfamily. A group of molecules appears to be evolutionarily derived from a primordial cell surface receptor. Depicted are only those members that are involved in immune reactions, i.e., antigen handling. Note the composition of polypeptide domains (homology units), a number of which are rather constant (c). Immunoglobulin (Ig) and T cell receptor (TCR) contain variable domains (v), the structures of which are encoded by genes resulting from gene rearrangement in individual lymphocyte maturation. MHC class I and II molecules contain polymorphic domains (p) whose structures are constant in the individual but have emerged from remarkable variations in phylogeny. N-linked carbohydrate sites are indicated by the symbol ⚲. *Not shown are the polypeptide chains γ and δ of the recently detected TCRγδ which are similar to the shown TCRαβ.*

erozygosity and codominant gene expression, it becomes obvious that nature can construct an enormous number of combinations of HLA molecules. Thus, it is very difficult to find two individuals who express completely identical HLA specificities, except among siblings and, possibly, among carriers of more frequent haplotypes.

Wherever it is impossible to obtain HLA identity between graft donor and recipient, tissue typing attempts to select combinations following certain rules:

1. For practical purposes, typing concentrates mainly on antigens encoded by the subregions A, B, and DR (see Fig. 1.2) using lymphocytotoxicity tests.
2. A maximum of subregion identity is sought.
3. No unequivocal evidence for major differences in various antigens' immunogenic strength has been obtained, but a large number of cross-reactivities of different grades have been established within the A, B, and DR antigen molecule groups, presumably based on partial epitope sharing or similarity.

Thus, certain HLA molecules are (evolutionarily) more related to each other, providing fewer immunogenic configurations. Taken together, not only non-MHC but also MHC incompatibilities comprise a broad range of variation that deserves much more consideration than it usually attracts.

Expression Patterns of MHC Molecules on Cell Surfaces

It has been stated that class I antigens are ubiquitous on nucleated cells, whereas class II antigen distribution is constitutively restricted, mainly to B lymphocytes, macrophages, and cells of the Langerhans and dendritic cell series. Such a generalization of ubiquitous vs restricted cannot be upheld. Class I antigens are not detectable on all cells in vivo, and the extent of class II antigen expression depends on a variety of physiologic and abnormal influences. For class II antigen expression the "tissue hormone"–like mediator molecules gamma interferon (up) and prostaglandins of the E class (down) appear to be capable of providing a "push-pull" effect, and various substances directly or indirectly upregulate (e.g., indomethacin, lipopolysaccharides) or downregulate (e.g., glucocorticoids, cyclosporine). Whereas gamma interferon (produced by activated T cells) is a potent inducer of both class II and I antigens, the alpha and beta interferons (produced by a variety of different cells) generally induce class I antigens only.

Interestingly, the physiologic, clearly nonimmunologic events that concur with appearance or increase of class II antigen expression are poorly appreciated. We have shown in rats that the number of class II antigen-positive islet beta cells increases significantly and continuously during syngeneic pregnancy, up to 85%. Others have reported the induction of these antigens in mouse breast epithelial cells in response to lactogenic hormone and lactation. In contrast, there are numerous reports on induced class II antigen expression on at least some cells of virtually every organ under a variety of abnormal conditions. They deal mainly with immunologic reactions, ranging from viral infections and autoaggression to graft rejection, and are mainly interpreted as the consequence of gamma interferon, released from the T lymphocytes involved.

Obviously, the biologic role of MHC molecule expression and its variations on a large variety of cells are still unclear. However, its immunologic importance for allograft rejection is clear [4,5]. All tissue grafts show strongly class I–positive vascular endothelial cells, whereas parenchymal cells, such as renal tubular cells or hepatocytes, have been reported to be only weakly positive; others, such as exocrine pancreas acinar cells or myocardial cells, are negative. For class II antigen expression, at the beginning of transplantation, interstitial macrophages and dendritic cells are the strongly positive cells, whereas vascular endothelial cells vary with strain and species from negative to moderately positive. Similar variations can be seen in certain parenchymal cells, such as renal tubular cells or pancreatic islet beta cells. A remarkable induction and increase of both class I and II antigen expression occurs as soon as the graft rejection reactions start, leading to an amplification loop, i.e., the graft contributes to its own destruction.

With regard to DR, DQ, and DP, the MHC class II subregions in the human, our knowledge of differences in expression in different organs under the various conditions is still very limited and certainly requires more study.

Basic Events in the Immune Response

A simplified outline of the cell interactions that take place in antigen presentation, recognition, regulation, and effector events is given in Figure 1.4.

Antigen Presentation

The immune system recognizes foreign antigens in two distinct ways. Whereas immunoglobulins can bind antigens directly, T cells recognize antigens only if they are presented to them together with MHC molecules or if they are allo-MHC molecules. The best-studied antigen-presenting cells (APC) are dendritic cells and macrophages showing three features: (1) uptake of the antigen, internalization, and processing if necessary, (2) expression of their own MHC class II molecules, and (3) secretion of amplification/

Figure 1.4
Cell interactions for immunologic recognition of and attack against grafts (simplified outline). Black triangles, MHC class II antigen; black squares, MHC class I antigen; dashed lines, second signal, such as IL-1; APC, antigen-presenting cells of the recipient. Lymphokine effects: B helper (IL-4) and T8 helper (IL-2), graft MHC expression (gamma IFN), macrophage activity (gamma IFN). Non-MHC antigens are not indicated; they are recognized and targeted with the help of MHC molecules.

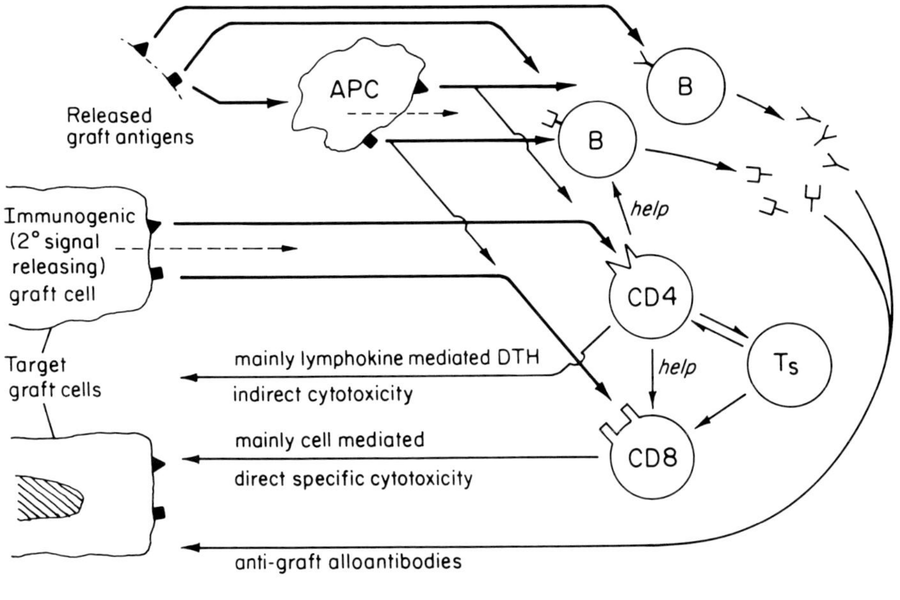

activation molecules, such as interleukin-1 (IL-1), which are required for T-cell activation [6,25,26,29,31,32].

Processing appears to involve cleavage of protein antigens into smaller peptides. Only certain fragments of a protein can serve as antigenic epitopes, determined by the requirement that peptides be able to bind to MHC molecules. Antigens are shuttled into endosomes, followed by strictly limited and regulated proteolysis, creating epitopes in association with MHC molecules and allowing re-presentation of these peptides on the APC surface. Presumably, shedding and neosynthesis of MHC is the main mechanism by which the system is renewed. Recent data have suggested that exogenous antigens would be mainly presented by class II molecules and endogenous antigens by class I.

The three-dimensional structure of the antigen-binding site of a human MHC class I molecule has been described (in crystals of purified HLA-A2; ref. 26), and a similar structure of class II molecules has been proposed. The basic structure of class I molecules is that of a groove formed between approximately parallel a-helices and a series of β-strands forming a β-pleated sheet as the floor. It is thought that foreign or self nominal peptides sit on top of that sheet and between the helices. Thus, our understanding of the molecular basis of alloantigen recognition has markedly improved within the last two years. However, the following is still unclear: Because an individual possesses only a limited set of different MHC molecules, each molecule of this set must have the ability to bind a large number of different peptides in order to ensure full immunocompetence. On the other hand, it has been shown that a single amino acid substitution in a human MHC class II molecule can selectively alter antigen presentation.

Which particular MHC class II-positive cells function as APC is still controversial. Some authors claim that the dendritic cells which appear to be by far most effective were observed, under many conditions, to be the only ones. Others hold that macrophages, B lymphocytes, and class II-positive vascular endothelial cells have similar potential. How far this potential depends on the metabolic state of a given cell has clearly been shown in B lymphocytes: Though resting B cells are competent to process antigen and to present it to T cells, a far more dramatic enhancement of this processing and presentation is observed under conditions where the surface immunoglobulin binds and internalizes antigen for subsequent processing (requiring only 1/1.000 of the antigen concentration under certain experimental conditions). At any rate, unprimed T cells require viable APC for activation, whereas primed T cells can be activated without. Viable APC are able to produce and release cytokines, such as interleukin-1 (IL-1) and IL-6, which may serve as second signals required for T activation.

The cell migration pattern in organ allografts represents another parameter which largely determines antigen presentation. Three types of presentation may be distinguished. (1) Bone marrow–derived, potentially mobile graft APC (so-called passenger cells) act locally on host T cells passing nearby, or they leave the organ and stimulate the T cells in the regional lymph nodes or spleen. Accordingly, allografts (e.g., kidney or thyroid) that were depleted of these "passenger cells" enjoyed markedly prolonged survival in nonimmunosuppressed recipients under certain experimental conditions. (2) Residential cells, such as vascular endothelial cells (which are class II-positive in humans and can easily be induced to become positive in rodents), have also been shown to activate T cells. (3) It has been convincingly demonstrated by Brent and others that host APC take up and present donor MHC class I as well as class II molecules, though this has been considered to be a less effective, "indirect" activation pathway of alloantigen response (see below).

Antigen Recognition

The central event is recognition by T lymphocytes, mediated by the T cell receptor (TCR) and assisted by a number of cell surface accessory molecules. Recently, particular progress has been made in the understanding of the structure and function of these molecules and of the maturation processes of T cells [4,7,27,33,38].

The TCR gene families are organized in a manner similar to the immunoglobulin light and heavy chain gene families. The mechanisms for generating diversity are also quite similar, such as multiple gene segments in germline DNA, combinatorial joining of gene segments, variation in junctional sites, random insertion of nucleotides (N) at the site of joining, and combinatorial chain association. Two sets of genes exist, αβ and γδ, encoding two different TCR expressed on different subpopulations of T cells. Each gene is composed of several genetic segments: V, D (lacking in α and γ), J, N, and the constant C, which rearrange to assemble a unique somatically functioning gene before a primary transcript can be made. The size of the germline repertoire of the V, D, and J segments varies strongly among the four genes (α–δ) and between species. But even where relatively few segments exist for rearrangement (as is the case for γ and δ), an enormous diversity can result from extensive junctional variation and from the random insertion of nucleotides.

The TCRγδ (TCR1), still unknown two years ago, can now be defined on the surface of T cells with the help of monoclonal antibodies specific for either the γ or the δ polypeptide chain of the heterodimer molecule. It is regularly associated with the chains of the CD3 complex, which are thought to be responsible for the transduction of the antigen-binding signal through the cell membrane to activate the T cell. Only 1% to 10% of the peripheral human T cells are TCR1 positive. Of these, some 2% are CD4 positive and approximately 20% are CD8 positive, i.e., carry the one or the other of two accessory molecules which are considered most important for TCRαβ-carrying cells (see below). The functional role of TCR1 is still obscure, but two interesting features merit mention: (1) Nude mice are able to generate $TCR1^+$ cells extrathymically (as demonstrated at the age of 8 weeks). (2) Various antibacterial reaction specificities have been shown and, in particular, specific MHC class I or class II alloantigen reactivities (without the requirement of CD8 or CD4 accessory molecules, suggesting particular affinities of TCR1 for these antigens).

The TCRαβ (TCR2) represents the major developmental pathway of T cells. It is also composed of two polymorphic, glycosylated polypeptide chains, noncovalently associated with the invariant protein complex CD3, all belonging to the immunoglobulin gene superfamily as shown in Figure 1.3. The time sequence of chain expression in ontogeny is γ, β, α. The thymic maturation is thought to include the following steps: (1) Bone marrow–derived prethymic precursors are $\alpha^-\beta^-CD3^-CD4^-CD8^-$ on their cell surfaces. (2) Intrathymically TCR$\alpha\beta$ low expressing, immature thymocytes develop which are $CD3^+CD4^+CD8^+$ and particularly sensitive to important selection processes comprising negative selection (deletion of strongly self-reactive clones via programmed, apoptotic cell death upon TCR activation by self-MHC expressing, marrow-derived thymus dendritic cells) and positive selection. (3) Positive selection allows maturation, mainly into two types of peripheral T cells, the TCR$\alpha\beta$ high expressing and either $CD4^+CD8^-$ or $CD4^-CD8^+$ cells. Thymus epithelial cells appear to be responsible for this selection process: MHC class I recognition on these cells leads to commitment toward the $CD8^+$ so-called cytotoxic/suppressor lineage, and class II recognition leads to commitment toward $CD4^+$ so-called helper/inflammatory lineage, thus yielding mature T cells with the broadly documental feature of self-MHC restriction of their antigen-specific reactivity. It is still difficult to understand how a single MHC molecule can act positively and negatively, either through quantitative (affinity) or, rather, qualitative MHC expression differences between thymus dendritic and epithelial cells.

CD4 (the murine L3T4), a monomeric 55 kDa cell surface glycoprotein, is misleadingly called a T helper cell marker. Recent data indicate that it is rather a coreceptor which is physically associated to the TCR, binds to a monomeric structure of an antigen-presenting MHC class II molecule, and strongly augments the intracellular signaling of the TCR/CD3 complex, probably by independent positive signals. Upon activation by antigen, $CD4^+$ T cells proliferate, as can be measured in mixed lymphocyte cultures. They release a range of lymphokines that can activate other cells. The role of IL-2 and its receptor on both $CD4^+$ and $CD8^+$ T cells has recently had a strong impact on immunology since they are absolutely required for proliferation and differentiation of these cells, including self-amplification loops. Other growth and differentiation factors are IL-3 for hemopoiesis, IL-4 for other T and B cells, IL-5 for B cells, etc. Furthermore, gamma interferon strongly upregulates MHC molecule expression and activates macrophages and other nonimmunologic cells to mediate delayed type hypersensitivity.

CD8 (the murine Lyt-2) is usually called the marker of the other of two mutually exclusive populations of peripheral T cells, which, analogous to CD4, appears to serve as a coreceptor which binds to antigen-presenting MHC class I molecules. $CD8^+$ cells appear to act preferentially as effectors rather than as activators. As cytotoxic effectors they can kill targets, e.g., cells with allogeneic or virus-determined surface structures, by direct cell-to-cell contact. They can release large amounts of gamma interferon. They also can play a role as suppressor cells (see below). However, it must be pointed out that a clear-cut distinction between $CD4^+$ and $CD8^+$ T cell specificities and functions cannot be upheld. Although the self-MHC restriction specificity, as described above, is high, exceptions to the rule have been described in both directions. Even more exceptions have been observed with regard to allo-MHC molecules, in that a $CD4^+$ T cell can react with an allo-MHC class I molecule and vice versa. Furthermore, $CD4^+$ cells can be cytolytic cells or suppressor cells, and $CD8^+$ cells can provide helper functions and secrete IL-2 and other lymphokines.

In general, it must be kept in mind that the rules which we discover apply to the conditions under which we observe them and that many misunderstandings simply result from premature generalization. Thus, the above described, well documented and generally agreed thymus epithelial–determined MHC restriction of T cells does not necessarily apply to MHC allogeneic hemopoietic chimeras, i.e., bone marrow graft recipients. Their T cells may become donor MHC restricted. More interestingly, in MHC fully allogeneic and nevertheless immunologically reconstituted (but donor-tolerant) mixed or split chimeras, APC of host origin have been shown by us [8] to cooperate with T cells of donor origin as well as with T cells of host origin in primary proliferative responses against third party MHC antigens, provided the APC and the T cells were collected from the chimera rather than from a normal rat of the bone marrow donor or recipient strain.

In addition to the TCR/CD3/CD4 or CD8 complex, a group of cell adhesion molecules may fulfill accessory functions in antigen recognition. Both APC and target cells for T cells have recently been shown to have specific counterstructures. Two ligand systems are already well defined: CD2 (T11, LFA-2) on T cells binding to LFA-3 (CD58) and LFA-1 (CL11α/CD18) on T cells binding to ICAM-1 (CD54). Virtually all of these molecules contain immunoglobulin-like domains, and thus also belong to the broader Ig supergene family.

Cellular Effector Mechanisms

The regular rejection of solid grafts in nonpresensitized recipients is mainly T cell determined [4,9,32,36]. Thymus-deprived animals, such as nude mice or adult thymectomized, lethally irradiated, bone marrow–reconstituted animals, do not reject skin allografts, for instance, and even accept xenografts in the absence of preformed, cytotoxic "natural" antibodies. There has been a long-standing debate on the question of the relative role of $CD4^+$ vs $CD8^+$ cells and on the relevance of various methodologic approaches to this question.

The first suggestion was that allografts were rejected by a delayed type of hypersensitivity (DTH) mechanism. In present terms this would mean the following: After an initiating interaction with the alloantigen, (mainly) $CD4^+$ cells act, not by releasing IL-2 and thus activating specifically allo-cytotoxic $CD8^+$, but instead by releasing other lymphokines that recruit and activate macrophages and other nonspecific effector cells. This process lacks the exquisite specificity of direct cytolysis; it can damage the recipient's own cells as well, and it remains unclear whether it is an essential process. However, there may be species variation, so that the rejection reactions in humans may cause more damage to the recipient's own tissue constituents than occurs in rodents.

There is as yet no assay available for in vitro analysis of DTH-like mechanisms. This contrasts with cell-mediated lymphocytotoxicity assays and with the in vitro measurement of lymphocyte proliferative responses (e.g., in the mixed lymphocyte culture), which are the most popular ones. But although these tests have contributed greatly to basic understanding, they have shed virtually no light on the phenomenon of graft rejection in vivo, in contrast to adoptive transfer analysis of in vitro defined T cells injected into thymus-deprived recipients. Still, the conclusiveness of demonstrations that the allograft rejection capacity of such T-cell-deficient animals could be restored by syngeneic $CD4^+$ cells came into question following the observation that the T-cell deficiency of these animals appears to be confined to the $CD4^+$ subset. Furthermore, cytotoxic T cells with specificity for MHC class II antigens arise from precursors of the $CD4^+$ phenotype.

A better understanding may be obtained by scrutinizing the quantitative effect of the adoptive inocula: cell transfer should restore rejection to normal if naive cells are used and to an accelerated rate if cells from a presensitized syngeneic donor are used. Furthermore, we should know the target antigen: usually, MHC class II alloantigens require $CD4^+$ cells, class I alloantigens require $CD8^+$ cells, and non-MHC alloantigens require association with self-MHC for recognition. Recent data from Singer's group [10] have shown the following: Reconstitution with isolated $CD8^+$ cells resulted in the rapid rejection of MHC class I–disparate skin allografts, whereas reconstitution with $CD4^+$ cells resulted in the rapid rejection of class II-disparate and of non-MHC-disparate grafts. Most important, by correlating these rejection responses with the functional capabilities of the pertinent T-cell populations, it was shown that mice rejected the skin allografts only if they contained both lymphokine-secreting and cytotoxic T cells that reacted specifically with the graft alloantigens. This set of data demonstrates again the limited value of the isolated description of phenotype markers, and it is consistent with the thesis, well supported by other recent findings, that cytotoxic effectors need help from lymphokine-secreting cells.

The expression patterns of MHC molecules in the grafted tissue determine the initiating recognition and the subsequent effector T-cell reactivities. In normal, freshly grafted tissue the $CD4^+$ cells are mainly, although probably not entirely, restricted to interstitial macrophages and dendritic cells, vascular endothelial cells, and, as far as they are present, B lymphocytes. As mentioned already, cellular rejection is accompanied by a marked increase in the expression of MHC class I and II on a number of cells in all tissues. For instance, in a rat kidney allograft, induction of class I antigens occurs much more rapidly (24 hr) than in a heart (72 hr); class II antigens are noted after three to four days in both organs. MHC expression may increase as much as thirty-fold within five days. Renal arteriolar endothelium, but not glomerular capillary endothelium, becomes selectively strongly positive for class II. It follows that not all cells would be or would become equally vulnerable to cytotoxic mechanisms and that the predominant sites of rejection are the sites of high MHC expression.

However, this supposition cannot be reversed by concluding from high MHC expression and concomitant allograft infiltration with $CD4^+$ and

$CD8^+$ cells that rejection will take place. Several recent studies have shown that preoperative donor-specific blood transfusion may lead to indefinite survival of rat renal allografts; these enhanced grafts even underwent an accelerated and extensive induction of both donor MHC class I and II antigen expression. The more rapid and substantial leukocyte infiltrate had phenotypes that were similar to those in unmodified grafts that are being rejected. Obviously, then, our present set of markers is still insufficient for safely distinguishing between cellular infiltrates that can cause rejection and those that cannot. It is possible that enhancing antibodies interfere with rejection. Also, it has not yet been investigated to what extent the $CD8^+$ cells that have been extracted from graft infiltrates and shown to cause cytotoxicity in vitro can differ from $CD8^+$ cells that suppress the complex event of graft rejection in vivo (so-called suppressor cells are in general $CD8^+$). We do not intend to discuss the complex nonspecific sequences that cause graft destruction and debris elimination in more detail here, but note that the initiating event is a clearly specific one requiring immunocompetent cells, as outlined above.

Therefore, it should not be surprising that apparently healthy allografts can also contain large numbers of cells with NK (natural killer) activity when tested in vitro. Most of these cells usually lack the above-mentioned T cell markers, have the morphology of large granular lymphocytes, and have cell membrane structures such as CD16 and Leu-19. Their activity may be defined as the capacity to lyse a variety of target cells, in vitro in particular established cell lines such as the human line K-562, without prior sensitization and independent of MHC restriction.

Humoral Effector Mechanisms

There are two major groups of humoral factors to be distinguished in transplantation immunology, the unspecific and the specific (antigen-reactive) ones. Among the first are the above-discussed interleukins, growth and differentiation factors for both T and B lymphocytes [31]. Seven interleukins (IL 1–7) have been identified to date. They are single chain polypeptides without structural homology to each other. A second group of immunologically unspecific but highly important humoral effectors comprise the mediators of inflammation, notably IL-1, gamma interferon, and tumor necrosis factor alpha. It is mentioned in the chapter on cellular effector mechanisms that even substantial cellular infiltration and MHC expression upregulation in an allograft can occur without cell injury. Thus, the hallmark of graft rejection is cell injury, both to endothelial and parenchymal cells, leading to functional impairment at the clinical level. There is now evidence that this injury is largely cytokine-dependent, and we will have to understand under which circumstances activation of macrophages and T lymphocytes leads to the release and effectiveness of these cytokines.

The specifically antigen-reactive humoral factors are the antibodies [11]. Humoral alloantibodies against MHC antigens are easily formed. The male-

production of cytotoxic alloantibodies and cytotoxic T cells, rather than by ample generation of suppressor T cells and antibodies capable of blocking antipaternal reactions. An increasing number of reports demonstrate that women with a history of chronic abortion enjoy normal pregnancies after inoculation with their partner's leukocytes (85% in our department). Furthermore, as astutely pointed out by Billingham, it appears that the systemic immunologic events become effective only under quite special local conditions. The maternal decidua plays an immunoprotective role, and the fetal trophoblast is an immunologically privileged site par excellence. The latter represents the continuous frontier tissue of the conceptus, which does not express MHC class II antigens (not even on interferon stimulation) or classic HLA-A, B, C alloantigens and synthesizes high local concentrations of a number of hormones purported to be immunosuppressive.

The immunobiologic features on which manipulative approaches can be based are outlined above. All considerations take into account that the various cell types in an organ may differ strongly in their immunogenicity, depending not only on their surface antigen expression but also on their potential to provide a second signal. Thus, as pointed out particularly by Lafferty, the antigen by itself is not the barrier to allotransplantation. Although the allograft response is one of the most violent immune reactions, even MHC class I and II molecules are relatively weak immunogens when isolated from the cell surface. Note also the simple in vitro observation that the stimulatory capacity of the stimulator cell in a mixed lymphocyte culture is a function of its metabolic activity.

For manipulation three aspects may be discussed in particular.

1. The passenger cell concept has led to a variety of approaches toward eliminating or inactivating those mobile, bone marrow–derived cells in a tissue that may be the predominant carriers of immunogenicity, such as lymphocytes, macrophages, and cells of the dendritic and Langerhans cells group. This has been achieved, for instance, by long-term tissue culture (of thyroid in Lafferty's classic experiments), by short-term hyperbaric oxygen (95% O_2) culture, by ultraviolet irradiation of cell suspensions or skin or by incubation with cytotoxic cell-specific or, if appropriate, anti-MHC class II antibodies (of pancreatic islets in our own studies). This approach has yielded very impressive allograft success in some cases and rather disappointing findings in many others. To our understanding, this does not invalidate the underlying concept but indicates that the relative role of the above passenger cells varies among the immunogenicity-providing pathways. However, any attempt at reducing the immunogenic load of a graft is desirable. In organ transplantation, this may even start with the elimination of organ-associated lymphoreticular components.

2. Other cell constituents of the graft may become capable of playing the role of "pre-APC." This mechanism was shown most clearly in recent experiments of ours with bone marrow. After appropriate lymphocyte depletion with cytotoxic antibodies (allowing the establishment of rat or mouse MHC fully allogeneic radiation chimeras), the residual hemopoietic cells

were unable to act as stimulator cells in T proliferation assays, although some of them were clearly MHC class II antigen positive; however, their immunogenic potential became fully restored after treatment with gamma interferon or noninterferon humoral factors. On the other hand, our recently developed cytotoxic monoclonal antibody K31 against an epitope located on human lymphocytes and certain myeloic lineage cells, uniquely allows elimination of those cells from human bone marrow which are immunogenic in T-cell proliferation assays after gamma interferon incubation. Hemopoietic cells are left untouched. The unaffected cells, nevertheless, increase their MHC class II expression about three-fold following the interferon incubation, but remain nonimmunogenic, presumably because of insufficient second signals [15]. Our present understanding is that such pre-APC may well become activated by the recipient after grafting unless they were eliminated beforehand, and it may well be assumed that in organ grafts vascular endothelial cells can play such a role.

3. Recipient APC should well be able to pick up and present graft antigen to recipient T cells. Interestingly, data indicate that this path may be less efficient and more vulnerable to immunosuppression. For example, the required immunosuppressive treatment of the recipient becomes much more effective if the graft has been deprived of passenger cells. The above studies clearly indicate that it is wise to interact at several defined points simultaneously (including the degree of histoincompatibility) to manipulate the immunogenicity of grafts as effectively as possible.

Modulation of Recipient Immune Responsiveness

The necessity of multifactorial approaches concerns both the graft and the recipient. Before examining the recipient, an interesting feature of nature deserves mention.

High or Low Responsiveness

In the 1970s much excitement was aroused by the discovery of so-called immune response (Ir) genes in the MHC gene region that regulate antigen-specific T cell activation. It is now clear that the products of these Ir genes are the MHC class I and II molecules themselves. This has been most clearly demonstrated in mice with minor changes in one of the MHC molecules only and a profoundly altered T-cell immune response repertoire. Similar observations are accumulating in the human with regard to the extent of T-cell responsiveness to certain virus infections that is determined by the MHC class II specificity. The molecular mechanism of these immunoregulatory functions of MHC molecules is still under debate (e.g., limited capacity of certain MHC molecules to interact with certain antigens? Lack of T-cell capacity to recognize certain MHC molecule-antigen combinations? Preferential induction of suppressor cells?) [4].

Reduction of Graft-vs-Host Reactions

GVHRs were first observed in lethally irradiated mouse recipients of bone marrow and of spleen cells from donors of different strains. They initially recovered, but after 3 to 6 weeks they developed a "secondary disease" and often died. It became clear that GVHR occurs when immunocompetent cells are injected into an allogeneic recipient who is immunosuppressed or into an immunogenetically nonreactive recipient (e.g., A cells into an (AxB)F1 hybrid recipient) [12].

Four factors affecting the incidence and severity of GVHR have been identified.

1. The degree of antigenic disparity between donor and recipient. Characteristically, bone marrow grafts between identical twins do not elicit GVHR, whereas in many species studied the risk of GVHR increases with the number of MHC locus incompatibilities from non-MHC different combinations onward.
2. The number of lymphocytes transferred. GVHR is associated with solid organ transplantation when a large portion of lymphoid tissue is an inherent component of the graft (e.g., spleen) or is attached to it. Our microsurgeons have shown in rat small bowel transplantation that careful removal of the attached mesenteric lymph nodes abolishes GVHR and that the remaining Peyer's patches are of minor relevance. Cell suspension grafts, mainly bone marrow grafts, have become the subject of a large variety of attempts to eliminate lymphocytes, especially T cells, as thoroughly as possible. This has met with variable success, as outlined below. The incidence and severity of GVHR has been correlated with the number of lymphocytes transfused both in animals and humans.
3. Microbial flora and infection. Germ-free mice suffer little or none of the typical clinical manifestations of GVHR. This has led some groups to attempt bacterial decontamination of prospective bone marrow graft recipients—without much success. Viral infections, particularly with cytomegalovirus, are feared because they can amplify GVHR. The mechanisms of this association are not clear. Cytoreductive treatment of a bone marrow recipient certainly facilitates new infections and reactivates latent ones. This may lead to the expression of MHC and non-MHC antigens on recipient cell surfaces, either directly or indirectly due to interferon production by T cells that are sensitized to the microbial antigens. In this way, recipient antigens at particular locations may become both trigger and target of GVHR-producing T cells.
4. Age of the recipient. Increasing recipient age is a major GVHR risk factor that is not understood. It is tempting to speculate that the infection load of an organism increases with age.

Bone marrow transplantation (BMT) is the clinical field in which GVHR prevention is of greatest importance. In addition to restricting to non-HLA histoincompability, attempts have centered mainly on eliminating or suppressing donor lymphocytes. An incomplete overview of these attempts is given in Table 1.1. For a full review see Muller-Ruchholtz [13].

The following comments may be made.

1. Many of these approaches have had to remain at the experimental stage.
2. The still dominant, clinically established approach consists in long-

Table 1.1
Approaches to prevention of graft vs host response in bone marrow transplantation

Type	*Comments*
In vivo	
Transplantation of fetal liver	Clinically limited to small children
Donor pretreatment: ALS, CSA, TLI	Mainly experimental
Host preconditioning: TLI	Experimental
Host posttreatment: CSA, MTX	Clinically established
In vitro, various	
Bone marrow culture	Experimental (selective stem cell proliferation)
Physical fractionation: density gradient or counterflow centrifugation	Experimental
Pharmacologic fractionation: MP	Experimental
Receptor fractionation: ER, SBA	Some success in SCID, trials in leukemia
In vitro, serologic (ab.-dependent)	
Elimination of host-specific lymphocytes: anti-idiotype ab., anti-IL2R ab.	Experimental
Elimination of various lymphocyte subpopulations	
Cell opsonization	Disappointing
Complement activation	Experimentally successful: ABS, ALS, SAL, Thy-1 ab. Clinically rewarding: CD2-8 ab. in various combin., Campath-1
Immunotoxin: ricin conjugate	Clinical trials
Magnetic immunomicrospheres: albumin, polystyrene/direct ab. or antiglobulin conjugated	Promising experimental and clinical trials

ab., antibodies; ABS, antibrain serum; ALS, antilymphocyte serum; CD, cluster of differentiation designation of the antigen; CSA, cyclosporine A; ER, erythrocyte (sheep) rosetting; IL2R, interleukin-2 receptor; MP, methylprednisolone; MTX, methotrexate; SAL, specified antilymphocyte serum; SBA, soybean agglutin; SCID, severe combined immunodeficiency disease; TLI, total lymphoid irradiation.

term cytostatic treatment of the recipient, which is in principle unsatisfactory.

3. The more elegant and promising approaches consist in depleting the bone marrow of lymphocytes in vitro without recipient post-treatment.
4. The most interesting and effective way to achieve this continues to be what we, in 1976, termed serologic dissection: elimination of the relevant lymphocytes with cell-specific antibodies.
5. The present clinical success is far from being satisfactory: according to a recent review by Gale's group of 31 reported trials in leukemia patients, T depletion reduced the incidence of GVHR from 45% to 11% in HLA-identical BMT and from 75% to 38% in HLA partially mismatched BMT, whereas the incidence of graft rejection increased from 1% to 13% and from 5% to 26%, respectively (with most data suggesting that this is due to immunologic rejection rather than to hemopoietic stem cell damage reaction). Some studies also showed an increased risk of relapse.

These comments require some explanation. For satisfying broad clinical applicability of BMT, transplantation across the MHC barrier should not be the major obstacle, and there should be no inverse correlation between GVHR and engraftment. Interestingly enough, this is not the case in adequate experimental models. Fifteen years ago we began to show in rats, shortly thereafter also in various mouse strain combinations, that specified antilymphocyte (SAL) serum-incubated, MHC fully allogeneic bone marrow allows restoration of lethally irradiated recipients to normal lymphoid tissue appearance and immune reactivity (including normal rejection of non-MHC allogeneic skin) within 6 to 7 weeks. This is without early or late GVHR or increased infection susceptibility (observation time in rats up to >600 days; in mice, up to >400 days), but with specific donor-recipient unresponsiveness in vivo and in vitro [14]. Similar findings from various laboratories have confirmed these observations in recent years. Therefore, we should feel obligated to fill the gap between the clinical and the experimental experience.

In this context we restrict ourselves here to three considerations with regard to an important and probably underestimated immunologic parameter that is not indicated in Table 1.1: antibody specificity.

1. We have shown that a subset of pre- or parathymic T cells can initiate antihost reactivity in MHC fully allogeneic BMT and that such BMT is thus successful only if the T-cell-depleting antibody reactivity crosses the prethymic-thymic border; interestingly, claims but no experimental data from the literature contradict this statement [28].

2. It is not clear how far a depletion protocol that saves the B lymphocytes will allow the transfer of cells that may both produce antirecipient antibodies and provide immunogenicity for residual recipient antigraft reactivity.

3. The immunogenic potential of bone marrow, as seen in T proliferation assays, is an additional factor which can be strongly reduced by the elimination of pre-APC [15].

These considerations may be seen in connection with the presently established clinical protocols: they aim at depleting mature T cells, and it has been shown that even monoclonal antibodies with broader specificities, such as Campath-1, do not reduce residual bone marrow immunogenicity [15].

Reduction of Host-vs-Graft Reactions

We would like to distinguish between means of broadly suppressing immune reactivity, thus facilitating alloengraftment, and approaches toward specifically reprogramming the reactivity repertoire of a graft recipient. The latter is dealt with in the next section under Specific Unresponsiveness. Certainly there are connecting links between these two paths (see below), but it should be clear that a continuous immunosuppressive regimen, implying increased susceptibility to infection, tumor incidence, and chronic drug toxicity, must be applied as long as no functional immunotolerance can be shown to exist [16]. If the dose has been reduced too far or if one of the factors disturbing the labile equilibrium, even such as infection, has gained weight, a rejection crisis may only be mastered with the help of strongly increased immunosuppression. Furthermore, much remains to be learned about the factors that maintain this equilibrium and that usually allow reduced dosage of immunosuppressive drugs after the first postgrafting phase. In other words: the more than 35-year-old descriptive term *graft adaptation* still awaits explanation.

There are six major approaches to immunosuppression.

1. GVHRs are known to be remarkable immunosuppressants, even at the subclinical level. They appear to be responsible, at least in part, for delaying immune reconstitution of BMT recipients. Interestingly enough, it has been repeatedly claimed that "some" GVHRs were required for bone marrow engraftment. We disagree and prefer to consider any possible reduction in graft immunogenicity, as outlined above, to be a first-line approach toward reducing HVGRs, not only in BMT.

2. Irradiation is one of the oldest immunosuppressive regimens. Total-body irradiation was applied to the recipients of the first kidney allografts in the middle 1950s, before the superiority of cytostatic drugs was discovered. In connection with its application before BMT we have noted a remarkable delay in the onset of immune suppression, even after a lethal irradiation dose: rats still rejected skin grafts at normal speed when sensitizing allogeneic cells such as bone marrow cells were injected intravenously 1 to 2 days after irradiation. Total lymphoid irradiation (TLI) also originated in tumor therapy: patients treated for malignant lymphomas with fractionated TLI had strikingly impaired cell-mediated immune responses. Subsequent experimental work indicated the emergence of nonspecific, non-T suppressor cells that may give rise to a subsequent state of specific unresponsiveness for allografts applied shortly after TLI. However, many of the essential parameters determining the functional outcome of TLI are not yet understood and are not under control, and therefore it has not been possible to establish transplantation tolerance in many experimental and clinical situations. The

current most interesting application is low-dose TLI to overcome host resistance in T-cell-depleted BMT.

3. Classic drug immunosuppression comprises mainly corticosteroids, antimetabolites (such as azathioprine and methotrexate), and alkylating agents (such as cyclophosphamide). In the 1950s, when experimental transplantation immunology broadened, the first drugs successfully used were corticosteroids. Meanwhile they have been shown to prevent transcription of IL-1 encoding mRNA, thus blocking the IL-1-dependent release of IL-2 from antigen-activated T cells.

Clinical transplantation essentially started in the early 1960s with cadaver kidney grafting when total body irradiation with its unacceptable side effects was replaced by the antileukemia drug azathioprine (plus steroids) following the demonstration in 1959 that its metabolite, 6-mercaptopurine, was immunosuppressive in animals. Its predominant effect is to block mitosis or proliferation of lymphoid cells by being incorporated into purine nucleotides and inhibiting the synthesis of DNA. Since antigen stimulation causes cell division and proliferation, the antiproliferative activity of azathioprine allows it to affect rapidly dividing activated T and B cells.

4. Cyclosporine A (CsA) was serendipitously discovered in 1972 to have immunosuppressive properties when it was being screened as an antibiotic. In the late 1970s it began to challenge the supremacy that azathioprine had enjoyed for nearly twenty years. The predominant effect of CsA appears to be interference with T-cell helper functions: it mainly blocks IL-2 release from activated T cells by blocking the transcription of the IL-2 gene, but it also inhibits the release of other lymphokines, including IL-4 and gamma interferon. Thus the indirect inhibition of the interferon-determined increase in MHC antigen expression appears to be another important path of action. In addition, experimental evidence suggests that CsA does not extensively interfere with the activation and proliferation of T-suppressor cells. It has now been established that CsA, with or without steroids, yields clinical organ graft survival rates superior to those achieved with azathioprine and steroids. The fact that CsA blood concentrations can be monitored with increasing precision and ease will add to its therapeutic efficacy and help to minimize its side effects, e.g., its nephrotoxicity.

Altogether, it appears that the various drugs, especially corticosteroids, azathioprine, and CsA, inhibit antigen-driven T-cell proliferation at distinct points in the activation cascade and that therefore combination drug protocols have benefits from synergistic effects. It remains to the clinician to handle properly the treatment of the individual organ graft recipient, including induction, maintenance, chronic dysfunction, and acute rejection crisis treatment with one or up to four drugs (in the latter case including antilymphocyte antibodies).

5. Antibodies may be very helpful for reducing HVGR, somewhat similar to their important role in reducing GVHR, as discussed above. However, the latter means short-term in vitro treatment, whereas HVGR in vivo treatment implies the long-known risk of adverse reactions when foreign species–derived antibodies are applied over extended periods. Therefore, and in

view of the remarkable efficiency of antilymphocyte antibodies, we predict that the golden age of their application is still to come, as soon as defined cocktails of monoclonal antibodies of human origin become available. In principle the same holds for a second group of antibodies, namely, those directed against graft donor antigens rather than against recipient lymphocytes.

Antilymphocyte antibodies of xenogeneic origin probably represent the oldest immunosuppressive agents. They were rediscovered by Woodruff in the early 1960s and were subsequently shown to be both potently immunosuppressive and useful for inducing tolerance in experimental animals. This phase was soon followed by the clinical use, which is still well established today, of antilymphocyte globulin (ALG) preparations from rabbit or horse for acute graft rejection crisis treatment requiring short-term application only. ALG has been challenged recently but obviously not yet replaced by the mouse monoclonal OKT3 antibodies, directed against the CD3 component of the above-described TCR/CD3 complex, which is present on virtually all mature T cells. Again, it is a potent agent for reversing established allograft rejection. Other monoclonal antibodies against leukocyte differentiation antigens become of increasing interest. They may be directed against lymphocyte cell surface structures which either directly or as accessory molecules are involved in antigen recognition, as described above. Such structures are TCR monomorphic epitopes, CD4, CD8, CD2, or LFA-1. However, they may also be directed against other differentiation antigens, such as CD5, CD7, etc. The former group is of special interest in that these antibodies may block the T cell functions without the T-cell-activating effects that have been observed under certain circumstances with anti-CD3 antibodies. More interestingly, blocking antibodies against surface molecules (such as CD4 and CD8) which transduce second signals (additional to the specific antigen recognition by the TCR) may even lead to specific unresponsiveness, as discussed below. Antibodies that have either no or only temporary effects may become potent killers of selective cell populations in the form of drug (e.g., daunomycin, idarubicin), toxin (e.g., ricin) or isotope (e.g., ^{131}J) immunoconjugates. Another trend in the selection of new monoclonal antibodies aims at limiting the reactivity to as few cells as possible. For example, antibodies directed at the IL-2 receptor provide selective reactions in that only T cells are subject to blockade or killing that strongly express this receptor because they are activated largely (though certainly not only) by the graft alloantigens.

Administering antibodies directed against graft rather than recipient antigens is an alternative. The fascinating results of anti-Rhesus blood group D prophylaxis are well known, and similar effects with other transplantation antigens have been sought in animals and humans. In 1956 Kaliss established that antigen-specific antibodies could protect tumor grafts from rejection, thus enhancing their growth in mice. Subsequently this enhancement expressed itself fairly well in renal grafts and some other parenchymal organ grafts in rats and mice but poorly in skin grafts and in other species. The often minute quantities of antibodies that are required do not support the simple explanation that the graft antigens are shielded from immune recognition; they may, on the other hand, explain the lack of injury to the graft, since these antibodies would be unable to activate complement or antibody-dependent cellular cytotoxicity (ADCC) reactions. Their protective effect may derive from a preferential elimination of mobile, highly immunogenic graft cells through opsonization (because the Fc fragment of the antibody appears to be required). More recently interest has arisen in monoclonal antibodies that are specific for MHC antigens, particularly the class II antigens of the graft. This extends the manipulation of graft immunogenicity.

6. Some recent developments in immunosuppressive drug research may be mentioned briefly. Although CsA was considered for several years to be the outstanding drug, FK506, a macrolide derived from a *Streptomyces* strain, was reported in 1987 as a potential breakthrough in immunosuppression. Another interesting substance under investigation is 15-deoxyspergualin, a derivative of spergualin. We and others have recently shown that it prolongs allograft survival in a variety of transplantation models, facilitates lasting specific immunotolerance after a short-term treatment, and reverses rejection. The mechanism of action of FK506 is similar to CsA, but the mechanism of deoxyspergualin is quite different. Its immunosuppressive activity may be due to a suppression of macrophage function. Altogether, we reemphasize that immunosuppression is an open-ended approach unless we find paths for converting nonspecific reduction of HVGR into specific immunotolerance in humans.

Specific Unresponsiveness

The necessity to distinguish clearly between a more or less broad reduction of HVGR and specific unresponsiveness (SUR) has been mentioned earlier in this chapter, and some of the early concepts and observations of immunologic tolerance have been described as well. These concepts implied the assumption that the specific inability to reject certain allografts was based on physical deletion of specifically reactive lymphocytes. During the 1960s and 1970s our understanding was increasingly broadened by the discovery of specifically suppressive immune reactions and, more recently, of functionally silencing mechanisms. The term SUR became familiar, and today it is mainly used synonymously with immunotolerance.

The literature is full of reports on induction of SUR in experimental models, and it provokes at least four basic comments:

1. Success in the induction of SUR does not necessarily imply its maintenance. The latter requires continuous, adequate accessibility of the antigens in question to the immune system.
2. Adequate specificity controls are remarkably often lacking. Only the demonstration of third-party graft rejection justifies the assertion of SUR. The proper choice of a third party is not easy: a moderately immunosuppressed graft recipient may reject only the third-party control graft

at a normal speed simply because it is more immunogenic, thus feigning SUR.

3. It remains to be shown that we can accomplish the most important step from reprogramming the allograft rejection repertoire of an adult experimental animal to reprogramming in humans (although we see no reason why it should not be possible).
4. Elimination of graft immunogenicity does not imply SUR. The latter must be demonstrated by the subsequent acceptance of an immunogenic allograft of the same origin.

Role of the Antigen and Its Presentation

Several years ago Mitchison suggested that we distinguish three functional types of antigen. *Nonimmunogenic antigens* evoke SUR in adult animals, e.g., bovine gamma globulin without adjuvant, in a nonaggregated state, injected into mice. *Weakly immunogenic antigens* elicit low-dose SUR, larger doses induce immunity, and still larger doses elicit SUR again, e.g., bovine serum albumin in mice. *Strongly immunogenic antigens,* such as most proteins, usually result in immunity.

MHC antigens are proteins on cell surfaces but are demonstrable in the serum as well. It appears that class II antigens are more immunogenic than those of class I, and the latter are certainly more so than non-MHC antigens. For example, Sachs [17] has recently shown in swine that kidney allografting led to SUR when the disparity involved only class I; skin was rejected in both class I and class II incompatible transplantation [17]. This observation indicates that the organ involved also plays a role. According to our experience, the immunogenicity of MHC fully allogeneic rat organs may be ranked in the following order: liver < heart or kidney < small bowel < pancreas or skin and, correspondingly, it is easiest to induce SUR in liver. This works in certain strain combinations even without additional treatment and in others after only two weeks of immunosuppressive treatment [18]. These differences are important and await elucidation. We may assume that they depend largely on the mechanisms of antigen presentation.

A number of recent model studies may be summarized as indicating that recognition of the antigen (in association with an APC) under nonmitogenic, second signal–free conditions can result in SUR. In this context, we consider those new paths which make use of the tools of modern molecular biology particularly interesting. One approach, recently described by the group of Morris, consists of MHC gene transfection. Another, followed by us, consists of the downregulation of the production of interleukins, such as IL-1, at the transcriptional level, by transfections in cells of cultured cell lines which originally were potent APC but continue to express their array of MHC cell surface mulocules, thereby potentially useful for pretreatment before organ transplantation. A variety of measures may facilitate these conditions, such as immunosuppressive drugs (see below) and the route of antigen application, apparently following the order lymphatic drainage < intravenously < into the portal vein.

Facilitating Role of Temporary Immunosuppression

The demonstration of the effectiveness of a short-term application of immunosuppressants for inducing of allograft SUR began in the 1960s. For example, in 1965 we showed that cyclophosphamide, given on days 2 and 1 before and 1 and 2 after a few hours of cross-transfusion between MHC-variant adult rats, initiated permanent SUR as documented by specific skin graft acceptance. It was later shown that cyclophosphamide was less effective in more strongly histoincompatible combinations, but its derivative ifosfamide proved to be much more potent at equicytotoxic levels although of similar efficacy in standard immunosuppression experiments with skin grafts [19]. This demonstrated for the first time that a drug's SUR-facilitating potential can be dissociated from its immunosuppressive potential. In 1970, Monaco started to show that antilymphocyte serum in combination with bone marrow injection yielded similar successes in SUR induction in mice. In 1972, we reported for the first time that total body irradiation followed by BMT without any additional recipient treatment allows the establishment of MHC fully allogeneic hemopoietic chimerism with lifelong SUR in rats, provided the graft was pre-T/T-cell depleted [13]. In the late 1970s, TLI began to attract major interest, as reported above. Recently it was impressively shown in a number of MHC-allogeneic rat organ models that a two-week treatment with, e.g., CsA following transplantation initiates lasting SUR [18]; although it may be mentioned that many of such models, at least in certain strain combinations with low responder recipients, appear to be "too easy" to be considered representative.

Specific Unresponsiveness Through Humoral Response Mechanisms

The administration of survival-enhancing xeno- and alloantibodies has been described above. Their effect is usually restricted to the simultaneously applied graft, thus not justifying the term SUR as it is explained above. However, as mentioned above, antibodies against T cell structures, such as CD4 and CD8, which transduce second signals (additional to the specific antigen recognition by the TCR) have recently been shown, by the group of Waldmann and by others, to be remarkably effective in the induction of SUR toward MHC class I and non-MHC alloantigens [39].

On the other side, active enhancement, i.e., the same phenomenon elicited by lasting alloantibody production of the graft recipient, may well provide a mechanism of SUR. Alternatively, both passive and active enhancement may help to initiate another SUR mechanism, similar to the immunosuppressive agents discussed above. This is supported by the observation that SUR following humoral enhancement can be transferred by cells.

Anti-idiotypic autoantibodies have also attracted considerable attention recently. They may be directed to the antigen-binding sites of antibodies or the T-cell receptor (TCR) of $CD4^+$ and $CD8^+$ T cells and initiate an antigen-specific abortive response. Very interesting experimental approaches by

Binz and Wigzell were difficult to reproduce, probably because of the multitude of receptors involved and because of a limited sharing of the receptor idiotypes by the antibodies and TCR involved in the rejection process [17].

Nevertheless, anti-idiotypic antibodies directed against anti-HLA reactivities of renal allograft patients have been observed and have recently been correlated with graft survival [20]. It must be pointed out, however, that rejecting recipients were shown to have antibodies as well, although differently functioning ones, be they antigraft response potentiating anti-idiotypic antibodies or blocking anti-anti-idiotypic ones. This puzzle may reflect our problems in understanding the lability and unpredictability of both the conversion from formerly positive to recently negative crossmatch and the usefulness of intentional pregraft blood transfusions in patients. Obviously, further research is needed.

Specific Unresponsiveness Through Cell-Mediated Response Mechanisms

Gershon and Kondo in 1970 were the first to notice specific T-suppressor cells (T_s) in mice whose humoral response to sheep erythrocytes was depressed after large numbers of these erythrocytes were injected. Since then we have learned much about T_s and their regulatory roles, be they antigen specific or anti-idiotypic, which must be clearly differentiated from nonspecific, "natural" suppressor cells of seemingly varied, still unclear origins. (The latter have recently attracted much interest in connection with TLI, as mentioned above.) Although it is presently common use to consider T_s to be $CD8^+$ cells (OKT8 or Leu-2 in humankind, Lyt-2 in mouse, and OX8 in rat, respectively), no strict relationship between these markers and cell function can be inferred. $CD4^+$ T cells and even macrophages, armed with T_s-derived humoral factors, have also been reported to suppress allograft reactions specifically. T_s function has been demonstrated in vitro by suppression of mixed lymphocyte reactions or cell-mediated lymphocytotoxicity and in vivo by adoptive transfer into syngeneic recipients.

According to recent analyses in several laboratories, three T-cell elements appear to be involved in specific suppression, forming a kind of idiotype–anti-idiotype network [21]. The first, T_s1, is an antigen-specific (i.e., idiotypic) induction phase-suppressing cell and is $CD4^+$ (i.e., MHC class II restricted) or not MHC restricted in its reactivity. The second, T_s2, is an anti-idiotypic, cyclophosphamide-resistant cell that has been named transducer/amplifier, and the third, T_s3, is an antigen-specific, cyclophosphamide-sensitive effector phase-suppressing cell. The last two cells were found to be $CD8^+$ and apparently MHC restricted. Interestingly, this network appears to also involve three specifically reactive factors that may be released from the cells.

The wide variety of manipulations in experimental animals, from rodents to nonhuman primates, to achieve functional SUR to skin, parenchymal organs, or bone marrow allografts are largely accompanied by the appearance of T_s. But, to the extent that SUR depends on suppressive reactivity, it is still as difficult to define the relative role of cell-mediated vs humoral mechanisms as in graft-rejecting immune reactivity. Furthermore, it appears from much experimental data, including our own, that temporary immunosuppressive manipulations may first be followed by a state of active nonspecific suppression, possibly associated with so-called natural suppressor cells, which then gives rise to a lasting state of SUR.

In spite of the general agreement on the existence of the phenomenon of cell-mediated SUR, there is an ongoing debate with regard to the existence of separate lineages of T cells performing functions different from those carried out by the other $CD4^+$ or $CD8^+$ subpopulations, thus requiring specific molecular structures [24]. Thus far there has been no convincing demonstration of such molecules on specific T_s. It is increasingly argued that the structures seen by these cells are in principle the same as those recognized by the other T cells (i.e., an MHC molecule holding a peptide in its groove) and that cell-mediated SUR should therefore be regarded as an operational term. The peptide may represent the variable, idiotypic region of another TCR, thus possibly turning a so-called T_s into an anti-idiotypic cytotoxic T cell. Of course, this explanation does not rule out alternative pathways of negative growth and function regulations between different cells. Humoral factors may again become involved, be they released specifically reactive molecules or secreted lymphokines antagonistic to another cell's crucial lymphokine.

Specific Unresponsiveness Through Inability to Respond

The state of SUR through inability to respond is basically different from the mechanisms described above which represent specifically downregulating immune responses. The original concepts of physical deletion of specifically reactive lymphocyte clones were almost entirely given up during the last two decades and had been increasingly replaced by suppressor cell concepts. It was only within the last few years that new experiments unequivocally established that many T cells bearing self-reactive receptors are clonally deleted in the thymus. Subsequently, it became apparent that two additional states of SUR through inability to respond can be observed at the level of peripheral T cells, namely functional silencing of clones (clonal anergy) with or without failure of activation by lack of costimulatory factors [30,34,37]. These discoveries were made possible by two methodologically new approaches: the use of newly raised monoclonal antibodies that can identify TCR of defined antigen reaction specificities, and the use of transgenic mice (i.e., the introduction of defined genes into the germline of an animal by microinjecting DNA into the pronuclei of fertilized eggs).

Clonal deletion was first proven by Kappler et al. [22]. They were able to show that particular T cells were selectively eliminated during the intrathymic maturation processes, namely, T cells carrying a TCR that uses a particular V beta gene segment (Vβ17a) and enables these cells to react strongly with a particular MHC class II molecule (I-E), but only if the animal's cells express this molecule themselves. Analogous data involving other, non-MHC transplantation antigens, such as Mls (see the chapter on non-MHC antigens) and H-Y (male sex-linked), have confirmed these findings.

The concept of functional silencing, also called clonal anergy, was introduced in the late 1970s by Nossal for antibody-producing B lymphocytes. The above-mentioned modern biotechnology allowed it to be proven for T cells. It could be shown that clonal deletion does not remove all autoreactive T cells, especially in the case of tissue-specific antigens not expressed in the thymus, but that such cells are present in the periphery and are nonreactive. For instance, mice failed to mount an immune response against an allogeneic (MHC class I) transgene product which they expressed not in the thymus but on pancreatic islet beta cells. More recently Miller et al. reported that the spleen cells from these transgenic mice do not kill target cells carrying the transgene product, whereas thymocytes from the same mice do. However, the unresponsiveness of these spleen cells could be reversed in vitro by providing IL-2 as costimulatory factor (second signal). On the other hand, Rammensee et al. described clonal anergy in mature T cells on immunizing adult Mls-1^b mice with Mls-1^a cells; the T cells were unable to produce IL-2 and to respond to exogenous IL-2, thus demonstrating another form of functional inactivation of mature T cells.

These recent observations have been mentioned in some detail in order to indicate the onset of "second generation transplantation biology through the molecular revolution" [35]. Only two years ago our insight into that which provides the basis for successful clinical transplantation was much more limited. The ultimate goal of transplantation immunology remains the induction of long-standing, true immunologic tolerance in the allografted patient. To achieve this we still have much to learn about the applicability of that which we observe in the laboratory to humans.

References

1. Klein J. Immunology, the science of self-nonself discrimination. New York: Wiley, 1982.
2. Milgrom F, Kano K, Zaleski MB. Transplantation immunology. In: Rose NR, Milgrom F, van Oss CJ, eds. Principles of immunology. New York: Macmillan, 1979;376–401.
3. Davies DAL. Non-MHC antigens and their relation to graft rejection. In: Calne RY, ed. Transplantation immunology. Oxford: Oxford University Press, 1984;159–68.
4. Hayry P, Koskimies S, eds. The state of the art of transplantation. Cellular and molecular mechanisms. Transplant Proc 1987;19:25–60.
5. Halloran PF, Wadgymar A, Autenried P. The regulation of expression of major histoincompatibility complex products. Transplantation 1986;41:413–20.
6. Unanue ER, Allen PM. The basis for the immunoregulatory role of macrophages and other accessory cells. Science 1987;236:551–7.

7. Allison JP, Lanier LL. Structure, function, and serology of the T-cell antigen receptor complex. Annu Rev Immunol 1987;5:503–40.
8. Wottge HU, Muller-Ruchholtz W. Dual basis for major histoincompatibility complex allogeneic cell-cell cooperation: T cell lymphocyte tolerance to Ia antigens and adaptive differentiation of macrophages. Transplant Proc 1987;17:982–4.
9. Mason DW, Morris PJ. Effector mechanisms in allograft rejection. Annu Rev Immunol 1986;4:119–45.
10. Rosenberg AS, Mizuochi T, Sharrow SO, Singer A. Phenotype, specificity, and function of T cell subsets and T cell interactions involved in skin allograft rejection. J Exp Med 1987;165:1296–315.
11. Meryman HT, ed. Transplantation: Approaches to graft rejection. New York: Alan R. Liss, 1986.
12. Barrett AJ. Graft-versus-host disease: a review. J R Soc Med 1987;80:368–73.
13. Muller-Ruchholtz W. Recent approaches to MHC (HLA)-allogeneic bone marrow transplantation without GVHR. Clin Immunol Newslett 1986;7:52–6.
14. Muller-Ruchholtz W, Wottge HU, Blank M, et al. Chimerism after elimination of immunocompetent cells and their precursors from bone marrow using specified antisera. In: Slavin E, ed. Tolerance in bone marrow and organ transplantation. Amsterdam: Elsevier, 1984;197–251.
15. Dreger P, Muller-Ruchholtz W. Reduction of immunogenicity of T-depleted bone marrow depends on additional depletion of accessory cells: implications for prevention of graft rejection. Transplantation 1989;48:in press.
16. Hayry P, Koskimies S, eds. Immunosuppression. Transplant Proc 1987;19:1833–2036, 2770–3.
17. Sachs DH. Specific immunosuppression. Transplant Proc 1987;19:123–7.
18. Thiede A, Deltz E, Engemann R, Hamelmann H, eds. Microsurgical models in rats for transplantation research. Berlin: Springer-Verlag, 1985.
19. Muller-Ruchholtz W. Beeinflussung Transplantations-immunologischer Reaktionen durch Cyclophosphamid und andere homologe Oxazaphosphorin-2-oxide. Drug Res 1974;24:1160–7.
20. Reed E, Hardy M, Benvenisty A, Lattes C, et al. Effect of anti-idiotypic antibodies to HLA on graft survival in renal allograft recipients. N Engl J Med 1987;316:1450–5.
21. Hutchinson IV. Suppressor T cells in allogeneic models. Transplantation 1986;41:547–55.
22. Kappler JW, Roehm N, Marrack P. T cell tolerance by clonal elimination in the thymus. Cell 1987;49:273–80.
23. Abe R, Hodes RJ. Properties of the Mls system: a revised formulation of Mls genetics and an analysis of T-cell recognition of Mls determinants. Immunol Rev 1989;107:5–28.
24. Batchelor JR, Lombardi G, Lechler RJ. Speculations on the specificity of suppression. Immunol Today 1989;10:37–40.
25. Berzofsky JA, Brett SJ, Streicher HZ, Takahashi H. Antigen processing for presentation to T lymphocytes: function, mechanisms and implications for the T-cell repertoire. Immunol Rev 1988;106:5–32.
26. Bjorkman MA, Saper MA, Samraoui B, et al. Structure of the human class I histocompatibility antigen, HLA-A2. Nature 1987;329:506–12.
27. Blackman MA, Kappler JW, Marrack P. T cell specificity and repertoire. Immunol Rev 1988;101:5–20.
28. Blank M, Gronau C, Sauer M, et al. Functional characterization of prethymic T cells committed to alloreactivity. Transplantation 1986;41:759–65.

29. Dinarello CA. Interleukin-1 and its biologically related cytokines. Adv Immunol 1989;44:153–206.
30. Hall BM. Transplantation tolerance: a 1988 perspective. Transplant Proc 1989;21:816–9.
31. Henney CS. The interleukins as lymphocyte growth factors. Transplant Proc 1989;21:22–5.
32. Kupiec-Weglinsky JW, Tilney NL. Lymphocyte migration patterns in organ allograft recipients. Immunol Rev 1989;108:63–82.
33. Kuypers TW, Roos D. Leukocyte membrane adhesion proteins: a review of functional and regulatory aspects. Res Immunol 1989;140:461–86.
34. Miller JFAP, Morahan G, Allison J. Immunological tolerance: new approaches using transgenic mice. Immunol Today 1989;10:53–7.
35. Nossal GJV. Second generation transplantation biology through the molecular revolution. Transplant Proc 1989;21:5–9.
36. Ritz J, Schmidt RE, Michon J, et al. Characterization of functional surface structures on human natural killer cells. Adv Immunol 1988;42:181–212.
37. Schwartz RH. Acquisition of immunologic self-tolerance. Cell 1989;57:1073–81.
38. Strominger JL. The $\gamma\delta$ T cell receptor and class Ib MHC-related proteins: enigmatic molecules of immune recognition. Cell 1989;57:895–8.
39. Qin S, Cobbold S, Benjamin R, Waldmann H. Induction of classical transplantation tolerance in the adult. J Exp Med, 1989;169:779–94.

2

Skin Grafts and Their Rejection

WAYNE W. HANCOCK
GEORGE F. MURPHY

Skin grafts are often a critical component in the management of patients who have suffered severe burns, trauma such as degloving injuries, or surgical procedures such as tumor resections. Skin grafts provide the coverage necessary to exclude infectious agents and maintain body fluids. Typically, if the wound is small, skin is harvested from another area of the patient's body. However, split-skin autografts are insufficient for management of large wounds, especially burns exceeding 50% of the total body surface. Such large wounds are currently treated using human cadaveric skin allografts, pigskin xenografts, or, increasingly, biosynthetic skin substitutes. Allografts and xenografts provide valuable, sometimes lifesaving coverage of denuded areas, but without continued and extensive immunosuppressive therapy, they are invariably rejected. Indeed, compared with vascularized organ allografts transplanted in the same animals, skin allografts appear to elicit a particularly potent allograft response [1–3]. Skin transplantation has received considerably less attention clinically than transplantation of solid organ grafts such as kidney, heart, lung, liver, and pancreas, in part because of this potent, often overwhelming allograft response.

Although the initial studies and impetus for skin grafts occurred during the management of injuries in wartime aviators and other military personnel, most studies of the skin graft response have been performed in experimental animals, particularly inbred rodents. The latter studies have provided some of the foundations of modern immunology, through recognition of histoincompatibility antigens, and have proved central to the development of clinical transplantation. Hence, this chapter begins with a review of the immunopathologic basis and associated histopathology of skin transplantation in experimental animals, emphasizing recent studies, followed by discussion of human skin graft rejection. We conclude with a synthesis of this knowledge and a discussion of current research that appears likely to lead to new clinical applications of skin allografts. The pathology of cutaneous graft-vs-host disease (GVHD) is discussed in Chapter 9.

Skin Allograft Rejection in Experimental Animals

Skin grafts, like grafts of muscle, bone, nerve, or blood vessels, are examples of nonprimarily vascularized grafts. Nonprimarily vascularized grafts generally show somewhat slower dynamics of rejection than vascularized grafts such as kidney, heart, lung, or liver. However, the principles of skin graft rejection are essentially the same as that of organ grafts [4]. Rejection can be conveniently divided into three stages [5]: (1) an *afferent stage* of drainage of antigenic material into afferent lymphatics, (2) a *central stage* of activation of the host immune system in regional lymph nodes, and (3) an *efferent stage* of attack and destruction of the graft by activated leukocytes that have migrated from regional lymph nodes through the efferent lymphatics, into the bloodstream, and hence into the graft itself.

Consistent with this schema, skin grafts placed in sites without lymphatic drainage [6], without a blood supply [7], or in animals deficient in T cells [8] enjoy prolonged survival. However, there are variations to this classic scheme. In particular, some degree of local immune activation (termed *peripheral sensitization*) does occur, as evidenced by the slower but seemingly inexorable rejection of skin allografts deprived of lympathic drainage [9].

Afferent Stage of Skin Allograft Rejection

This initial stage involves activation of host inducer–helper T (T-h) cells either directly by interaction with donor antigen presenting cells (APC) or following uptake and processing of graft transplantation antigens by host APC, as occurs for conventional antigens (Fig. 2.1). As with rejection of other vascularized allografts, major histocompatibility complex (MHC) antigens play a key role in the initiation and pathogenesis of skin allograft rejection. However, even after complete matching of MHC and blood group antigens, and despite negative mixed-lymphocyte reactions between donor and recipient, untreated skin grafts in humans and in animals are eventually rejected, although the delay may take up to 20 days for HLA-identical siblings [10]. This is presumably the result of allostimulation by non-MHC, or so-called minor histocompatibility antigens, including keratinocyte-specific alloantigens [11].

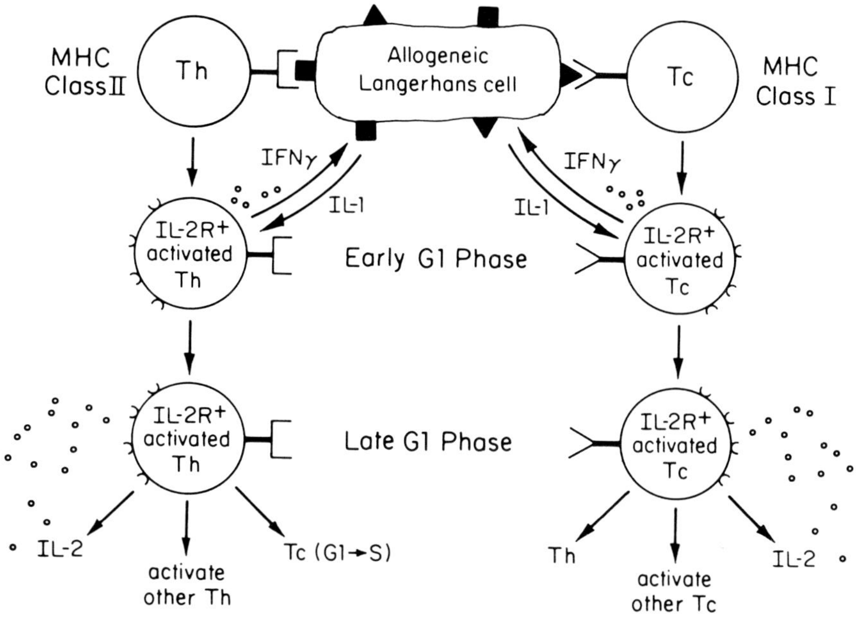

Figure 2.1
Diagram of T-cell activation in response to a skin graft; the events shown may occur within the skin graft itself or within regional lymph nodes. In this model, an allogeneic cell such as an epidermal LC expresses class I and class II alloantigens and can interact directly with host T cells; alternately, ingestion, processing, and antigen presentation to Th can occur through host APC such as macrophages. Unlike conventional MHC restriction wherein T cells are activated in the presence of host class II antigen complexed with antigen, alloantigens on LC may appear sufficiently similar to antigen plus self-MHC antigen for direct stimulation of Th and Tc to occur. Th activation begins with direct binding of Th to a class II alloantigen-bearing LC. On binding to the alloantigen, the Th enters the early G1 phase of the cell cycle, with expression of receptors for IL-1 (IL-1R) and IL-2 (IL-2R) and production of IFN-γ. IFN-γ boosts both IL-1 production and MHC antigen expression by LC. IL-1 stimulates the IL-1R$^+$ (and IL-2R$^+$) Th to move into the late G1 phase and begin to synthesize and release IL-2 and additional lymphokines. IL-2 release provides an autocrine signal for Th replication and also stimulates activation (S phase) and clonal expansion of adjacent antigen-specific T cells, including Tc. Tc may be activated directly by LC class I alloantigens, as shown on the right side of the diagram, with analogous events occurring to that depicted for Th activation. As discussed in the text, macrophages and other cells are recruited and the combined onslaught of various DTH and Tc cells leads to skin graft destruction.

Major Histocompatibility Complex Skin Alloantigens The MHC locus located on chromosome 6 encodes a series of immunogenic and extraordinarily polymorphic glycoproteins termed class I molecules (human HLA-A and B antigens) and class II molecules (human HLA-D and DR antigens) [12]. Class I alloantigens are densely expressed on the membranes of keratinocytes and may be detected on Langerhans cells but not on melanocytes by immunoelectron microscopy [13]. Unlike class I antigens, class II alloantigens are normally restricted to the membranes of epidermal Langerhans cells (LC) and their dermal precursors (termed indeterminate cells), acrosyringeal epithelial cells, dermal macrophages, and, in humans, unlike most experimental animals, vascular endothelial cells.

The importance of both class I and class II alloantigens to the pathogenesis of skin allograft rejection can be understood by reference to the passenger leukocyte theory of graft rejection, first proposed by Snell in 1957 and popularized by Lafferty et al. [14]. According to this theory, class II antigen-rich "stimulator" cells are found in all tissues and, in the presence of a costimulatory factor such as interleukin-1 (IL-1), activate host T-h cells. Such activation may result either from direct interaction of T-h cells with foreign antigen on the surface of stimulator cells or by indirect activation following phagocytosis of allogeneic cells and processing by host macrophages [15]. On activation, T-h cells produce interleukin-2 (IL-2) and other lymphokines that attract and activate cytotoxic T cells (T-c) and macrophages. T-c cells generated in this response are typically directed against class I antigens; hence rejection involves interaction of T-h, T-c, and other cells.

An important feature of this theory has been to explain the success of in vitro culture in modifying the antigenicity of various tissues. Thus, in vitro culture of skin [16,17] and many other tissues results in loss of class II antigens, though class I antigen expression is unaltered. Grafts of such cultured tissues are generally not rejected, even in the absence of immunosuppression, and this is interpreted as the result of loss of stimulator cells. Importantly, allografts do appear to retain their antigenicity since even established grafts are soon rejected if the hosts are challenged with spleen cells syngeneic to the graft.

Non–Major Histocompatibility Complex Skin Alloantigens Skin allografts elicit a potent host immune response; e.g., certain rat strain combinations will accept a kidney allograft, but not a skin allograft, from the same donor [1]. This may result from expression of non-MHC skin-specific alloantigens, which are thought to occur in various species, including humans [11,18]. In the mouse, such epidermal alloantigens serve as targets for T-c cells [19]. H-Y antigens are a special class of non-MHC antigens relevant to the pathogenesis of murine skin graft rejection, since in some strain combinations, female mice will reject syngeneic male skin grafts [20]. However, the overall significance and biochemical characterization of H-Y and other non-MHC or minor antigens remains elusive [5,20].

Skin Antigen Presenting Cells Using various models and strain combinations, three types of skin antigen presenting cells (APC) have been established: epidermal LC, keratinocytes, and, at least in the mouse, epidermal Thy-1^+ dendritic cells.

LC have been the most extensively studied skin APC; they possess class II antigens, express surface receptors for IgG and complement, produce IL-1, and have potent alloactivating and antigen-presenting capabilities [21–24]. Indeed, recent studies [25] have shown that LC are 100 to 1000 times more efficient than keratinocytes in inducing skin allograft rejection; thus injection of as few as 100 class II^+ LC results in accelerated skin graft rejection.

Conversely, in vitro depletion of LC from keratinocyte cultures results in indefinite survival of murine keratinocyte grafts, unlike freshly dispersed epidermal cells, which include small numbers of class II^+ LC and are readily rejected [26]. These studies support the widely held view that LC function as passenger leukocytes and thereby play a dominant role in initiating skin allograft rejection [25], even though their depletion in certain models does not always prevent generation of T-c [27] or murine skin graft rejection [28].

In contrast to LC, keratinocytes are thought to function as APC only under highly specialized circumstances, if at all [29,30]. Based on the passenger leukocyte theory, this may be because keratinocytes normally lack class II antigens. Keratinocytes, however, do produce immunologically relevant cytokines, including IL-1-like thymocyte activating factor (ETAF) [31]. ETAF has similar pleiotropic effects to IL-1, including induction of fever; neutrophil chemotaxis; induction of thymocyte, keratinocyte, and fibroblast proliferation; T and B cell activation; and increased fibroblast collagenase synthesis, muscle proteolysis, and production of hepatic acute phase reactants. Recently, Ansel et al. [32] showed constitutive keratinocyte production of messenger RNA for IL-1, which was upregulated by exposure to lipopolysaccharide (LPS) or ultraviolet light and downregulated by cell differentiation, suggesting that ETAF/IL-1 plays a role in normal skin homeostasis. Other skin-based cytokines may also act on the immune system; e.g., murine keratinocytes reportedly produce IL-2-like factors that support the growth of T cells [33].

Thy-1^+ dendritic cells are Ia^-, bone marrow–derived cells that display natural killer (NK) cell functions in vitro [34]. Their role in induction of alloimmunity is currently highly speculative, as is that of skin endothelial cells, although some types of vascular endothelial cells can function as APC at least in vitro [35].

Central Stage of Skin Allograft Rejection

Although the systemic nature of the host immune response to a skin allograft has long been recognized [36], few details are known regarding the precise events associated with T-cell activation within draining lymph nodes. Compared with contralateral lymph nodes, the weight of draining lymph nodes doubles, the numbers of intranodal lymphocytes increase 5- to 6-fold, and there is a 4-fold increase in blastogenesis detectable 6 to 8 days after transplantation, just before skin graft rejection [37]. In addition, the proportion of lymphocytes bearing receptors for IL-2 (IL-$2R^+$) increases from 3% to 11% during unmodified acute skin graft rejection [38].

Effector Stage of Skin Allograft Rejection

There is little evidence for humoral immunity in the rejection of skin allografts [5]; this section summarizes current views regarding the cellular mechanisms of skin graft rejection.

Delayed-Type Hypersensitivity Response to a Skin Allograft Histologic similarities between the cellular infiltrates of classic delayed-type hypersensitivity (DTH) reactions and skin graft rejection have long been noted [39]. Moreover, studies in T-cell-deficient rats [40] and mice [41] showed that animals reconstituted with syngeneic cells of the T-h phenotype rejected skin grafts, whereas rodents reconstituted with cells of the T-c phenotype maintained their skin grafts.

However, these transfer experiments have been regarded as inconclusive for two main reasons [5]. First, phenotypically and functionally distinct T-c cells have been identified and isolated from rejecting grafts and spleens of T-h-reconstituted animals, indicating either persistence of T-c-cell precursors in animals thought to have been rendered T-cell deficient or contamination of the T-h innocula used. Second, it is now recognized that phenotypic identification of T cells does not necessarily correlate with a particular T-cell function. Thus, although T-c cells directed against class I antigens typically have the CD-8$^+$ phenotype, class II-specific T cells with the T-h phenotype (CD-4$^+$) have been described [5] and may be important to the pathogenesis of rejection, as described below. Hence, data based on the use of monoclonal antibodies (mAbs) and cell-transfer experiments suggest but do not prove a dominant role for a DTH response in skin allograft rejection.

Cytotoxic T Cells and Skin Allograft Rejection Several lines of evidence suggest a role for T-c cells in skin allograft rejection. Using skin grafts from allophenic mice into parental strain recipients, Mintz and Silvers [42] showed that melanoblasts and hair follicles expressing syngeneic H-2 antigens survived, while those expressing allogeneic H-2 antigens were destroyed. This result was consistent with specific destruction of discrete cells rather than widespread, nonspecific destruction. Subsequently, Tyler et al. [43] showed that intradermal injection of various murine T-c clones directed against a minor skin-specific antigen caused local skin necrosis only in strains expressing the relevant minor antigen. In addition, using a skin graft model in adult thymectomized mice, Cobbold et al. [44] showed that administration of an anti-Lyt 2$^+$ mAb directed against murine T-c cells and their precursors prolonged skin graft survival. Similarly, using sublethally irradiated inbred rats, Mason et al. [45] found that skin grafts across minor MHC barriers survived longer when animals were reconstituted with inocula depleted of T-c than in rats receiving whole unfractionated innocula.

In experimental models, T-h cell activation can lead to lymphokine-mediated induction of class II antigens and augmentation of class I expression on graft vascular endothelial cells [46], keratinocytes, and hair follicles [45]. Recently, gamma interferon (IFN-g)–mediated augmentation of class I expression and induction of class II expression on cultured human keratinocytes was demonstrated [47]. Interestingly, cultured human keratinocytes appeared resistant to lysis by T-c cells unless class I expression was increased by exposure to IFN-g [47]. Decreased expression of class I antigens by cultured keratinocytes, compared with their in vivo counterparts, may contribute to the enhanced survival of allogeneic cultured keratinocyte grafts. In addition, induction of class II antigens on keratinocytes stimulated proliferation of T lymphoblasts but not resting cells [47], suggesting that class II expression by keratinocytes can amplify but not initiate an allograft response in vivo.

Induction of class II antigen expression explains what had previously appeared as anomalous results. Thus, Woodward et al. [48] reported widespread skin graft rejection in recombinant mice differing only at class II loci, although in these strains class II antigens are normally present only on epidermal LC. Activation of host T-h cells by donor skin LC leads to lymphokine production and induction of class II antigen expression on graft vasculature and keratinocytes. These class II$^+$ cells are then targets for the host immune response, including T-c directed against class II molecules.

Morphologic and Immunohistologic Studies of Experimental Skin Allograft Rejection

The sequential histologic features of rat skin allograft rejection studied in untreated or cyclosporine (CsA)-treated rats [49] are typical of skin allograft rejection in rodents and are very similar to the known features of human skin allograft rejection [50,51].

Macroscopic Appearance Skin graft rejection is noted visually by erythema, followed progressively by dry scaling skin, vesicle formation, serous ulcerations, scabbing, and necrosis.

Light Microscopic Appearance Few changes were seen in the histology of rat skin allografts for 5 to 6 days after transplantation. However, by day 6, endothelial cells lining the graft microvasculature exhibited focal degeneration and hypertrophy that resulted in occasional obliteration of the lumina, similar to that described in human skin allograft rejection [50]. Thus, although rejection may be initiated by class II antigens expressed by cells in both the epidermis and dermis, the early cellular injury that characterizes the effector stage is focused at the dermal microvasculature. An inflammatory infiltrate, although present through all levels of the grafts, was particularly prominent around affected vessels and consisted of a mixture of lymphocytes and macrophages. Degranulated mast cells were also frequently encountered. In contrast to isograft controls and CsA-treated animals, a marked increase in the numbers of inflammatory cells was seen by days 8 to 10 (Table 2.1). At this time, vascular lesions were most prominent, with marked hypertrophy and necrosis of endothelium and widespread occlusive thrombosis. By day 10, all grafts showed widespread signs of rejection, with coagulative necrosis of the epidermis and the cells of the dermis. Vascular thrombosis and extracellular edema were extensive within the dermis, and numerous lymphocytes and macrophages were observed in association with the remaining intact vessels of the graft bed.

Table 2.1
Morphologic and immunohistologic features of rat skin allograft rejection (days 8 to 10)[a]

Histologic features	*Untreated allografts*	*CsA-treated allografts*	*Isografts*
Endothelial damage	3+	±	−
Thrombosis	3+	−	−
Fibrin deposition	2+	−	−
Mast cell degranulation	2+	−	−
Helper T cells	3+	2+	2+
Cytotoxic T cells	3+	±	1+
TF + macrophages	3+	±	1+
Ia + endothelial cells	2+	−	−
Ia + epidermal cells	3+	+	+

Source: Adapted from Guillen FJ, Hancock WW, Towpik E, et al. Transplantation 1986;41:734–9.

[a]Graded semiquantitatively as absent (−) or present to a trace (±), minor (1+), moderate (2+), or marked (3+) extent. mAb markers included W3/13 (T cells), W3/25 (helper T cells), OX-8 (cytotoxic T cells), Al-3 (procoagulant molecule tissue factor, TF), and OX-4 (Ia antigens).

Ultrastructural Appearance Transmission electron microscopy of allografts confirmed the microvascular injury seen by light microscopy. At days 6 to 8, before graft necrosis, allograft venules and arterioles showed endothelial cell swelling and vacuolization, disruption of cell membranes, nuclear pyknosis, focal areas of endothelial cell sloughing, and luminal thrombosis. Vascular lesions were invariably accompanied by vasocentric mononuclear cell infiltrates and fibrin deposition. Focal endothelial swelling was also seen in some vessels from CsA-treated allografts, but necrosis and thrombosis were never observed. Endothelial alterations were not seen in isografts. Ultrastructural examination of the infiltrating mononuclear cells confirmed identification of macrophages with primary and secondary lysosomes as well as lymphocytes, small numbers of which had the morphologic features of large granular lymphocytes.

Immunohistology Unlike isograft or CsA-treated controls (see Table 2.1), dermal vessels of untreated day 10 allografts were surrounded by large numbers of mononuclear cells bearing the leukocyte common (OX-1^{+}) and Ia-(OX-4^{+}) antigens. Dermal endothelial cells were variably Ia^{+}, consistent with lymphokine-induced activation. Infiltrating mononuclear cells consisted of equal proportions of lymphocytes and macrophages. More than 90% of the lymphocytes expressed the membrane phenotype of T-c cells (OX8^{+}, W3/13^{+}), whereas over 90% of the intragraft macrophages were labeled using the activation marker Al-3 (Fig. 2.2). The latter mAb (A1-3) is directed against the procoagulant molecule tissue factor (TF) [52,53], and

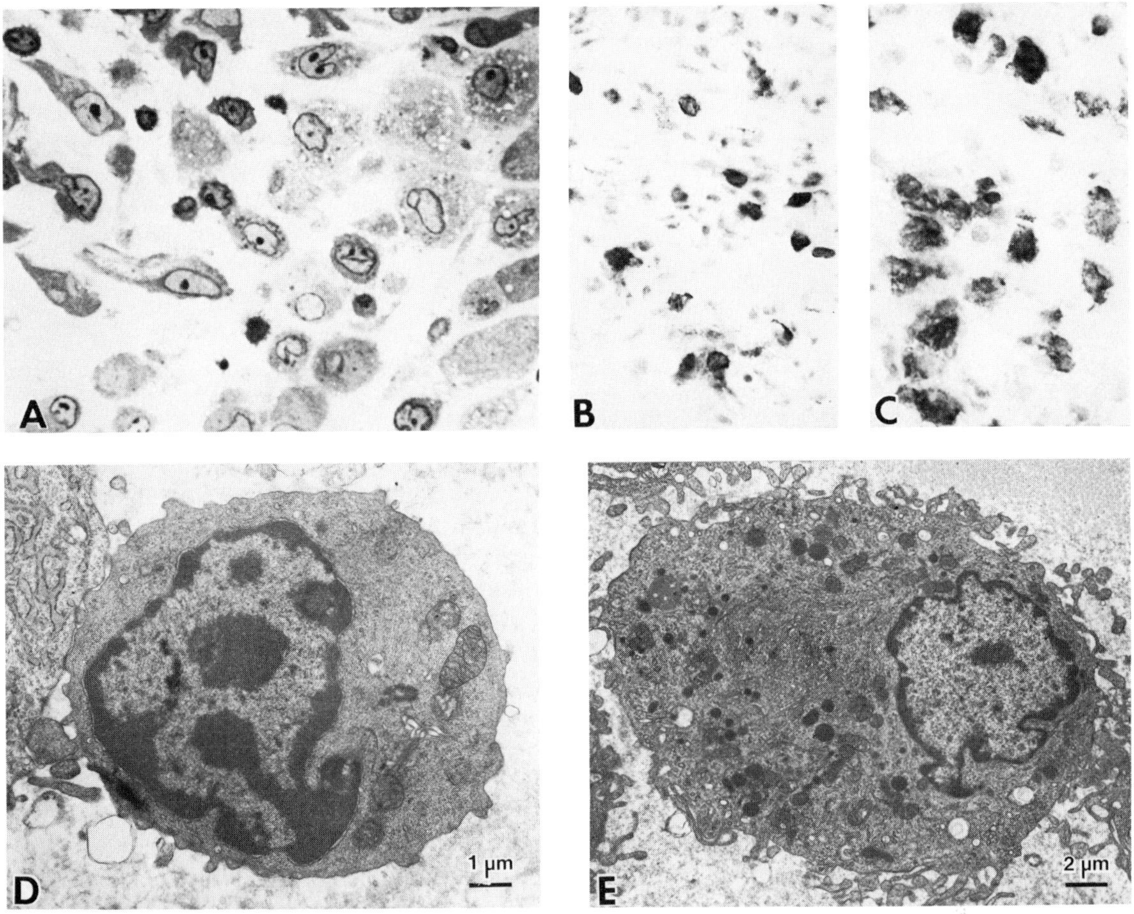

Figure 2.2
Cells composing the inflammatory infiltrates in experimental cutaneous allograft rejection consist of (A) small lymphoid cells and larger, macrophage-like cells by light microscopy. The smaller cells label with OX-8 (B), whereas the larger cells are reactive with A1-3 (C). Ultrastructurally, the smaller cells have characteristics of lymphocytes, whereas the larger cells contain numerous lysosomes and cytoplasmic organelles typical of monocyte/macrophages. These cells appear to be effectors of the endothelial injury seen in early skin allograft rejection.

the presence and distribution of Al-3^{+} macrophages corresponded histologically with that of fibrin deposits.

In summary, untreated rat skin graft rejection is associated sequentially with perivascular accumulation of T cells and activated macrophages expressing the tissue factor procoagulant molecule, followed by hypertrophy and necrosis of endothelium, occlusive thrombosis, and eventually coagulative necrosis of the epidermis and dermis. By contrast, the vascular changes, mononuclear cell activation, fibrin deposition, and graft rejection are all prevented by treatment with CsA.

Prolongation of Experimental Skin Allograft Survival

Historically, corticosteroids, cyclosphosphamide, 6-mercatopurine, azathioprine, bredinin, antilymphocyte serum, and various mAbs have shown only limited success in prolonging skin graft survival, often in association with undesirable morbidity or mortality [37]. In contrast, Borel et al. [54] showed that CsA significantly and effectively prolonged experimental skin graft survival. Similar results were subsequently reported in several animal models: thus, parenteral or oral [49,55–59] or topical CsA [60] all prolong skin allograft in rodents. However, unlike the long-term survival achieved with primarily vascularized allografts after even short courses with CsA, continuous low-dose maintenance doses of CsA are necessary to achieve long-term skin graft survival [37].

The mechanism of action of CsA is complex. Initially, CsA was perceived as predominantly inhibiting T-h cell function, as shown by inhibition of IL-2 and IFN-g gene transription. However, CsA is also known to affect APC [61]. In particular, cultured murine skin LC pulsed with CsA shows a direct and marked reduction in APC capability, which is not due to diminished IL-1 production, increased PGE synthesis, or decreased membrane Ia expression [62]. The finding that topical CsA can also prolong rat skin allograft survival [60] is consistent with local immunosuppressive effects on skin APC. Regardless of topical, oral, or parenteral CsA administration, some degree of cell infiltration, loss of hair follicles, follicular cysts, and hyperkeratosis are consistently observed after moderate to long-term CsA use [63].

A new drug, FK506, derived from *Streptomyces tsukabaensis,* appears even more potent than CsA in suppressing the mixed lymphocyte culture (MLC) of both human and murine cells and inhibiting the release of several lymphokines, including IL-2, IFN-g, and IL-3. Inamura et al. [64] reported that FK506 was as effective as CsA in prolonging rat skin allograft or xenograft (mouse→rat) survival at one-hundredth the dose of CsA. However, as with CsA, skin grafts were rejected once maintenance drug therapy was stopped. This and other studies suggest that FK506 may well prove of future clinical value in skin and organ transplantation.

Skin Allograft Rejection in Humans

The first systematic studies of any form of human allograft rejection were reported by Gibson and Medawar [65] in their classic observations of acute skin graft rejection in wartime burn patients (particularly aviators). However, most subsequent studies of skin graft rejection have relied on experimental animal models, as reviewed above. This section deals with data relevant to understanding, treating, and preventing skin allograft rejection in humans.

Using normal human volunteer subjects, Dvorak et al. [50] performed detailed and classic ultrastructural studies of unmodified skin allograft rejection. Rejection was associated with microvascular damage to the graft and the graft bed in conjunction with extravascular fibrin deposition and infiltration by mononuclear cells. These morphologic results were consistent with skin rejection resulting from a cell-mediated immune response against MHC antigens expressed on the dermal vasculature, causing endothelial injury, vascular occlusion, and graft ischemia.

An analysis of the mononuclear cells present in these tissues, using anti-T cell mAbs and enzyme histochemistry, was subsequently reported by Bhan et al. [51]. Early and focal signs of injury were seen in the small vessels of the graft and graft bed at days 5 to 6 after transplantation, particularly those vessels surrounded by small cuffs of lymphocytes. Progressive endothelial injury, necrosis, and sloughing extended to nearly all small vessels by days 8 to 10. Coagulative necrosis of skin grafts and superficial areas of the graft bed followed at days 10 to 12. Both $CD4^+$ and $CD8^+$ cells were identified; the perivascular mononuclear cell cuffs consisted predominantly of $CD4^+$ T cells and esterase-positive mononuclear phagocytes, while $CD8^+$ cells were more numerous in the epidermis and around hair follicles. Two mechanisms for graft destruction were suggested: (1) direct lysis of small numbers of epidermal cells by $CD8^+$ T cells and (2) damage to the microvascular endothelium, leading to secondary graft infarction, possibly as a result of the action of $CD4^+$ cells or other cells that had been recruited, such as macrophages. Moreover, since both studies reported considerable microvascular damage to the graft bed as well as to the graft itself, such immunologically nonspecific damage is similar to that seen in DTH reactions, rather than the precise cell-to-cell lysis expected with T-c effector cells.

Therapeutic Advances in the Use of Skin Grafts to Treat Burn Patients

Skin Allografts Small to moderate-sized burns are widely managed by excision of necrotic tissue and immediate closure of wounds with split-thickness skin autografts [66]. However, wound closure in patients with extensive burns is complicated by the limited availability of tissue for autografts. Once donor sites are harvested, weeks may pass before sufficient healing has occurred such that further autografts may be prepared. Currently, pig or cadaveric split-thickness skin allografts or various synthetic membranes are used without immunosuppression for temporary wound coverage during healing of donor sites; these allografts are rejected by 10 days. It is especially in this group of severely burned patients that advances in skin transplantation may prove lifesaving. In particular, efforts to overcome the shortage of skin available for immediate wound coverage in such patients are necessary to improve survival rates and to decrease scar formation, risk of infection, and length of hospitalization.

In 1974, Burke et al. [67] first showed that the immunosuppressive agents azathioprine, antithymocyte globulin, and corticosteroids could be used to prolong cadaveric skin allograft survival in burn patients for 30 to 60 days. Subsequent clinical trials in severely burned patients using cadaveric skin allografts and combined immunosuppression with azathioprine and antithymocyte globulin showed a decrease in mortality from 100% to 40% [68,69].

However, problems of sepsis in such immunocompromised hosts led to abandonment of this approach.

Recently, Achaeur et al. [70] showed that short-term treatment with CsA led to long-term survival of skin allografts from several donors used to treat a single patient with multiple and widespread burns. CsA allowed survival despite MHC and blood group antigen mismatches, and permanent allograft survival with no signs of rejection were noted after 3 years of follow-up [59]. This result was extended by detailed studies of the success of maintenance low-dose CsA and skin allografts in treatment of thermal injuries in rats [58,59], including full-thickness burns to 75% of the body.

Cultured Keratinocyte Grafts Unlike freshly dispersed epidermal cells, cultured human epidermal cells do not express class II antigens [17] and no longer stimulate allogeneic mixed lymphocyte cultures [16]. Hammond et al. [26] have shown that such in vitro culture leads to depletion of class II$^+$ LC. Together, these studies have led to renewed interest in grafting of keratinocytes, following culture and expansion in vitro, as an alternative approach to split skin grafts.

Cultured keratinocytes may be used as autografts [71] or allografts [72]. The immediate application of keratinocyte autografts is limited by the time taken after the burn for expansion of cells in culture, typically 3 to 5 weeks if large areas of coverage are required. This major disadvantage might be overcome if allogeneic-cultured epithelial cells could be used, since these could be grown in advance, cryopreserved, and stored in skin banks. In the study by Hefton et al. [72], long-term survival of cultured keratinocyte allografts without immunosuppression in three patients was reported. Larger confirmatory studies in humans [73,74] and in rodents [26] have occurred. Whether the successful results in humans were actually due to allograft survival or possible host reepithelialization is unclear. However, the study by Hammond et al. [26] provided good evidence that graft survival in a murine model was not due to reepithelialization.

Recently, Aubock et al. [10] reported a detailed analysis of the intragraft events associated with human allogeneic epidermal cell grafts depleted of LC by culture techniques. In the latter study cultured keratinocyte allografts in 11 patients showed only slightly prolonged graft survival (mean survival of 14.5 days) over that generally noted with standard split-skin allografts (10 days). Rejection was associated with a DTH-type histologic response in the dermis, with large numbers of CD4$^+$ T cells and macrophages as well as an influx of CD8$^+$ T cells into the epidermis where discrete single-cell necrosis of keratinocytes was observed. Interestingly, host LC were also present by rejection. Rejection was postulated as due (1) to shedding of skin antigens into the lymphatics and presentation by host APC to T-h [15] or (2) by uptake of these antigens by repopulating LC and subsequent antigen presentation to host T cells.

Clearly, further studies are necessary to clarify the conflicting accounts on the success of cultured keratinocyte grafts. Nevertheless, initial successes with allografting of cultured keratinocytes and the recent observation that long-term skin allograft survival can be achieved using low-dose CsA are of major clinical significance. In particular, the combination of allografts and CsA may provide the critical means for immediate and long-term wound coverage in severely burned patients and the beginning of a new phase of clinical skin transplantation.

References

1. White E, Hildemann WH. Allografts in genetically defined rats: difference in survival between kidney and skin. Science 1968;162:1293–8.
2. Sakai A, Yakushiji K, Mashimo S. Lymphocyte stimulation by allogeneic tissue cells in rats: with special reference to differential survival of skin and kidney allografts. Transplant Proc 1980;7:74–7.
3. Birinyi LK, Baldwin WM III, Tilney NL. Differential effects of heterologous antisera on the survival of cardiac and skin allografts in rats. Transplantation 1981;32:336–9.
4. Hancock WW. Analysis of intragraft effector mechanisms associated with human renal allograft rejection: immunohistological studies using monoclonal antibodies. Immunol Rev 1984;77:61–84.
5. Mason DW, Morris PJ. Effector mechanisms in allograft rejection. Annu Rev Immunol 1986;4:119–45.
6. Barker CF, Billingham RE. The role of afferent lymphatics in the rejection of skin homografts. J Exp Med 1968;128:97–102.
7. Medawar PB. Immunity to homologous grafted skin. III. The fate of skin homografts transplanted to the brain, to subcutaneous tissue, and to the anterior chamber of the eye. Br J Exp Pathol 1948;29:58–61.
8. Miller JFAB. Effect of neonatal thymectomy on the immunologic responsiveness of the mouse. Proc R Soc Lond Ser B 1962;156:415–19.
9. Tilney NL, Gowans JL. The sensitization of rats by allografts transplanted to alymphatic pedicles of skin. J Exp Med 1971;133:951–7.
10. Aubock J, Irschick E, Romani N, et al. Rejection, after a slightly prolonged survival time, of Langerhans cell-free allogeneic cultured epidermis used for wound coverage in humans. Transplantation 1988;45:730–7.
11. Steinmuller D, Tyler JD. Cross-priming reveals similar tissue-restricted CTL-defined alloantigens on mouse, rat and human epidermal cells. Transplant Proc 1983;15:238–41.
12. Klein J. The major histocompatibility complex of the mouse. Science 1979; 203:516–20.
13. Bronstein BR, Murphy GF, Harrist TJ, et al. Location of HLA-A,B,C antigens in dendritic cells of normal human skin: an ultrastructural study. J Invest Dermatol 1983;80:481–4.
14. Lafferty KJ, Prowse SJ, Simeneovic CJ, Warren HS. Immunobiology of tissue transplantation: a return to the passenger leucocyte concept. Annu Rev Immunol 1983;1:143–54.
15. Sherwood RA, Brent L, Rayfield LS. Presentation of alloantigens by host cells. Eur J Immunol 1986;16:569–74.
16. Hefton JM, Amberson JG, Biozes DG, Weksler ME. Human epidermal cells no longer stimulate allogeneic lymphocytes after growth in culture. J Invest Dermatol 1981;6:308–12.
17. Morhenn VB, Benike CV, Cox AJ, et al. Cultured human epidermal cells do not synthesise HLA-DR. J Invest Dermatol 1981;76:32–8.

for the treatment of thermal injury. I. Extensive graft survival with low-level long-term administration and prolongation in a rat burn model. Transplantation 1988;45:8–12.

59. Black KS, Hewitt CW, Smelser S, et al. Cyclosporine and skin allografts for the treatment of thermal injury. II. Development of an experimental massive third-degree burn model demonstrating extensive graft survival. Transplantation 1988;45:13–16.
60. Lai CS, Wesseler TA, Alexander JW, Babcock GF. Longterm survival of skin allografts in rats treated with topical cyclosporine. Transplantation 1987;44: 83–87.
61. Palay DA, Cluff CW, Wentworth PA, Ziegler HK. Cyclosporine inhibits macrophage-mediated antigen presentation. J Immunol 1986;136:4348–53.
62. Furue M, Katz S. Cyclosporine inhibits accessory and antigen-presenting cell functions of epidermal Langerhans cells. Transplant Proc 1988;20:87–91.
63. Hewitt CW, Black KS, Aguinaldo AM, et al. Pathological alterations in the skin component of composite tissue and skin allografts treated with cyclosporine. Transplant Proc 1988;(Suppl 2);1003–4.
64. Inamura N, Nakahara K, Kino T, et al. Prolongation of skin allograft survival in rats by a novel immunosuppressive agent, FK506. Transplantation 1988; 45:206–9.
65. Gibson T, Medawar PB. The fate of skin allografts in man. J Anat 1943;77: 299–302.
66. Burke JF, Quinby WC Jr, Bondoc CC. Primary excision and prompt grafting as routine therapy for the treatment of thermal burns in children. Surg Clin North Am 1976;56:477–80.
67. Burke J, May JW, Albright N, et al. Temporary skin transplantation and immunosuppression for extensive burns. N Engl J Med 1974;290:269–73.
68. Burke JF, Quinby WC, Bondoc CC. Immunosuppression and temporary skin transplantation in the treatment of massive third-degree burns. Ann Surg 1975;182:183–5.
69. Delmonico FL, Cosimi AB, Russell PS. Temporary skin transplantation for the treatment of extensive burns. Ann Clin Res 1981;13:373ff.
70. Achauer BM, Hewitt CW, Black KS. Long-term skin allograft survival after short-term cyclosporine treatment in a patient with massive burns. Lancet 1986;1:14–15.
71. Gallico GC, O'Connor NE, Compton CC, et al. Permanent coverage of large burns with autologous cultured human epithelium. N Engl J Med 1984;311: 448–51.
72. Hefton JM, Madden MR, Finkelstein JL, Shires GT. Grafting of burn patients with allografts of cultured epidermal cells. Lancet 1983;2:428–30.
73. Thivolet J, Faure M, Demidem A, Mauduit G. Long-term survival and immunological tolerance of human epidermal allografts produced in culture. Transplantation 1986;42:274–80.
74. Madden MR, Finkelstein JL, Staiano-Coico L, Hefton JM. Grafting of cultured allogeneic epidermis on second- and third-degree burn wounds on 16 patients. J Trauma 1986;26:955–9.

3

Renal Transplantation

FRED SANFILIPPO

Pathologic Evaluation of the Renal Allograft

Historical Perspective

Transplanted kidneys have been evaluated by biopsy for more than 20 years to help determine causes of graft dysfunction and to guide clinical management of the transplant recipient. Initial biopsy studies in the mid to late 1960s were focused largely on two goals: to identify patterns of rejection that correlated with ultimate graft outcome [1–7] and to characterize the immunologic mechanisms involved in allograft rejection [8–13]. These and other early ultrastructural and immunohistologic studies of renal allografts [14,15] extended previous experimental work suggesting that a wide range of pathologic changes could be seen in transplanted tissues and that their associations with graft function and outcome would often be unpredictable.

Continued progress in the clinical management of renal transplant recipients during the 1970s and early 1980s led to a decline in the use of biopsy to evaluate allograft dysfunction at some centers. Several factors contributed to this phenomenon, including the fear of complications from the biopsy procedure, the development of numerous noninvasive tests thought to have good predictive value in diagnosing the causes of allograft dysfunction, increased confidence in using clinical signs and symptoms to direct therapy, and the perception that allograft biopsy findings were often of limited value. Interestingly, the available literature clearly demonstrates that each of these considerations is largely unfounded.

For example, the major complication of renal allograft biopsy is gross hematuria, which has been reported to occur in less than 10% of all cases and is usually self-limited [16–21]. In the more severe cases of hematuria, treatment with selective embolization [22] or aminocaproic acid [23] has proved highly effective. Other serious complications are even less frequent but can include pseudoaneurysm or hemorrhage, both of which can be treated by embolization [24,25]; obstruction secondary to blood clots, which can be treated by catheterization [26]; and arteriovenous fistulae [27]. Graft loss due to biopsy complications is exceedingly rare; in reports on large series where complications from biopsy were clearly enumerated [21,26,28–31] only 1 of 454 biopsies (0.2%) ultimately led to graft failure. Similarly, in a recent single-center review of complications involving 420 allograft biopsies performed over 11½ years, none involved graft loss [32].

The limited risks associated with renal allograft biopsy appear to be far outweighed by the significant benefits that have been reported. Numerous studies have documented the value of routine renal allograft biopsy evaluation in guiding therapy [28–37] and have demonstrated that biopsy findings provide diagnoses that are clinically unsuspected in 42% to 46% of cases [30,31,36]. Moreover, although a substantial number of serologic, cellular immune, and urine assays have been suggested to be of diagnostic value in evaluating renal allograft dysfunction [38,39], none has been able to provide a means of diagnosis that is as uniformly quick and accurate. Radiologic measures of assessing renal allograph dysfunction also appear to have limited diagnostic value; recent studies indicate that neither sonography [40] nor magnetic resonance imaging [41] provides a sensitive or specific means of diagnosing the cause of allograft dysfunction. Thus, current evidence indicates that use of renal allograft biopsy for determining the cause of renal allograft dysfunction provides: (1) a low and acceptable risk of transient graft injury and minimal risk of graft loss, (2) useful diagnostic information that leads to significant changes in therapy in approximately half the cases biopsied, and (3) information that (as yet) no alternative test can provide with equivalent speed or diagnostic sensitivity and specificity.

Indications and Potential Utility

Renal transplant biopsy is most often used to evaluate allograft dysfunction in three different situations occurring at characteristic periods (Table 3.1). First, biopsy is frequently indicated when there is initial impairment or delay in graft function, a situation that may persist for varying lengths of time following transplant surgery and that is usually associated with poorer graft survival [42–44]. Although dysfunction in this setting is most commonly associated with acute tubular necrosis (ATN) due to organ recovery or preservation injury, delayed graft function may also be a manifestation of early

Table 3.1
Common indications for renal allograft biopsy with major differential diagnoses

Initial graft nonfunction/dysfunction: Delayed graft function
Acute tubular necrosis
Perfusion injury
Hyperacute graft rejection
Surgical-urologic complications
Endogenous donor kidney diseases
Concomitant acute allograft rejection
Rapid decline in normal graft function: Acute dysfunction
Acute rejection
Acute cyclosporine vasculopathy/nephrotoxicity
Drug or serum sickness reactions
Infections
Vascular-ureteral complications
Early recurrent diseases
Acute transplant glomerulopathy
Malignant hypertension
Intravascular coagulopathy
Other de novo or acquired renal disease
Slow decline in normal graft function: Chronic dysfunction
Chronic rejection
Chronic cyclosporine nephrotoxicity
Recurrent renal diseases
Transplant glomerulopathy
Arterionephrosclerosis
Other de novo or acquired renal disease

allograft rejection, surgical complications, obstructive lesions, or endogenous donor disease. The development of rejection during a period of post-transplant ATN is often difficult to assess, since renal graft function is already impaired. The increased risk of masked rejection during periods of delayed function has been suggested by the higher incidence of delayed function in patients with immunologic risk factors such as prior graft rejection or significant presensitization and by the poorer ultimate graft survival associated with initial allograft dysfunction [42–45]. Thus, renal allograft biopsy evaluation during periods of delayed graft function is often useful in distinguishing ATN from other causes of delayed function as well as in identifying the presence of occult rejection.

A second common indication for allograft biopsy is the rapid deterioration of graft function, especially in a previously well-functioning transplant. This usually occurs during the first weeks or months following transplantation and is most often the result of acute rejection, nephrotoxicity from the use of cyclosporine (CsA), or infection. Acute allograft dysfunction may also be due to other causes such as urologic or renovascular complications, malignant hypertension, drug reactions, and de novo or early recurrent glomerulonephritis. The evaluation of acute graft dysfunction is the most frequent indication for renal transplant biopsy, and such biopsies tend to be the most difficult to interpret, since the major diagnostic considerations have overlapping pathologic features and may be present concomitantly. However, prompt evaluation of acute dysfunction is especially important, since early treatment of rejection reactions is more likely to reduce immune-mediated damage and lead to recovery.

The third major indication for biopsy is a slow progressive decline in renal allograft function, usually seen at later times (months to years) following transplantation. This generally presents a differential diagnosis of chronic rejection vs other etiologies such as recurrent disease, chronic CsA nephrotoxicity, transplant glomerulopathy, and arterionephrosclerosis. The ability to discriminate among these and other possibilities is important in determining prognosis and directing appropriate therapy.

Because immune-mediated rejection provides a significant risk of dysfunction at any time after transplantation, the ability to determine the extent and type of rejection that may be present is vital for the proper management of immunosuppressive therapy. As has been demonstrated in numerous studies, patient morbidity and mortality following kidney transplantation are most associated with complications due to antirejection therapy [46,47]. Thus, quantitative and qualitative pathologic evaluation of the allograft biopsy to exclude the presence of rejection or to identify rejection reactions that are unlikely to be reversed (e.g., humorally mediated vascular rejection, very severe acute cellular rejection) is of significant importance to prevent unnecessary treatment.

Methods of Evaluation

Although cytologic evaluation of fine-needle aspiration biopsies (see Chapter 12) or exfoliative cells in urinary sediment [48–50] may be useful adjuncts in monitoring renal transplants for the development of rejection, histologic examination of allograft biopsy specimens remains the best means of evaluating kidney transplant pathology. Concern for potential sampling error in evaluating small biopsy sections [51] has been addressed by recent studies that compared findings on biopsy with changes in nephrectomy specimens [37,52]. These studies have verified that isolated renal allograft biopsies provide representative information about the presence of most rejection reactions. However, some sampling bias may lead to overestimation of rejection, such as with superficial biopsies where subcapsular inflammation secondary to perirenal reactions such as "healing-in" of the organ can be mistaken for cellular rejection.

In addition to routine histologic examination, ultrastructural and immunohistochemical analyses often play an important role in renal allograft biopsy evaluation. Electron microscopy is particularly helpful in identifying the occurrence or recurrence of certain glomerular diseases. Similarly, immunofluorescence labeling is useful in identifying the presence of immunoglobulin and complement components for the diagnosis of humorally mediated rejection or immune complex deposition in certain recurrent, de novo, or acquired nephropathies. Immunohistologic labeling with monoclonal antibodies to a variety of phenotypic, activation, and other cell surface markers has also been of significant value in the evaluation of renal allograft biopsies [53,54]. In particular, phenotypic evaluation of inflammatory cell infiltrates has provided useful information in qualitatively evaluating the nature of rejection reactions and in discriminating rejection from inflammatory reactions often seen with CsA toxicity. Likewise, immunopathologic studies to identify activation markers on infiltrating cell populations, the increased expression of HLA or other antigens on renal parenchymal cells, and the production of inflammatory mediators may eventually prove to have important diagnostic use.

To allow for these procedures, routine handling of renal allograft biopsies typically includes dividing the specimen for appropriate fixation and processing for histologic, electron microscopic (EM), and immunohistochemical analyses. The general need of frozen tissue for immunohistochemical studies also provides material for potential histologic evaluation by frozen section on an immediate basis. Frozen section staining of kidney allograft biopsies by routine hematoxylin-eosin (H&E) and periodic acid–Schiff (PAS) stains has been particularly useful at our center in providing rapid diagnosis in a substantial number of cases. Indeed, we have provided frozen section evaluation on almost 60% of all renal transplant biopsies performed during the last 3 years.

In preliminary studies, we have found that the ability to identify or exclude rejection by frozen section diagnosis has a high correlation with the subsequent diagnosis based on complete histologic and immunohistochemical evaluation. Frozen section diagnosis is particularly useful in permitting prompt intervention during rapidly progressive or severe changes in graft function, such as in discriminating hyperacute rejection from perfusion injury or vascular-urologic complications and in distinguishing aggressive acute rejection from other causes of dysfunction. Recent technical advances in tissue fixation and processing have also led to methods whereby high-quality histologic sections can be prepared in less than 90 minutes, providing an alternative means for rapid evaluation of transplant biopsies [55].

Although immediate routine post-transplant ("1-hour") biopsies have not been found to be especially useful [56], we have found that a biopsy of the donor kidney taken before transplantation is crucial in identifying occasional donor organ abnormalities and often is helpful in the interpretation of subsequent post-transplant biopsies. Typically, a small wedge biopsy of renal cortex is taken immediately before the transplant procedure is completed and is evaluated for unusual organ procurement-preservation injury as well as any endogenous donor kidney disease. In addition, the degree of underlying irreversible injury such as glomerulosclerosis and interstitial fibrosis often provides a useful indicator of eventual baseline graft function. Since serum creatinine levels are especially inaccurate in identifying modest renal functional impairment [57], an otherwise unexplained rise in creatinine following transplantation may reflect this type of preexistent donor injury superimposed on mild post-transplant rejection or CsA nephrotoxicity.

Occasionally, a donor biopsy may also identify preexisting glomerulopathy [58,59], which can be invaluable in discriminating transmitted from de novo, recurrent, or acquired disease. Since in the majority of cases pretransplant donor biopsies show only variable degrees of reversible tubular injury, we routinely screen formalin-fixed H&E sections and hold further processing for special stains, immunohistology, or EM as indicated. By this approach, we are able to minimize costs, prospectively identify the presence of donor renal injury or disease, and have important reference material available to aid in the evaluation of subsequent post-transplant biopsies that show changes of uncertain etiology.

Donor Kidney Pathology

Transmitted Donor Kidney Disease

The majority of kidney transplants performed in the United States involve the use of organs from cadaver donors who are brain dead due to acute traumatic injury. Thus, two possible situations can lead to the unknowing use of donor kidneys that may have endogenous disease: (1) the presence of occult donor nephropathy undetected by examination or history and (2) disease acquired during donor management before organ recovery. With live donor transplantation, the ability to evaluate renal function and donor history thoroughly minimizes these risk factors.

Undetected infection and malignant tumors are the most potentially life-threatening native donor diseases that can be transmitted by kidney transplantation into the immunosuppressed host [60]. The combination of acute trauma, maintenance on life-support systems, and frequent use of steroidal anti-inflammatory agents promotes the risk of donor infection with opportunistic organisms. Thus, with the limited time often available for organ recovery and use, the transmission of fungal, bacterial, parasitic, and viral infections by cadaver kidney transplantation sometimes occurs. Unfortunately, positive identification of a transmitted organism by culture of organ flush or perfusate solutions is often made too late to prevent overwhelming sepsis in the recipient. The most frequent infectious disease transmitted by renal transplantation is cytomegalovirus (CMV) infection, with a majority of seronegative recipients who receive kidneys from seropositive donors [61,62] becoming seroconverted. Although human immunodeficiency virus (HIV) testing of potential organ donors is now standard practice before transplantation, the risk of false-negative results due to factors such as short donor infection incubation time [63] or massive transfusions during donor management [64] provides a low but finite risk of HIV transmission. The transmission of tumors by renal transplantation is also uncommon, but most reported cases involve donors with extrarenal malignancy with a high percentage of such recipients developing widespread disease [65].

In addition to infectious organisms and tumors, a variety of undetected renal diseases can be present in transplanted kidneys. Unless a donor biopsy is taken before transplantation and the cause of recipient native renal failure clearly established, it is difficult to be certain whether many renal diseases developing after transplantation are transmitted, recurrent, or de novo (see below).

In our own large series of pretransplant donor biopsies, we have identified a number of donor abnormalities unsuspected on cadaver donor evaluation, including cases of IgA nephropathy [59], microvascular thrombosis (Fig. 3.1), arterionephrosclerosis, starch granule microemboli (Fig. 3.2), and several cases with atypical preservation injury. Other reports have also identified glomerulopathy [58] or other disorders [66,67] in donor biopsy specimens. The identification of glomerular or microvascular thrombosis in pretransplant donor kidneys can greatly help in the evaluation of early graft dysfunction, especially in differentiating transmitted diseases from perfusion injury or accelerated rejection. Although donor intravascular coagulopathy is often a contraindication for kidney donation, good graft function has been reported with appropriate therapy [67].

Figure 3.1
Disseminated intravascular coagulopathy in a pretransplant donor kidney. A. Histologic appearance of glomerular microthrombi (Masson ×325). B. Immunofluorescence staining for fibrinogen (×200).

A *B*

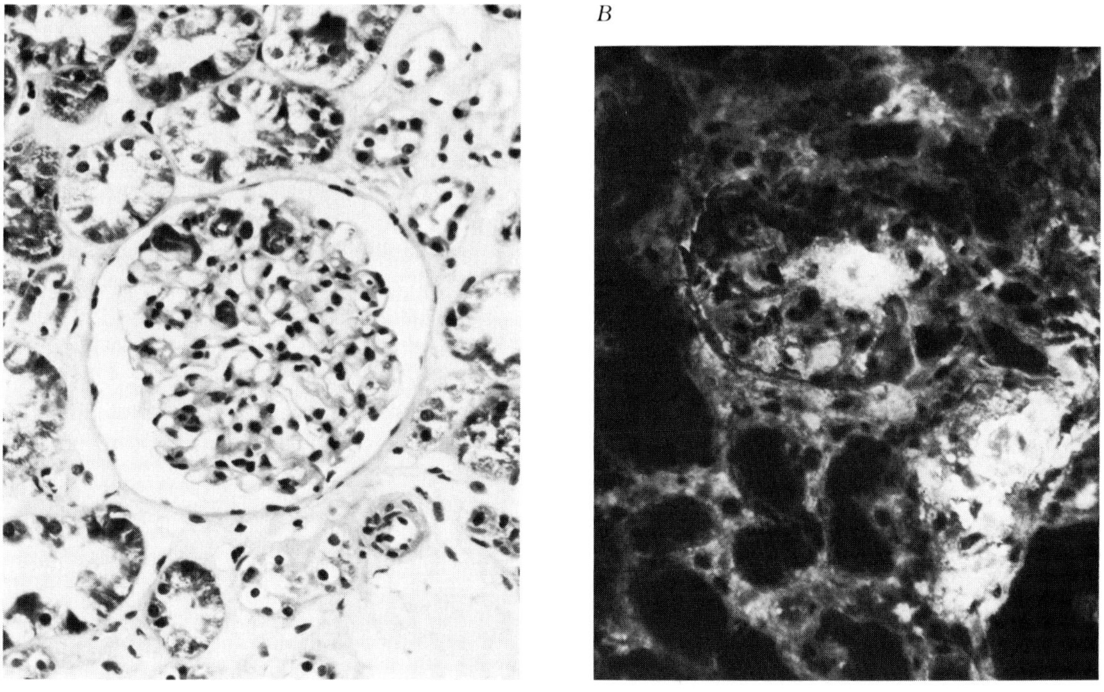

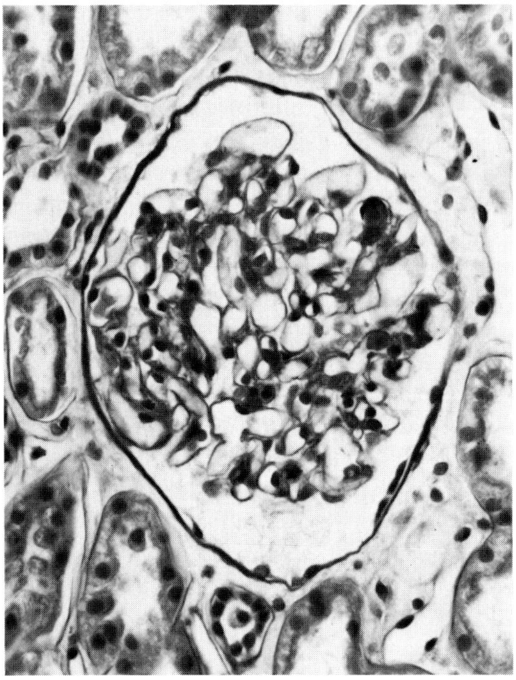

A

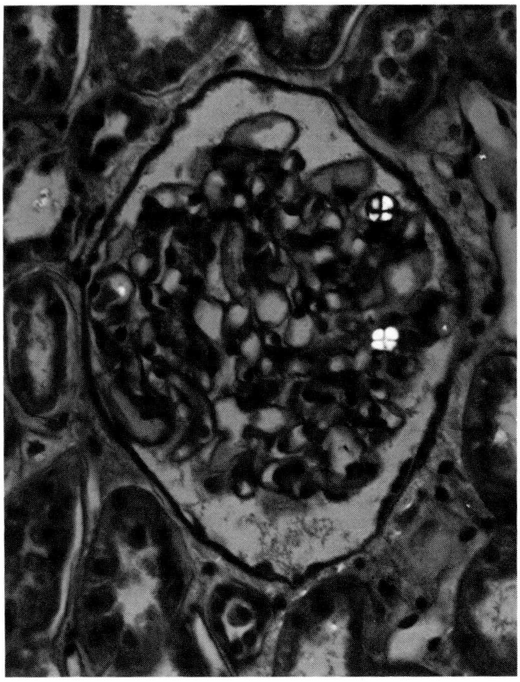

B

Figure 3.2
Starch granules in a pretransplant donor kidney. A. Histologic appearance within glomeruli (PAS ×400). B. Polarization of the same section.

The degree of irreversible interstitial fibrosis and glomerulosclerosis in donor organs may also affect the observed decline in graft function, potentially exaggerating the apparent degree of chronic rejection or CsA toxicity seen in post-transplant biopsies. However, the presence of a new host environment and the use of maintenance immunosuppressive therapy may inhibit or even reverse the progression of some donor kidney diseases, as has been reported with diabetic nephropathy [68]. Certain vascular, ureteral, or structural anomalies are also not necessarily a contraindication to transplantation but should be identified to the pathologist who is asked to interpret an allograft biopsy of such a transplanted organ. For example, small anomalous renal vessels may become occluded and lead to segmental allograft injury, which is usually detectible by radiographic studies but can be potentially misleading if biopsied.

Surgical Complications

There are two stages during which the donor kidney may be injured by surgical procedures: during the donor nephrectomy–organ recovery process and during transplantation into the recipient. Surgical and urologic complications associated with kidney transplantation have been well described [69,70] and most often involve vascular or ureteral damage resulting in obstructive lesions. Renal artery thrombosis can result from vessel damage due to surgical manipulation or endothelial injury due to improper cannulation [71] and may lead to focal cortical necrosis and infarction. Renal vessel occlusion can also be due to stenosis resulting from improper vascular anastomosis, external pressure causing kinking, or scarring from trauma or endothelial-intimal damage. Transplant renal artery stenosis can cause primary renovascular hypertension that often is successfully treated by angioplasty or revascularization surgery. The pathologic changes seen on biopsy in this setting can be variable. Indeed, several cases with documented renal artery stenosis, hypertension, and graft dysfunction in our own series have shown minimal vascular reaction or juxtaglomerular apparatus hyperplasia. However, renal artery vs vein obstruction can usually be distinguished by biopsy on the basis of finding predominantly ischemic injury, cortical necrosis, and infarction with the former versus predominantly congestive, thrombotic, and hemorrhagic changes (Fig. 3.3) with the latter.

Other surgical complications include lacerations resulting in focal hemorrhage and superficial trauma with focal subcapsular thrombosis and

Figure 3.3
Changes seen with major renal vessel injury. A. Renal vein thrombosis; note sparing of arteries (H&E ×100). B. Infarction due to renal artery occlusion; note band of subcapsular inflammation and partial sparing of cortex (H&E ×100).

A *B*

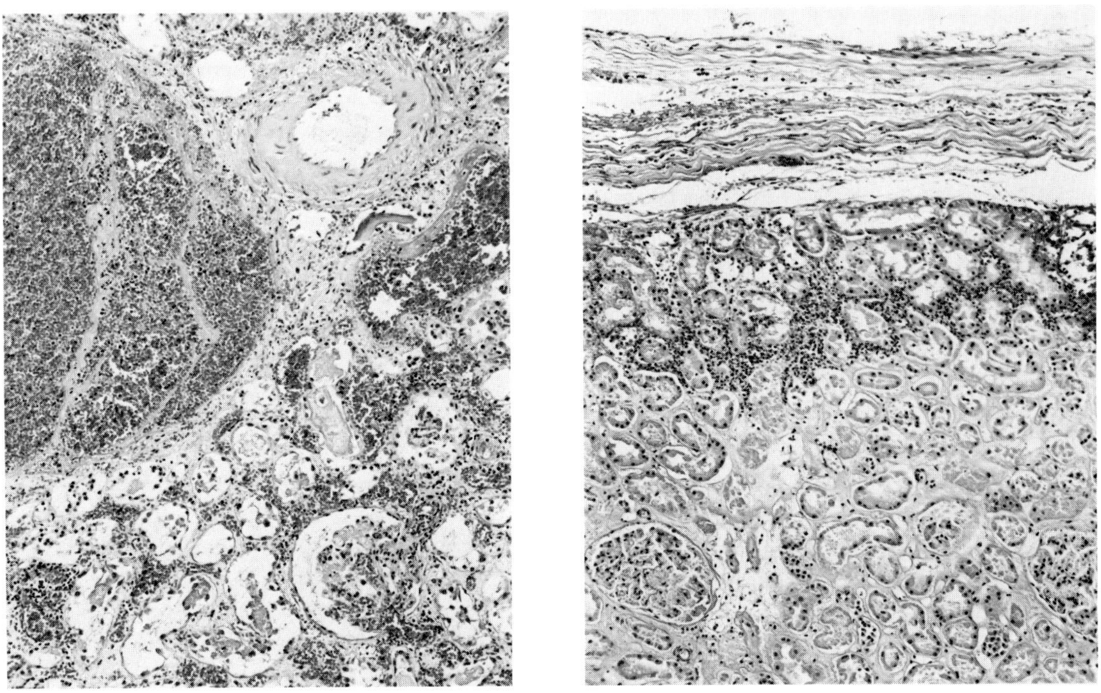

inflammation. Contamination of flush or perfusate solutions with starch granules from surgical gloves may present as microemboli (see Fig. 3.2), but in our experience, and that of others [72], they have not been associated with significant graft dysfunction.

The most serious urologic complications include ureteral infarction due to surgical compromise, injury, or thrombosis of the ureteral vasculature; ureteral injury or stricture leading to obstructive uropathy; ureteric fistula usually resulting from improper donor nephrectomy; lymphocele development providing a risk of infection or ureteral-vascular compression; and vesicoureteric reflux resulting from complications in the neocytostomy procedure.

Organ Preservation Injury

Initial graft nonfunction or delayed graft function following renal transplantation is relatively common, occurring in up to 30% to 40% of transplant recipients in most large reported series [42, 43]. In a majority of cases, initial dysfunction is transient and usually attributed to ATN associated with donor organ recovery and preservation. Preservation of donor kidneys during the interval between donor removal and recipient implantation is generally by hypothermic "cold storage" or mechanical pulsatile perfusion. Although no significant differences in ultimate graft survival have been associated with preservation method [73], the higher incidence of delayed graft function with cadaveric versus live-related donors is considered to be largely the result of prolonged preservation time. Indeed, recent studies involving the immediate use of cadaver donor kidneys suggest that the superior results seen with live donor transplantation may be more the result of decreased donor organ preservation time than increased histocompatibility with the recipient [74].

The common histologic and ultrastructural manifestations of donor kidney preservation have been well described by a number of investigators. Changes are most prominent in tubules and glomeruli [75–81] and appear to be largely the result of ischemic and osmotic injury associated with hypothermic and perfusion preservation methods. Tubular changes are not uncommon before and immediately following renal transplantation and range from mild dilation and epithelial cell vacuolization, especially of the proximal tubules, to more severe changes including frank ATN with epithelial cell necrosis and sloughing [79,80]. A mild interstitial inflammatory reaction with edema and leukocyte infiltration can also be seen, especially when ATN is present [82].

In our own series of more than 200 pretransplant donor biopsies performed over the past 10 years, we have generally found a range of modest tubular and glomerular histologic changes that, in the absence of frank ATN or other specific donor disease or abnormality, do not correlate with graft function in the early post-transplant period, nor with long-term outcome. Likewise, prospective immunofluorescence labeling of over 50 consecutive donor biopsies demonstrated a pattern of mild glomerular mesangial and arteriolar deposition of IgM and C3 in the majority of cases, the intensity of which did not predict immediate graft function or later outcome.

Occasionally, a severe form of preservation injury develops that is felt to be the result of mechanical damage to vascular endothelial cells by pulsatile perfusion [75,83,84]. In such cases, extensive microvascular and glomerular thrombosis are seen shortly after transplantation, with a variable but often intense accumulation of neutrophils in peritubular capillaries, glomeruli, and small vessels (Fig. 3.4). In our own limited experience with this disorder, pretransplant donor biopsies have usually revealed nonspecific histologic and immunofluorescent changes, although striking findings have been seen in several cases immediately after transplantation, characterized by extensive C3 and fibrinogen localization along peritubular capillaries and glomeruli (see Fig. 3.4).

Differential Diagnosis

The differential diagnosis of early graft dysfunction (see Table 3.1) includes transmitted donor diseases (e.g., infection, intravascular coagulopathy), sur-

Figure 3.4
Perfusion injury seen 1 hour after transplantation. A. Peritubular capillary with PMN and subendothelial reaction (×3300). B. Localization of C3 in peritubular capillaries (×250).

A *B*

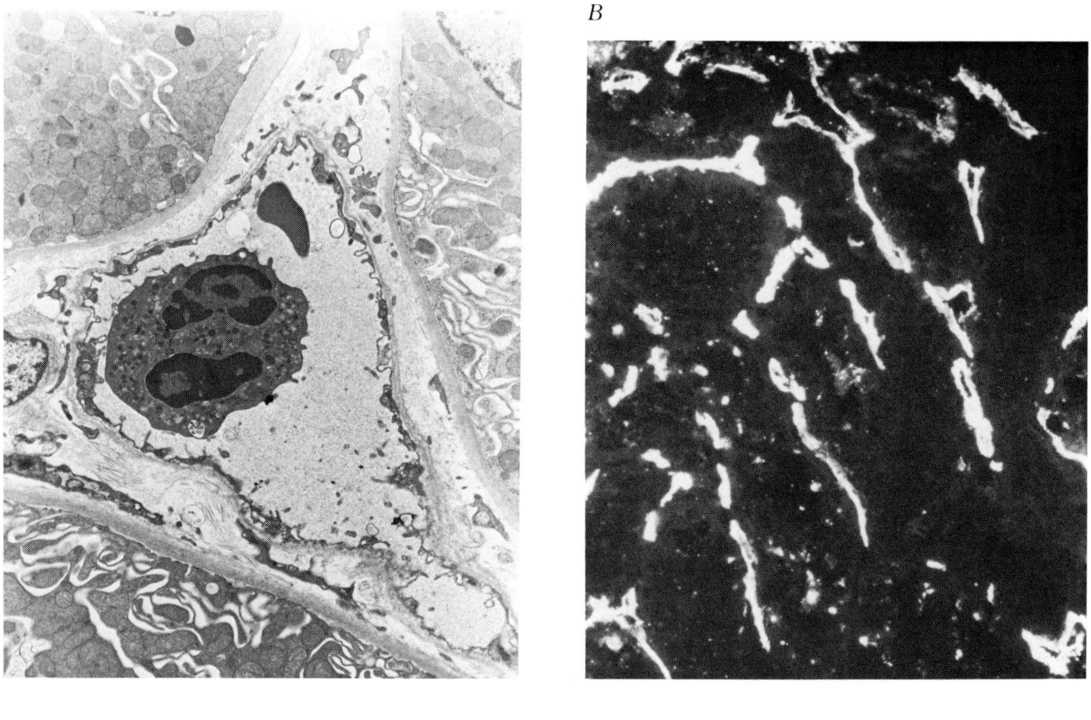

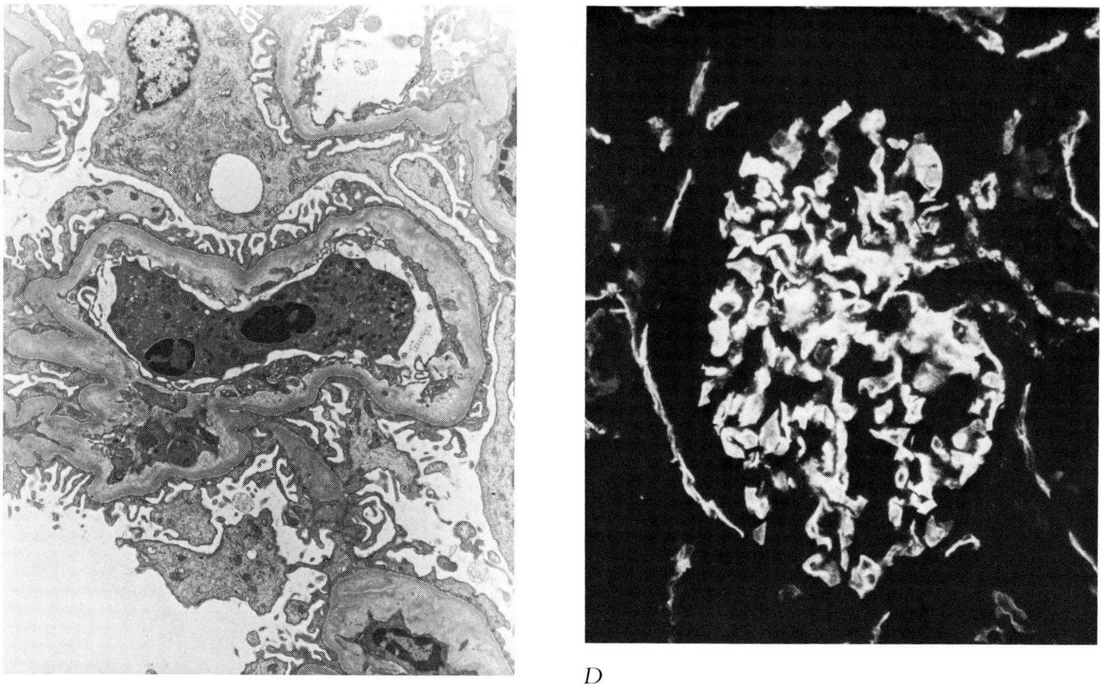

C

D

Figure 3.4 *(continued)*
C. Glomerular capillary loop with PMN and subendothelial reaction (×3300). D. Localization of C3 along glomerular capillary loops (×250). This organ had initial delayed function with full recovery.

gical complications (e.g., vascular occlusion, obstructive uropathy), organ preservation injury (e.g., ATN, severe perfusion injury), and early host-related problems (e.g., hyperacute rejection, acute CsA toxicity, infection). The presence of tubular epithelial cell necrosis with no more than mild edema, congestion, and inflammatory cell infiltration helps establish the diagnosis of ATN. Alternatively, microvascular or glomerular thrombosis with (or without) edema, congestion, and inflammatory cells (predominantly neutrophils) suggests severe preservation injury. However, the additional presence of interstitial hemorrhage, frank cortical necrosis, or vascular reaction (endothelial swelling, intimal proliferation, medial edema, fibrinoid necrosis, inflammatory cell infiltration) signifies the more ominous diagnosis of hyperacute rejection (see below). Cortical necrosis, especially in the absence of significant inflammation, suggests renal artery obstruction (e.g., stenosis or thrombosis), whereas hemorrhagic necrosis with extensive congestion suggests renal vein obstruction. Intravascular coagulopathy and acute CsA nephrotoxicity may appear similar to perfusion injury but usually exhibit less inflammatory cell involvement, while obstructive uropathy presents with tubular expansion, casts, and dilatation of Bowman's space with early compression of glomerular tufts.

As mentioned above, the availability of a pretransplant donor biopsy is of particular help in differentiating potential causes of immediate or early graft dysfunction. In addition, the identification of early acute rejection in biopsies taken of grafts with delayed function is important in guiding the use of antirejection therapy during the early post-transplant period.

Renal Allograft Rejection

General Concepts

Immune Mechanisms Host responses to a renal allograft involve a variety of immunologic, physiologic, and biochemical processes that can lead to a wide range of pathologic manifestations: alloimmune responses can be antibody- or cell-mediated; involve vessels, interstitium, tubules, or glomeruli; and exhibit acute or chronic inflammatory reactions. Although the immunobiology of human allograft rejection has been reviewed in detail elsewhere [85–87], several aspects of host immune responsiveness in general, and alloimmunity in particular, help to characterize the various pathologic changes seen with rejection.

1. The major antigens that can provoke (and act as targets for) host reactions are the major histocompatibility complex (MHC) antigens (HLA in humans) and major blood group ABO antigens [85,88], although other antigens such as vascular endothelial cell (VEC) antigens [89,90] may also play a role, especially in antibody-mediated reactions [91,92].
2. The major cells in the graft that stimulate host immune reactions are vascular endothelium, dendritic cells, and passenger leukocytes, which can exhibit several common features as antigen presenting cells (APC): they may express class II (as well as class I) MHC antigens, they can produce cytokines that support helper T cell activation, and they can directly stimulate alloreactive T cells in vitro.
3. The clonotypic receptor of T cells recognizes antigens in association with self-class I or class II HLA determinants [93,94]; so-called MHC restriction or associative recognition.
4. A high frequency of host T cells recognize foreign MHC antigens due to the cross-reactive recognition of alloantigen (non-self MHC) by T cells specific for various unrelated antigens [95].
5. Various regulatory T-cell populations affect the magnitude and type (e.g., humoral, cellular) of immune responses generated against specific antigens.
6. Inflammatory cell responses, including those in allograft rejection, can involve the release of cytokines (e.g., interferon-γ from T cells) that upregulate donor graft MHC antigen expression [96], potentially exacerbating the rejection reaction.

Thus, allografts present a highly immunogenic challenge to the host, allowing for the direct stimulation of various T cell populations and a means for continuous propagation of host rejection responses. Indeed, the strength of alloimmune responsiveness is well demonstrated clinically by the level of immunosuppression needed to prevent rejection in an unmodified host.

Beyond these general considerations, the specific nature of the inflammatory response by an individual host to a particular donor is extremely complex and only partially understood. The state of host immunity at the time of transplant plays a significant role in determining allograft responsiveness, as does the antigenic composition of the donor organ. Thus, host responses may be preferentially directed against antigens and cells expressed on larger vessels resulting in "vascular" types of rejection, or they may involve responses to interstitial dendritic cells or antigens on peritubular capillaries, causing "interstitial" patterns of rejection.

The nature of the host response can also vary depending on host immune factors such as the nature of prior antigen exposure, the extent of antigenic disparity with the donor, the type of immunosuppressive therapy used, and the patient's general medical status. For example, prior graft rejection or pretransplant blood transfusions can cause sensitization to HLA antigens, but the risk of subsequent renal allograft rejection is generally increased with the former and reduced with the latter [97]. Host responses to donor kidneys may also be affected by the extent of HLA incompatibility [98,99], the type (class I vs class II) of HLA disparity [100,101], and the level of HLA antigen expression [102,103]. Alternatively, host exposure to donor HLA antigens may in some cases lead to stimulation of specific inhibitory responses involving suppressor T cells [104,105] or anti-idiotypic antibody [106,107]. The use of T cell specific immunosuppression (e.g., heterologous anti-T-cell monoclonal or polyclonal antibody) can also influence the manifestation of a rejection response, as can a concomitant inflammatory stimulus such as infection.

Classification of Intragraft Reactions In addition to the potential variability in host immune responses, the mechanisms leading to ultimate inflammatory injury and graft dysfunction involve complex in situ interactions that can further provide variation in the pathologic manifestations of allograft rejection [86,108,109]. It is therefore perhaps not surprising that the traditional classification of renal allograft rejection is based more on clinical presentation than immunologic or pathologic mechanisms and has remained largely unchanged since first described in detail more than 20 years ago by Porter [3]. By this classification, the simple categorization of rejection as hyperacute, acute, or chronic provides a framework that is still useful, although more precise definitions considering particular morphologic features and presumed immunologic reactions often provide greater diagnostic and prognostic value.

The clinically defined categories are supplemented by descriptions based on the pattern of involvement of target structures (vascular, interstitial, tubular, glomerular) and the general nature of the inflammatory reaction. Characteristics of humoral rejection typically include neutrophil infiltrates, edema, hemorrhage, and necrosis, while cellular rejection is usually manifested by mononuclear inflammatory cell infiltrates. Since the pathologist sees inflammatory patterns rather than immunologic mechanisms, the descriptive terms *acute* and *chronic* are customarily used to classify these inflammatory types. This leads to an unfortunate ambiguity of terminology, since the same modifiers are used to describe the clinical rate of rejection; one can (and frequently does) see rejection reactions that are clinically acute (rapid) but histologically chronic. However, the use of pathologic modifiers in describing clinically defined rejection reactions is of practical as well as didactic use, since certain types of reaction (especially humorally mediated acute inflammation) are less responsive to standard immunosuppressive antirejection agents [110]. A summary of the major subdivisions of clinical rejection categories by predominant location (vascular, interstitial), type of inflammatory reaction (acute, chronic), and presumptive immunologic response (humoral, cellular) is presented in Table 3.2.

Even detailed classification methods using all currently available criteria can be inexact in terms of clinical correlation, since other conditions may exhibit very similar findings, and certain reactions are simply not understood. The immunologic basis for acute and chronic inflammatory responses is certainly more complex than being simply "humoral" or "cellular." Likewise, classification based on the immunopathologic types of response and injury such as that described by Gell and Coombs [111] only partially describes common renal allograft reactions. By this nomenclature [86,108,111], hyperacute and acute vascular rejection are generally classified as Type II (antibody-mediated) reactions, while acute interstitial rejection usually represents a Type IV (cellular-delayed-type hypersensitivity) reaction. However, "vascular" rejection may involve Type IV responses, "interstitial" rejection may involve Type II responses, and Type I (anaphylactic) and Type III (immune-complex) reactions can also be expressed with either vascular or interstitial types of rejection. Perhaps the best example of

Table 3.2
Relationships among clinical, pathologic, and immunologic characteristics of allograft reaction

Clinical (temporal) classification	*Pathologic category* — *Predominant location*	*Pathologic category* — *Inflammatory reaction*	*Predominant immunologic response*
Hyperacute	Vascular	Acute	Humoral
Acute	Interstitial	Chronic	Cellular
	Interstitial	Acute	Humoral-mixed
	Vascular	Chronic	Cellular
	Vascular	Acute	Humoral
Chronic	Interstitial	Chronic	Cellular
	Vascular	Chronic	Humoral-mixed

how even detailed immunologic and pathologic evaluation of renal allograft reactions can be totally inaccurate is demonstrated by experimental studies of graft enhancement in animals. Recent work has demonstrated that histologic and immunopathologic changes identical to those seen with severe acute irreversible rejection can be found in grafts of animals with no renal functional impairment and indefinite graft survival [112–114]. Clearly, the functional activity of inflammatory cells and their products correlates more with graft injury than just their mere presence as observed by biopsy.

Hyperacute Rejection

Clinical Features Hyperacute renal allograft rejection represents the best characterized form of rejection in terms of clinical expression, immune mechanisms, and pathologic findings. Clinically, hyperacute rejection usually presents as an abrupt loss of allograft function within minutes to hours following vascular anastomosis, with anuria and the striking gross changes of cyanosis, erythema, and edema. Initial studies in the 1960s demonstrated a strong association between hyperacute rejection and the presence of preformed circulating antibodies in the recipient directed against donor HLA or ABO antigens [11,115,116]. However, not all patients with circulating antidonor HLA [116] or ABO [117] antibodies develop hyperacute rejection, and occasional cases that are clinically and pathologically characterized as hyperacute rejection demonstrate no detectable antidonor antibodies in recipient serum or allograft eluates.

Since the late 1960s, routine pretransplant screening and crossmatching of recipient sera with donor red cells and lymphocytes has dramatically reduced the incidence of hyperacute rejection. However, the recent increase in patients who are highly sensitized (largely due to prior graft loss, as well as pretransplant transfusion policies), has caused a reevaluation of crossmatching techniques, with an increased emphasis on maximizing diagnostic specificity (i.e., reducing biologic false-positive results) rather than simply increasing analytic sensitivity (i.e., reducing false-negative reactions). Recent studies have suggested that positive crossmatches that are due to certain antibodies (e.g., autoreactive, cold reactive) or that are directed toward certain target antigens (e.g., surface IgM on B cells, Lewis and Rh blood group antigens) appear to provide minimal if any risk of rejection. Moreover, maneuvers to reduce preformed antibody or host immunity such as thoracic duct drainage, plasmapheresis, immunoadsorption, and total lymphoid irradiation may prevent hyperacute rejection in some cases.

Of perhaps greatest impact to transplanting highly presensitized patients in the past decade has been the finding that the natural loss of antidonor reactive antibodies is associated with a diminished risk of hyperacute rejection [118,119]. Thus, some patients with a positive donor crossmatch using past or historical serum samples, but who have a negative crossmatch with recent or current pretransplant samples, are now considered to be acceptable for transplantation at many centers. However, at present, the predictive values of negative as well as positive crossmatches are not absolute for any technique regardless of its analytic sensitivity or specificity.

Pathologic Features The pathologic changes seen with hyperacute rejection are generally consistent with an acute inflammatory, humorally mediated reaction directed at the vasculature. Initial antibody binding to vascular endothelial cells activates the complement and coagulation cascades, resulting in the predictable sequential changes of polymorphonuclear leukocyte (PMN) chemotaxis and intravascular-glomerular thrombosis, which in turn leads to congestion and edema, inflammatory injury of the vasculature and glomeruli with hemorrhage and necrosis, secondary ischemic tubular injury, and ultimately frank cortical necrosis. By immunofluorescence, deposits of immunoglobulin, complement components, and fibrinogen may be seen along vessels and within glomeruli (Fig. 3.5). Often, by the time a biopsy is obtained, tissue injury is advanced enough to preclude the distinct localization of immunoglobulin. Ultrastructurally, striking changes involving glo-

Figure 3.5
Hyperacute allograft rejection. A. Renal cortex with vascular, interstitial, and glomerular PMN infiltrates and acute inflammation with congestion and hemorrhage (H&E ×130). B. Ureter with adventitial vascular and interstitial acute inflammation (H&E ×130). C. Localization of IgG in interlobular artery (×250). D. Localization of IgG in glomerulus (×250).

A *B*

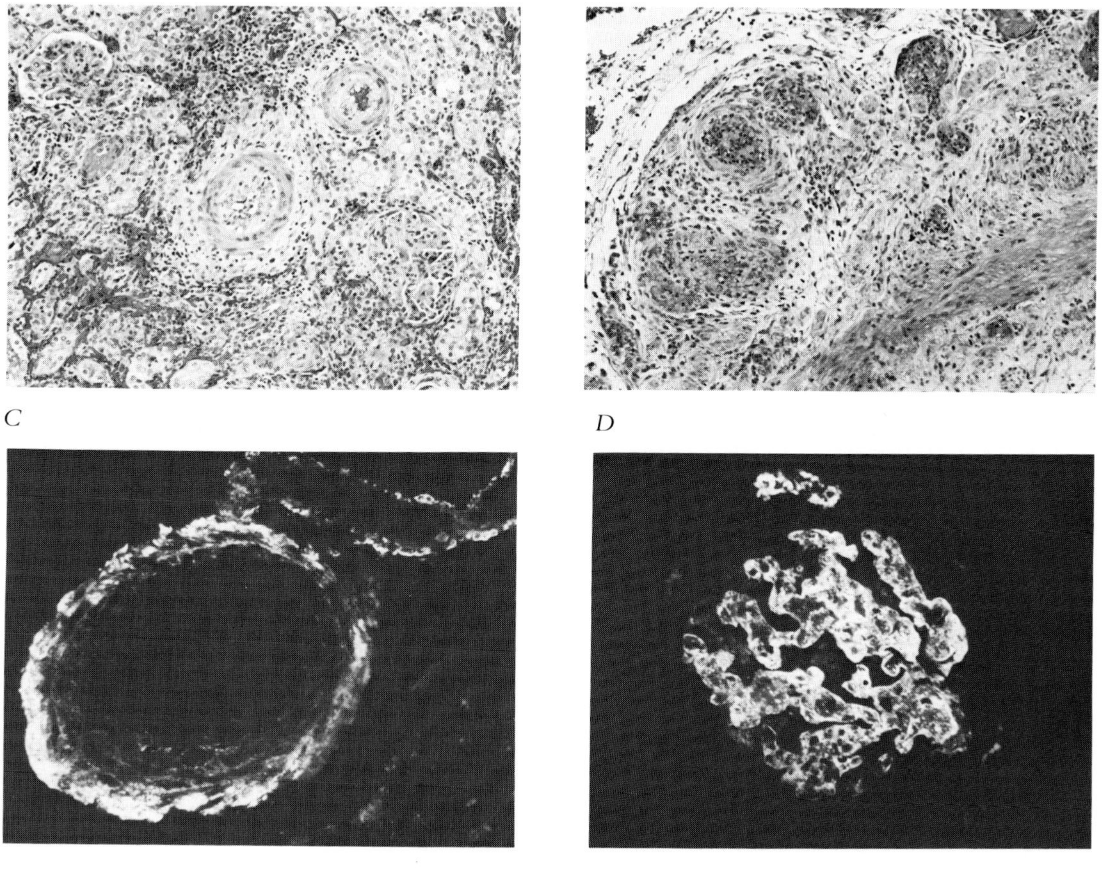

merular capillary loops and the microvasculature may also be seen. Typically, the initial PMN influx occurs within the first several minutes, followed quickly by microvascular-glomerular thrombosis, with the full manifestation of cortical necrosis seen within hours. In some cases, however, this process may begin up to a few days after transplantation or may present as a more prolonged sequence, clinically representing an accelerated form of acute rejection. Since these forms of "humoral-vascular" rejection are essentially irreversible and provide a risk for disseminated intravascular coagulopathy or a nidus for infection, prompt diagnosis and graft removal are important.

Differential Diagnosis Although the diagnosis of hyperacute rejection is usually made visually by the surgeon shortly after release of the vascular clamps, a number of conditions may cause acute loss of graft function within the first few days after transplantation. As discussed above, perfusion injury can lead to a similar clinical and pathologic picture, but it is often reversible and generally exhibits microvascular-glomerular thrombosis before subsequent PMN accumulation, which also is usually milder than that seen in hyperacute rejection. The reversed sequence and reduced injury seen with perfusion injury presumably is the result of the initial activation of coagulation pathways following physical endothelial cell injury and exposure of basement membrane components, as opposed to hyperacute rejection, where the initial reaction involves complement activation from antibody binding, resulting in the release of fragments with chemotactic (C5a) and anaphylatoxic (C3a and C5a) activities. Thus, compared with hyperacute rejection, reversible perfusion injury usually has prominent microvascular thrombosis and less PMN infiltration with minimal or only focal hemorrhage. However, later phases of severe, often irreversible perfusion injury are essentially indistinguishable from hyperacute rejection histologically and by immunofluorescence, since abundant fibrin deposition and serum protein accumulation can be seen in vessels and glomeruli.

Other lesions that may mimic hyperacute or accelerated acute rejection include acute CsA vasculopathy, microvascular coagulopathy, renal artery or vein thrombosis with occlusion and infarction, and ureteral obstruction. The acute vascular form of CsA toxicity will be discussed below; it generally presents as a microvascular-glomerular thrombotic lesion without significant PMN infiltrate or hemorrhage and tends to preferentially involve arterioles and smaller arteries [120]. Microvascular thrombosis can also be due to transmission from a donor with intravascular coagulopathy [67], the precipitation of cold-agglutinins in the hypothermic kidney [121], or the development of post-transplant coagulopathy. As with perfusion injury, these lesions generally exhibit prominent microvascular thrombosis with delayed and less inflammatory cell accumulation, but unlike hyperacute rejection, there is usually minimal hemorrhage or cortical necrosis.

Acute infarction due to severe renal artery or vein occlusion generally can be distinguished from hyperacute rejection, even in late biopsies of essentially necrotic kidneys, based on the paucity of underlying inflammatory cell infiltration relative to the severity of the injury. Often, the immediate subcapsular cortex will be viable and exhibit a margin of inflammatory cells at the border of the infarct (see Fig. 3.3B). Finally, ureteral obstruction due to donor ureter injury, infarction, physical compression, or occlusion at the implantation site may be associated with tubular dilatation, interstitial edema, congestion, and enlargement of Bowman's space, but generally not the thrombotic and inflammatory cell reaction seen with hyperacute rejection. Since the ureter can also be injured as a result of rejection reactions, especially those involving the ureteral vasculature (see Fig. 3.5B), obstructive changes may also be present during rejection.

Acute Rejection

Clinical Features and Classification In contrast to the fairly consistent clinical and pathologic findings seen with hyperacute rejection, acute renal allograft rejection may exhibit a variety of clinical presentations and a wide range of histologic changes on biopsy. Acute rejection occurs most frequently between the first week and several months after transplantation and is suggested clinically by a rapid decline in renal function, graft swelling and tenderness, decreased urine output with proteinuria, and fever. However, acute rejection may occur within a few days or as late as years after transplantation and can vary in severity, speed of onset, and expression of signs and symptoms. Moreover, even in the most classic clinical presentation of acute rejection, a wide range of pathologic changes may affect the interstitium, vasculature, glomeruli, and tubules and can vary in intensity as well as pattern. Thus, the classification of "acute rejection" is at best poorly defined and generally used to include any immune-mediated host rejection reaction that occurs rapidly and is not identified as hyperacute or chronic.

Since the rationale for establishing classification schemes is based clinically on their diagnostic and prognostic value, there is some justification for using this categorization of renal graft rejection. Clinically, hyperacute and chronic rejections proceed with fairly well-defined courses that are essentially irreversible by antirejection therapy, whereas many forms of acute rejection are indeed reversible, especially if treated early. Thus, the major emphasis in evaluating acute rejection by biopsy is to identify the presence or absence of prognostic features that justify the use of antirejection therapy.

Several approaches have been used in an attempt to classify types of acute rejection. As discussed above, our current understanding of how immune reactions lead to graft dysfunction is incomplete and, in many cases, does not provide good clinical-pathologic correlations even in well-defined animal models. The disappointing prognostic value of immunologic monitoring in clinical renal transplantation bears this out in humans. In addition, it is becoming clear from recent animal studies that classic in situ immunopathologic reactions per se are not necessarily associated with tissue injury [112,114,122,123], supporting the observation that significant cellular infiltration [82] and the presence of donor-specific alloreactive T cells [105] in human renal allografts do not necessarily indicate rejection reactions that are associated with graft dysfunction. Nevertheless, certain pathologic fea-

Table 3.3
Major types of clinically acute renal allograft rejection

Interstitial: Chronic inflammatory (cellular) type

Features: Most common, best prognosis, severe reaction is often present with other types

Pathologic findings: Interstitial mononuclear cell infiltration and edema; tubulitis and prominent diffuse peritubular infiltrates if severe

Differential diagnosis: CsA toxicity, chronic rejection, ATN, viral infection, obstruction, perirenal inflammation

Interstitial: Acute inflammatory type

Features: Pure form is rare, poor prognosis, often is present with interstitial-cellular or vascular-humoral types

Pathologic findings: Interstitial PMN and eosinophil infiltration, edema, and congestion; thrombosis and focal hemorrhage if severe

Differential diagnosis: Drug reaction, pyelonephritis, serum sickness

Vascular: Acute inflammatory (humoral) type

Features: Poor prognosis, similar to hyperacute rejection, often involves the microvasculature and glomeruli

Pathologic findings: Arteritis (predominantly endothelial, intimal), glomerulitis, small vessel vasculitis, congestion; necrotizing arteritis and glomerulitis, thrombosis, hemorrhage, cortical necrosis if severe

Differential diagnosis: Vascular occlusion, intravascular coagulopathy, vasculitis, acute CsA vasculopathy, malignant hypertension, hemolytic-uremic syndrome

Vascular: Chronic inflammatory type

Features: Pure form uncommon, poor prognosis, generally spares the microvasculature

Pathologic findings: Transmural mononuclear cell arteritis, congestion; thrombosis, hemorrhage, cortical necrosis and infarction if severe

Differential diagnosis: Recurrent or de novo arteritis (e.g., polyarteritis, Wegener's, rheumatoid, lupoid vasculitis), CsA nephrotoxicity, hypertensive vasculopathy

ATN, acute tubular necrosis; PMN, polymorphonuclear leukocyte; CsA, cyclosporine.

tures of inflammatory renal allograft reactions appear to be useful in identifying several distinct forms of acute rejection and predicting host response to treatment [124].

The most common pathologic descriptions of acute rejection generally involve two categories: (1) interstitial rejection, which is often referred to as "cellular" rejection and appears predominantly as tubulointerstitial nephritis, and (2) vascular rejection, which is often referred to as "humoral" rejection and appears predominantly as arteritis. Unfortunately, this classification scheme has several shortcomings. First, from a prognostic standpoint, while interstitial rejections tend to show a better response to antirejection therapy than do vascular rejections, this is not always the case. Second, as discussed earlier from a mechanistic standpoint (see Table 3.2), interstitial reactions can involve humoral responses while vascular reactions can involve cellular responses, such that the common inference that interstitial rejection is cellular and vascular rejection is humoral does not always hold. Third, from a histologic standpoint, interstitial and vascular rejections may demonstrate predominantly chronic or acute inflammatory reactions, representing qualitative (and presumably mechanistic) distinctions with potential prognostic value. For these reasons, we have used a classification scheme that defines four types of acute rejection (Table 3.3) based on the pathologic expression of inflammation (acute, chronic) and predominant pattern of involvement (vascular, interstitial). We have found this scheme to be useful in evaluating allograft biopsies in a variety of settings [125,126].

Pathologic Features The classic morphologic changes seen with acute allograft rejection were described in detail by Medawar in studies of rabbit skin transplants more than 40 years ago [127] and suggested that cellular immunity plays a dominant role in acute rejection reactions. Indeed, mononuclear cell infiltration of the interstitium is the most frequent lesion associated with acute rejection in human renal allografts, and the *interstitial-chronic inflammatory* (*cellular*) type of acute rejection exhibits this feature as its predominant characteristic (Fig. 3.6). In addition to being the most common type of acute rejection, it has the best prognosis. In its "pure" form, the histologic features of interstitial-cellular rejection include interstitial edema and diffuse peritubular and intratubular infiltrates of lymphocytes, lymphoblasts, and monocytes-macrophages. Mononuclear cell aggregates may also be present and most typically are periglomerular or perivascular.

The severity of interstitial-cellular rejection is generally associated with the degree and type of peritubular infiltrates (see below), the extent of tubulitis and tubular injury, and the presence of features associated with other types of acute rejection, such as vascular involvement and infiltration with eosinophils and neutrophils. Immunofluorescence findings are generally nonspecific with variable interstitial localization of fibrinogen and, in some cases, C3 deposition along tubular basement membranes. As with all forms of acute rejection, the presence of thrombosis, interstitial hemorrhage, and cortical necrosis is ominous.

The ability to predict severity and outcome of interstitial-cellular rejection reactions by evaluating the intensity and phenotype of specific infiltrating leukocyte populations by immunohistochemical labeling has remained controversial despite numerous studies in recent years. Several studies have challenged the notion that the presence of leukocyte infiltration per se is associated with clinical manifestations of rejection [82,128–130], while others have alternatively implicated macrophages [131], eosinophils [132],

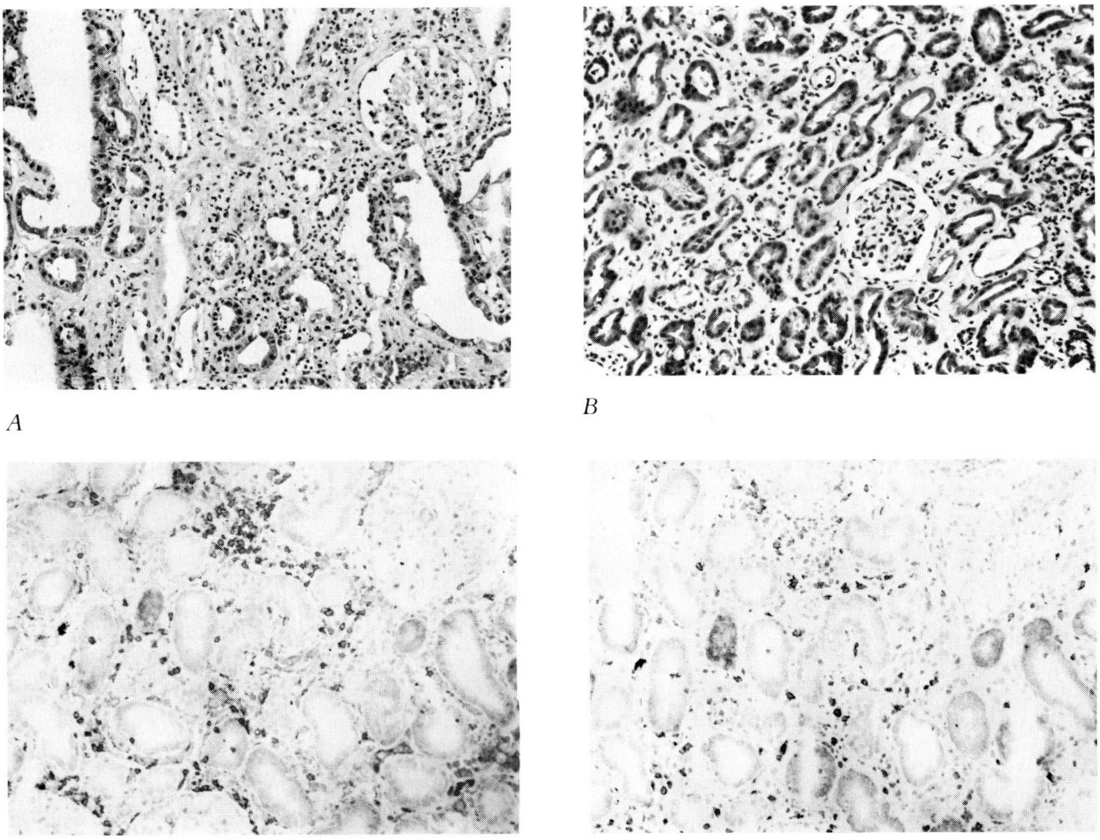

A B C D

Figure 3.6
Acute allograft rejection, interstitial-chronic inflammatory (cellular) type. A. Frozen section appearance with interstitial widening, mononuclear cell infiltration (H&E ×170). B. Histologic appearance on permanent formalin fixed section (H&E ×170). C. Immunoperoxidase labeling of a serial frozen section for CD4$^+$ T cells (Leu 3a ×170). D. Immunoperoxidase labeling of a serial frozen section for CD8$^+$ T cells (Leu 2a ×170). Note the relatively increased infiltrate of CD4$^+$ cells in the focal cell cluster compared with the more diffusely distributed pattern.

Leu7$^+$ natural killer (NK) cells [133], CD4$^+$ (T-helper-inducer) cells [134], or CD8$^+$ (T-cytotoxic-suppressor) cells [135] as most predictive of severe rejection.

Clearly, several clinical factors may have a significant influence on the intensity or predominant phenotype of cellular infiltrates expressed during severe interstitial-cellular rejection reactions, including the selective effects of various immunosuppressive agents on different cell populations [110], the presence of concomitant intragraft inflammatory reactions (e.g., infection, drug reactions), and the nature of donor HLA antigen disparity, which may predispose to responses by MHC class I (CD8$^+$)- versus class II (CD4$^+$)-

restricted T cells [100,101]. Moreover, the identification of T-cell populations by immunohistologic labeling must be qualified by several technical considerations such as the expression of CD4 on some non-T-cell populations including monocytes-macrophages and dendritic cells [136], the presence of double-labeled $CD4^+$ $CD8^+$ T cells [137], and the inexact correlations between T-cell phenotype and function.

In our own immunohistologic studies of renal allograft biopsies we initially found that the relative ratio of T cell subpopulations in different areas and patterns varied with the overall intensity of the infiltrate, such that $CD4^+$ cells predominate in aggregates and perivascular areas while $CD8^+$ cells predominate in diffuse peritubular infiltrates [138]. Thus, without stratification for pattern (i.e., diffuse peritubular, aggregate, perivascular), the overall level of mononuclear cell infiltration and phenotype showed no significant association with irreversible rejection [126]. However, by considering the infiltration of different phenotypically defined cell populations in each pattern, as well as various potential confounding variables using multivariate analysis, we found that a relative increase in $CD8^+$ T cells in the diffuse peritubular pattern was associated with the highest relative risk of irreversible rejection [125,126]. These findings are supported by other studies that associate interstitial $CD8^+$ T cells with acute cellular rejection [135,140,141]. In addition, we have found that the degree of diffuse interstitial $CD8^+$ T-cell infiltration provides a useful diagnostic means of discriminating acute rejection from CsA toxicity and of identifying acute rejection when present with toxicity [139]. However, these findings must be qualified by the considerations mentioned above and the results of others who have not found these associations [130,142,143], albeit without consideration of cell infiltrate pattern and location.

The related but distinct and less common type of interstitial rejection termed *interstitial–acute inflammatory* rejection involves acute inflammatory changes in the interstitium, characterized by the presence of significant PMN and eosinophil inflammatory cell infiltration, edema, and congestion. Immunofluorescence may demonstrate fibrinogen and C3 along peritubular capillaries. This type of rejection is usually seen with the interstitial-cellular or vascular-humoral forms and has a poor prognosis [132]. In its severest form, thrombosis in peritubular vessels with interstitial hemorrhage is seen. It is tempting to speculate that the reaction in interstitial-acute inflammatory rejection may involve predominantly humoral responses to peritubular capillary endothelium and perhaps dendritic cells, or preferential stimulation of alloreactive T cells that release lymphokines that act on eosinophils (e.g., interleukin 5) or PMNs.

Analogous to these patterns of interstitial rejection, two patterns of predominantly vascular involvement may be seen in acute rejection. The more common type parallels the changes seen with hyperacute rejection but occurs beyond 2 days after transplantation. This *vascular–acute inflammatory* (*humoral*) form of acute rejection presumably represents a host antibody response resulting in rejection directed primarily against arteries and arterioles. Its occurrence in the early post-transplant period has also been re-

[125,126,135,139–141]. In addition, tubular epithelial cell injury tends to be more accentuated with CsA toxicity than rejection when considered relative to the degree of interstitial inflammation, and class II HLA antigen expression on tubular epithelium may be more pronounced with rejection than CsA toxicity [149]. The presence of isolated glomerular and vascular endothelial changes, especially with superficial fibrinoid or hyaline reaction in the absence of other vascular changes, may also indicate acute CsA vasculopathy. Obstructive uropathy may present with interstitial edema and inflammatory cell infiltration but can usually be distinguished from rejection on the basis of prominent tubular dilatation, expansion of Bowman's space, and relatively mild inflammatory changes.

Pyelonephritis can usually be distinguished from interstitial–acute inflammatory rejection by the presence of PMNs and white blood cell casts within tubules, while serum sickness reactions to heterologous agents such as horse antithymocyte globulin (ATG) typically demonstrate diagnostic immunofluorescence and ultrastructural findings of glomerular and vascular immune complex deposits. However, reactions to drugs and dyes can lead to interstitial and vascular inflammatory reactions that may be difficult to distinguish from acute rejection.

For vascular forms of acute rejection, the differential diagnosis of the acute inflammatory (humoral) type is similar to that discussed above for hyperacute rejection and includes vascular occlusion, thrombosis, acute CsA vasculopathy (see below), and vasculitis. Primary or secondary forms of vasculitis such as polyarteritis nodosa, Wegener's granulomatosis, and those associated with rheumatoid arthritis or systemic lupus erythematosus may also present as vascular–chronic inflammatory acute rejection. However, they usually can be distinguished on the basis of more focal vessel involvement, the presence of proliferative glomerulonephritis on biopsy, as well as the clinical manifestations of extrarenal involvement. Vascular lesions associated with hemolytic-uremic syndrome (HUS), intravascular coagulopathy, or severe CsA vasculopathy generally will exhibit intimal and endothelial reactions with fibrinoid change, only modest involvement of the muscularis, and absent or minimal PMN or mononuclear inflammatory cell infiltration of vessel walls. Sclerotic or hyalinotic vascular lesions associated with the not infrequent complication of post-transplant hypertension can usually be distinguished from both forms of vascular rejection by the relative paucity of intravascular acute or chronic inflammatory cells. Malignant hypertension may present with more striking vascular changes, similar to those of HUS, and can be distinguished on the same basis.

In general, a discordant expression of inflammatory changes in the renal cortex provides the most useful means of diagnosing nonrejection-related reactions. For example, causes other than rejection should be strongly considered with isolated changes such as vascular thrombosis, sclerosis, or hyalinosis; severe ischemic tubular epithelial injury, tubulitis, tubular dilatation, atrophy, or casts; reactive glomerular changes (proliferation, endothelial, or mesangial swelling); and interstitial edema or fibrosis.

Chronic Rejection

Clinical and Pathologic Features Chronic rejection is classified clinically as the gradual but progressive impairment of renal allograft function in the absence of other specific disease. Typically, chronic rejection occurs later than 6 months to 1 year after transplantation, and dysfunction is reflected by increasing serum creatinine and proteinuria. The pathologic changes generally associated with chronic rejection are those of chronic inflammatory reactions involving the larger vessels and interstitium (Fig. 3.8).

The predominant vascular change seen with chronic rejection is marked myointimal proliferation of arteries and large arterioles that in later stages appears as dense fibrointimal thickening with scarring and foam cell accumulation. Endothelial cell swelling, disruption, and reduplication of the internal elastica; hyalinosis; and medial thickening and fibrosis are commonly seen, and modest inflammatory cell infiltrates may be present. Even at early stages there is significant luminal narrowing that likely contributes to the development of secondary ischemic injury involving tubules, glomeruli, and

Figure 3.8
Chronic allograft rejection. A. Interstitial pattern with fibrosis, mononuclear cell infiltration, loss of tubules, and relative sparing of glomeruli (H&E ×130). B. Vascular pattern with occlusive arterial fibrointimal reaction (H&E ×130).

A *B*

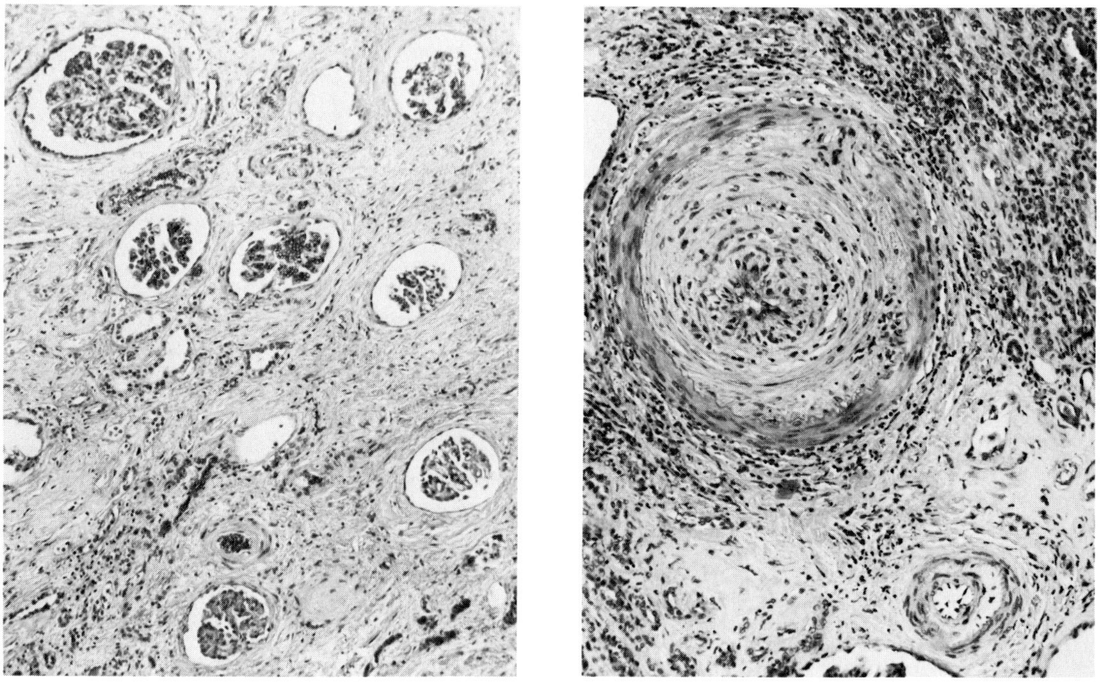

interstitium. Immunofluorescence typically demonstrates vascular staining with IgM and C3, especially in hyalin deposits.

The prominent interstitial change present in chronic rejection is fibrosis with relatively mild mononuclear cell infiltration but significant tubular atrophy. Although chronic interstitial rejection can present independently of chronic vascular rejection, they are most often seen together. Ischemic glomerular changes including capillary basement membrane thickening and wrinkling, increased mesangial matrix, and, in some cases, tuft collapse and hyalinosis may be seen with chronic rejection, but the degree of glomerular sclerosis generally appears to be less than expected, considering the degree of vascular and interstitial sclerosis present. Controversy exists over the appropriate classification of the various glomerular changes that can be seen with chronic rejection, since it is unclear whether they are the result of primary immune-mediated allograft responses, types of de novo glomerulopathy, injury due to hyperfiltration, or simply secondary reactions to chronic vascular and interstitial rejection. For purposes of organization, these glomerular lesions will be discussed below under Transplant Glomerulopathy.

Differential Diagnosis Since chronic vascular and interstitial rejection are essentially irreversible, their diagnosis is important for avoiding unnecessary antirejection immunosuppressive therapy. Several disorders can present with clinical and pathologic features similar to forms of chronic rejection, including mild acute rejection, hypertensive arterionephrosclerosis, chronic CsA toxicity, vesicoureteral reflux, and renal artery or vein stenosis. Chronic rejection can generally be distinguished from mild acute rejection based on the predominance of sclerotic vascular and interstitial lesions relative to the modest degree of inflammatory cell infiltration. Acute rejection can usually be identified when simultaneously present with chronic rejection, but occasionally chronic rejection may be masked by the presence of significant acute rejection. In such cases, sclerotic vascular or interstitial changes may sometimes be attributed to resolution of previous acute rejection episodes rather than due to ongoing chronic rejection.

The value in identifying chronic rejection in the presence or absence of acute rejection has been demonstrated by the significant differences observed in response to antirejection therapy given for rejections occurring more than 1 year after transplantation [150]. In this study, over 90% of patients with only acute rejection responded, compared with 30% for patients with only chronic rejection. However, over 75% of patients with both acute and chronic rejection showed some response. Since acute rejection reactions are frequently the cause of late graft dysfunction as a result of patient noncompliance with therapy, acute infections, or other precipitating causes, biopsy diagnosis and appropriate antirejection treatment are often indicated [151]. Although transplant nephrectomy specimens from patients with chronic rejection will often show significant acute rejection, this is often due to cessation of immunosuppression therapy before graft removal.

Hypertensive arterionephrosclerosis is difficult to distinguish from chronic vascular rejection but may show relatively greater hypertrophic changes in the media than intima, whereas intimal damage generally predominates in chronic rejection. Chronic CsA toxicity often has more striking fibrinoid and hyalinotic vascular changes and tends to exhibit less fibrointimal dysplasia than chronic vascular rejection. Nevertheless, we have found that the accelerated interstitial fibrosis and ischemic tubular reactions seen in long-term renal allografts of patients receiving CsA are difficult to distinguish from the changes of chronic interstitial rejection [152]. The morphologic manifestations of renal artery stenosis at late times after transplantation are also variable. For example, we have seen cases with minimal vascular or interstitial changes despite significant renal artery occlusion and graft dysfunction that was reversed on revascularization by surgery or angioplasty.

Renal Allograft Nephropathy

Cyclosporine Nephrotoxicity

Clinical Features The introduction of CsA as an immunosuppressive agent has had a profound effect on clinical organ transplantation since the early 1980s. In cadaver renal transplantation, the use of CsA has been generally demonstrated to improve graft survival and reduce the need for steroids, thus lowering infectious complications. In one-haplotype matched living–related transplantation, CsA therapy may obviate the need for pretransplant donor-specific blood transfusions and their associated potential risks of donor sensitization and exclusion [153]. The immunosuppressive activity of CsA involves a variety of effects on different immunocompetent cell functions [154], including T-helper-cell lymphokine production, T-cytotoxic-cell IL-2 receptor expression, and antigen presentation by macrophages, all key elements in regulating specific host responsiveness. The apparent benefits of CsA are reflected in its current use in the United States; between 1986 and 1988 more than 70% of cadaveric and 25% of one-haplotype live donor transplant recipients were treated with CsA as reported by available transplant registry data.

Unfortunately, CsA therapy has also been associated with specific toxic complications, including lymphoproliferative disorders at high doses, hepatotoxicity, and nephrotoxicity. The effects of CsA nephrotoxicity are clearly dose and patient dependent and most strikingly involve a reduction in glomerular filtration rate. This is demonstrated clinically by a rise in serum creatinine or decrease in creatinine clearance, often with oliguria, hyperchloremia, and a decreased renal blood flow. The physiologic effects of CsA on renal function are multifactoral [155] and involve alterations in the production of various vasoactive and thrombogenic lipid mediators such as prostaglandin E_2, thromboxane A_2, and platelet activating factors [156]. CsA also appears to directly affect vascular endothelial cell production of (and sensitivity to) various inflammatory mediators. In renal allograft recipients, the nephrotoxic potential of CsA may be compounded by several factors, including denervation, ischemic vascular and tubular injury due to organ preservation, and inflammatory injury due to rejection.

Classification Several classification schemes have been used to categorize the clinical features associated with CsA nephrotoxicity [155,156]. For the purpose of correlation with the pathologic classification used below, the major clinical syndromes can be grouped into 3 types: *acute CsA vasculopathy, acute CsA nephrotoxicity,* and *chronic CsA nephrotoxicity* (Table 3.4).

Acute CsA vasculopathy occurs with the least frequency but has the most dramatic clinical presentation. Its presentation includes signs and symptoms similar to HUS, including thrombotic vasculopathy and glomerulopathy, thrombocytopenia, and bilirubinemia [120,157]. Indeed, CsA is generally contraindicated for patients with HUS because of the associated high risk of recurrence. Acute CsA vasculopathy appears most likely to occur in the early post-transplant period, especially in patients with initially impaired graft function. Although a serious complication, this reaction is potentially

Table 3.4
Classification of cyclosporine nephrotoxicity

Acute CsA vasculopathy
Clinical features: Rapid onset, usually early after transplantation; thrombocytopenia, uremia
Pathologic features: Thrombotic angiopathy and glomerulopathy without significant inflammatory cell infiltration; congestion without significant hemorrhage
Differential diagnosis: Vascular-humoral or hyperacute rejection; perfusion injury, HUS, DIC, malignant hypertension
Acute CsA nephrotoxicity
Clinical features: Acute dysfunction, early post-transplant
Pathologic features: Isometric tubular vascuolization; patchy interstitial edema and mild mononuclear cell infiltration; arteriolar endothelial swelling and intimal thickening
Differential diagnosis: Acute rejection, acute tubular necrosis
Chronic CsA nephrotoxicity
Clinical features: Slow, progressive dysfunction, late post-transplant; often self-limited
Pathologic features: Interstitial fibrosis with mild mononuclear cell infiltration; marked arteriolar hyalinosis; focal tubular atrophy; variable glomerular changes
Differential diagnosis: Chronic rejection, arterionephrosclerosis, diabetic nephropathy, prior acute rejections

CsA, cyclosporine; HUS, hemolytic-uremic syndrome; DIC, disseminated intravascular coagulation.

reversed by prompt diagnosis and CsA withdrawal [120]. Many centers prefer to delay the start of CsA treatment until good allograft function is obtained, thus avoiding the potentially exacerbating toxicity of CsA in this setting.

Acute CsA nephrotoxicity typically presents as acute renal functional impairment several weeks after transplantation, usually in association with elevated serum CsA levels and without graft tenderness or fever [158,159]. In most cases, functional impairment is reversed by lowering CsA dosage. In contrast, *chronic CsA nephrotoxicity* generally presents as a slow, progressive decrease in renal function 6 months or more after transplantation. Withdrawal of CsA and conversion to alternative therapy has been employed with some success to prevent the progression of chronic CsA toxicity, although this provides the risk of "break-through" rejections. Recent studies suggest that allograft impairment with chronic CsA toxicity is stable after the first year post-transplant [160].

A

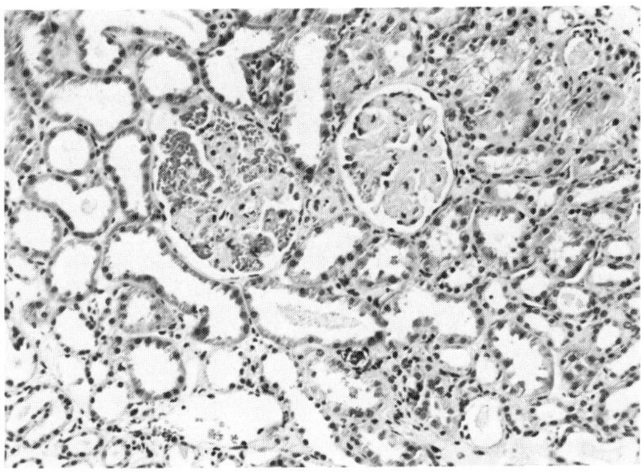

Figure 3.9
Acute cyclosporine vasculopathy. A. Glomerular congestion and microthrombosis without significant interstitial changes (H&E ×170). B. Microthrombosis of glomerular afferent arteriole (H&E ×250).

B

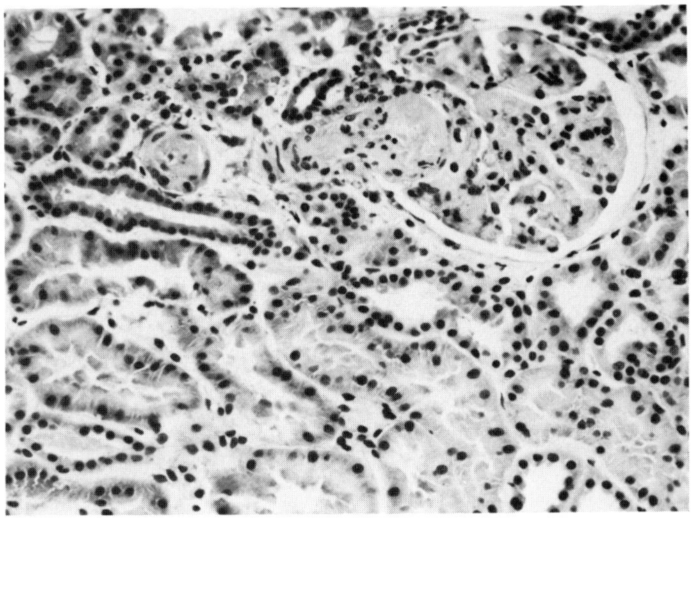

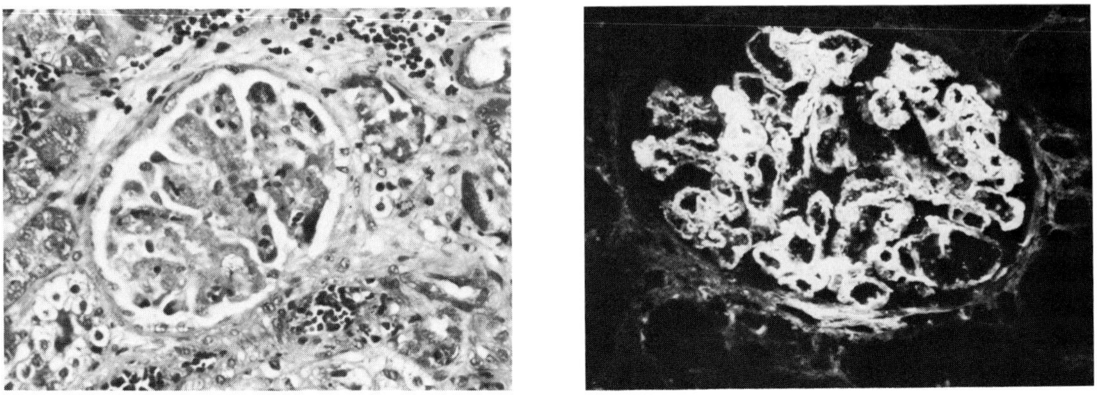

C D

Figure 3.9 *(continued)*
C. Glomerular microthrombi without significant PMN infiltration or hypercellularity (MAS ×325). D. Localization of fibrinogen within glomerular microthrombi (×250).

Pathologic Features CsA toxicity can cause a variety of pathologic changes within the renal allograft involving the vessels, tubules, interstitium, and glomeruli [120,139,148,152,155–165]. Using the clinical classifications described above, certain morphologic features are predominant for each. In acute CsA vasculopathy, the pathologic findings are similar to HUS [120,157] and best characterized by the presence of platelet and fibrin thrombi in vessels and glomeruli with minimal inflammatory cell infiltration (Fig. 3.9). The degree of tubular and interstitial reaction varies but may include epithelial disruption, luminal dilatation with casts, congestion, and edema.

In acute CsA nephrotoxicity, the most striking changes involve the tubules and vessels (Fig. 3.10). Tubules can show striking epithelial cell vacuolization, often in an isometric pattern with giant mitochondria, large lysozomal inclusions, and microcalcification [161–165]. However, the range of tubular changes substantially overlaps with that of acute rejection [166,167]. A variable degree of early interstitial fibrosis with patchy edema and minimal inflammatory cell infiltrates is also common. Vascular changes typically involve arterioles, with endothelial cell swelling, intimal thickening, variable hyalinosis, and mucoid or insudative deposits that together may result in significant luminal occlusion. Glomeruli may show endothelial cell swelling and mild ischemic changes, essentially indistinguishable from the changes observed in a variety of transplant glomerulopathies. Inflammatory cell infiltration within vessels is minimal or absent.

Chronic CsA toxicity (Fig. 3.11) is characterized by a greater progression of the lesions seen with acute toxicity. The typical changes observed include significant interstitial fibrosis with modest inflammatory cell infiltration and marked arteriolar hyalinosis. Tubules show variable atrophy, and glomerular changes may range from mild mesangial hypercellularity and widening to focal segmental or global sclerosis.

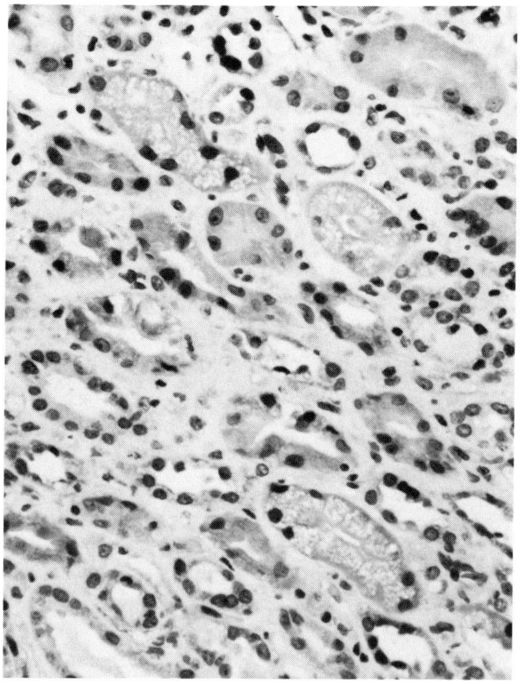

Figure 3.10
Acute cyclosporine nephrotoxicity. Isometric epithelial vacuolization of convoluted tubules (H&E ×325).

Differential Diagnosis Since the morphologic changes seen with any type of CsA toxicity are essentially nonspecific and may suggest several potential etiologies, the diagnosis of CsA toxicity is usually by exclusion. For acute CsA vasculopathy the major differential diagnoses include vascular-humoral

Figure 3.11
Chronic cyclosporine nephrotoxicity. A. Arteriolar hyalinosis (H&E ×170). B. Localization of serum protein (IgM) within glomerular afferent arteriole (×250).

A *B*

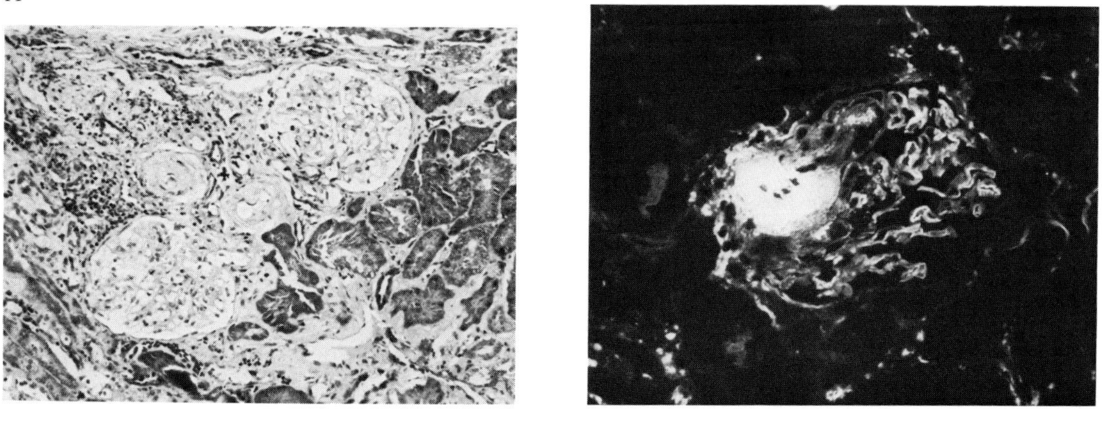

(or hyperacute) rejection, perfusion injury, de novo or recurrent HUS, disseminated intravascular coagulation (DIC), and malignant hypertension. The changes of HUS, DIC, and malignant hypertension on allograft biopsy are not readily distinguished from acute CsA vasculopathy, and their diagnosis is largely made in the context of clinical findings. However, differentiation from vascular-humoral hyperacute rejection is possible histologically and of considerable importance, since immediate cessation of CsA can lead to rapid reversal and return of good renal function [120], whereas vascular-humoral–hyperacute rejection is normally unresponsive to treatment and an indication for graft removal.

Features distinguishing acute CsA vasculopathy from vascular forms of humoral rejection include the absence of significant PMN infiltration in vessels, glomeruli, and the interstitium; minimal or absent hemorrhage; less striking congestion; and the less frequent involvement of larger arteries. However, serum protein localization in vessels and glomeruli may give an immunofluorescence picture similar to that often seen with vascular-humoral rejection (compare Figures 3.5D and 3.9D). The elevated PMN infiltration usually seen with perfusion injury will usually allow differentiation of this diagnosis, although as demonstrated for HUS, CsA can aggravate or potentiate various types of thrombotic angiopathy, including that resulting from perfusion injury.

Differentiation of acute CsA nephrotoxicity from acute rejection provides one of the most difficult (and common) challenges in renal pathology. Indeed, initial suggestions that specific tubular, interstitial, or vascular morphologic features could provide a definitive diagnosis have been largely unsubstantiated [166,167]. Morphologic evaluation generally focuses on diagnosing acute CsA toxicity by the exclusion of rejection and other causes of dysfunction, and the identification of at least some of the histologic changes associated with CsA toxicity. The presence of acute rejection will often mask the histologic changes of acute CsA toxicity, and in some cases toxicity may mimic mild rejection.

We have found that two means of immunopathologic evaluation are potentially helpful in differentiating CsA toxicity from mild acute rejection. First, phenotypic evaluation of cellular infiltrates often can distinguish acute rejection of the cellular-interstitial type from acute CsA toxicity. The predominance of $CD8^+$ T cells in diffuse interstitial peritubular infiltrates is more characteristic of acute interstitial-cellular rejection, and the $CD4^+$:$CD8^+$ cell ratio in this pattern has been proposed to help distinguish rejection from toxicity [126,139,148]. Indeed, we have followed patients with documented successive episodes of acute rejection and toxicity (and, in one case, further rejection episodes) who demonstrated a good correlation of the CD4:CD8 cell ratio in the diffuse peritubular (but not focal aggregate) pattern of infiltration with the diagnosis of rejection vs CsA toxicity [139]. Second, the identification of CsA deposition by immunohistologic labeling of FNAB specimens [168] or biopsies [159,169] has provided useful information in helping to identify CsA toxicity, even in the presence of concomitant acute rejection. Clinical parameters, such as elevated serum CsA levels and the absence of fever or graft tenderness, can serve as important factors in establishing the diagnosis of CsA toxicity [158,159].

In chronic CsA toxicity the major differential includes chronic rejection, prior acute rejections, arterionephrosclerosis, and diabetes. As with acute toxicity, most of the features associated with chronic CsA toxicity are not diagnostic. We have found that the tubular changes in chronic toxicity are essentially nonspecific but that a subtle increase in interstitial fibrosis can be detected at 6 months or more after transplantation by quantitative morphometry but not by routine histologic grading [152,170]. Prior acute rejection or nephrosclerosis may lead to the focal or striped pattern of fibrosis that has been suggested to be associated with chronic toxicity [163], while the focal or segmental glomerulosclerosis sometimes associated with toxicity can also be seen in renal allografts of patients not receiving CsA who have chronic rejection, transplant glomerulopathy, or recurrent disease. Likewise, the hyalinotic arteriolar lesions commonly present in chronic CsA toxicity can also be seen with chronic rejection, arterionephrosclerosis, and diabetes. However, the pattern of intercapillary nodular glomerular sclerosis seen in diabetes usually can be distinguished from the segmental tuft sclerosis seen with chronic CsA toxicity.

Transplant Glomerulopathy

Transplant glomerulopathy (TGP) is a term that has been used to describe a variety of lesions without necessarily differentiating specific etiologies or distinctive morphologic characteristics. Initial descriptions of TGP focused on changes seen in the glomeruli of long-surviving allografts that exhibited variable dysfunction, most often with proteinuria [14,171–174]. TGP was initially characterized by expansion of the lamina rara interna, epithelial foot process effacement, and mesangial widening. However, more recent studies [175] suggest that these changes represent the later stages of a glomerulopathic process that may begin relatively early after transplantation and progress at a somewhat variable rate. In this context, TGP could be considered a type of glomerular rejection that may have both acute and chronic phases, analogous to the difference in vascular or interstitial changes present in acute versus chronic rejection. In the early phase of TGP, glomerular enlargement, endothelial and mesangial cell swelling, and glomerular basement membrane abnormalities appear, accompanied in some cases by variable deposits of predominantly IgM and fibrinogen [145,146,175,176]. Endothelial cell swelling may become severe and even exhibit necrosis, while mesangial reactions in the acute phase may include hypercellularity and widening.

The pathogenesis of TGP remains controversial and includes several possible etiologies. A report in 1981 suggested that the changes now used to characterize acute TGP were due to cytomegalovirus (CMV) infection [177]. Subsequent studies, however, have generally not supported this conclusion [178–180], and it appears more likely that these changes represent an early (or acute) form of TGP. Virtually all the morphologic features of TGP can be seen independently of any evidence of CMV infection and are often present in association with vascular or interstitial rejection reactions. However, they may also develop in the absence of any other type of rejection. The prognosis of TGP is generally poor, although there is substantial variation in the time of acute onset (months to years) and the rate of progression. Thus, it is possible that as with vascular or interstitial reactions, glomerular rejection may involve acute (early or rapid) and chronic (late or indolent) phases mediated by acute (predominantly humoral) or chronic (predominantly cellular) types of inflammatory responses.

Other similar forms of transplant glomerulopathy certainly may occur, especially secondary to vascular or interstitial rejection. Ischemic glomerular changes may be seen with any rejection reaction and can range from capillary loop thickening and wrinkling with mesangial widening, to tuft collapse and sclerosis. It is interesting to note, however, that even when severe chronic rejection is present, glomeruli may only be minimally affected, supporting the notion that glomerular rejection may exist as an independent entity rather than solely as a secondary manifestation of vascular or interstitial rejection.

Recurrent Diseases

A variety of changes are commonly seen in the renal allograft and can generally be categorized as *transmitted donor diseases,* resulting from endogenous disease in the donor kidney before transplantation; *rejection reactions,* caused directly or indirectly by host anti-donor alloimmune-mediated injury; *recurrent diseases,* caused by a recurrence of the original native kidney disease leading to renal failure; and *de novo and acquired diseases,* resulting from processes (typically of iatrogenic or infectious etiology) not included in the other three.

Transmitted donor diseases have been discussed above and can involve primary donor nephropathy or donor kidney injury acquired during the process of donor management, organ recovery, organ preservation, or transplantation surgery. *Rejection reactions* include the various vascular, interstitial, glomerular, and tubular changes previously discussed that are associated with immune responses against donor antigens.

Recurrent diseases most often include the systemic or renal disease that contributed to original native kidney failure. Native host systemic diseases that may recur in renal allografts include diabetes mellitus, vasculitis, systemic lupus erythematosus (SLE), amyloidosis, oxalosis, cystinosis, HUS, thrombotic-thrombocytopenic purpura (TTP), and Fabry's disease.

Although a significant number of patients with diabetes receive renal transplants, the reported rate of recurrence within the graft is low [181–183]. However, a true assessment of the recurrence rate may be difficult to determine due to similarities in the diabetic changes of nodular intercapillary glomerulosclerosis and vascular hyalinosis with those of chronic allograft rejection and transplant glomerulopathy. The availability of CsA has had a significant impact in increasing the success (and frequency) of renal transplantation for patients with diabetic nephropathy, such that more transplanted diabetics maintaining long-term allografts are being followed. To date, the modestly reduced graft survival seen in diabetics appears more likely related to systemic factors (e.g., cardiovascular complications) than dysfunction due to recurrent disease.

The differential diagnosis of recurrent diabetes includes chronic rejection, chronic CsA nephrotoxicity, and arterionephrosclerosis. The sclerotic and hyalinotic vascular and glomerular changes seen in recurrent diabetes may also be associated with these other lesions. Likewise, the nonspecific linear glomerular basement membrane (GBM) pattern seen with diabetes by immunofluorescence labeling for most serum proteins is also often seen in allograft biopsies of patients without diabetes. However, in early lesions, the observation of GBM thickening (without wrinkling) and the presence of intercapillary nodular sclerosis (without tuft collapse) helps differentiate diabetes from other lesions.

Patients with SLE receive transplants less frequently than do diabetics but have a very low reported recurrence rate [184,185]. Although initial studies suggested a virtual absence of SLE recurrence in renal allografts [185], occasional cases have been reported even in patients receiving CsA [186–189]. The degree of renal dysfunction associated with recurrent SLE appears to vary, but the typical immunofluorescence and ultrastructural findings of glomerular immune complex deposition in all the various forms of SLE makes the diagnosis of recurrent lupus nephritis relatively straightforward regardless of type.

Systemic diseases with renal dysfunction secondary to deposition or accumulation of particular products, such as in amyloidosis [186,190], oxalosis [186,191], Fabry's disease [192], and cystinosis [193], have a variable rate of recurrence and are relatively easy to identify. However, the inflammatory changes associated with recurrence may often make evaluation of concomitant rejection, especially of the interstitial-cellular type, difficult.

Systemic diseases may also exhibit predominantly vascular or glomerular features such as inflammatory reactions (e.g., Wegener's granulomatosis, polyarteritis nodosa, Henoch-Schönlein purpura); thrombotic microangiopathy (e.g., HUS, TTP, malignant hypertension); or sclerotic-hyalinotic changes (e.g., arterionephrosclerosis, progressive systemic sclerosis, PSS) that may recur in transplants and mimic changes seen with vascular rejection or CsA toxicity [194–198].

Vasculitis is most often confused with the humoral and less common cellular types of acute vascular rejection but can often be distinguished by the presence of segmental proliferative glomerular changes, which do not frequently occur with vascular types of rejection. The thrombotic microangiopathies may mimic lesions seen with vascular rejection and CsA toxicity (compare Figs. 3.1, 3.5, and 3.9). They can often be differentiated from rejection by the lack of inflammatory cell infiltration and hemorrhage but are generally difficult to distinguish from acute CsA vasculopathy.

Arterionephrosclerosis may "recur" in the allografts of patients with a history of hypertension and arises de novo in a significant number of transplant recipients without a prior history of hypertension but who become hypertensive following transplantation [196]. The hypertensive sclerotic and hyalinotic changes seen in vessels and glomeruli, along with interstitial fibrosis, are often difficult to distinguish from chronic vascular rejection or chronic CsA toxicity. However, the presence of only minimal inflammation and relatively pronounced medial (rather than intimal) hypertrophy suggests arterionephrosclerosis. The presence of prominent mucoid intimal thickening and, in some cases, adventitial fibrosis suggests recurrent PSS (especially in the absence of vascular rejection), but may appear similar to the hyalosis and changes seen with chronic CsA nephrotoxicity.

The recurrence of glomerulonephritis (GN) in renal allografts is not uncommon but varies in incidence for different diseases [184,185,199–202]. For example, type II membranoproliferative GN (dense deposit disease) has a very high recurrence rate (reported at greater than 70%), while type I membranoproliferative GN has a somewhat lower rate at 10% to 60%. IgA nephropathy is reported to recur in approximately 50% of cases. Other reported recurrent glomerulopathies include focal segmental glomerulosclerosis (FSGS), membranous GN, and anti-GBM disease. The standard histologic, immunofluorescence, and ultrastructural criteria generally used to diagnose these diseases can usually identify their presence in an allograft, even with some degree of underlying or superimposed rejection. However, the variable glomerulosclerotic changes often seen with acute and chronic rejection can make distinction of recurrent from de novo or transplant-associated FSGS difficult. Nevertheless, the clear recurrence of FSGS demonstrated in some patients has afforded the opportunity to examine the development of this disease, albeit in immunosuppressed allograft recipients [203,204].

In most cases, the degree of renal dysfunction associated with recurrent GN is milder than anticipated by morphologic appearance. This is perhaps most striking in some cases of recurrent anti-GBM disease, where even high titers of antibody are not associated with significant proliferative changes or nephritis. Presumably, the effects of chronic immunosuppression reduce the development of inflammatory reactions. Similarly, a significant number of patients with Alport's syndrome develop antibodies following transplantation to glycoproteins missing from their native GBM. Such patients may demonstrate IgG anti-GBM deposition by immunofluorescence but show a variable degree of inflammatory glomerular reaction [205,206].

De Novo and Acquired Diseases

In many cases, the categorization of a disease affecting a renal allograft as "de novo" or "acquired" is arbitrary and merely the result of uncertainty or exclusion of the other major categories of transmitted, alloreactive, and recurrent diseases. Nevertheless, a number of relatively common disorders can be included in this category, such as drug reactions, infections, renovascular or urologic disease, hypertensive nephropathy, and primary allograft GN.

As discussed above, CsA currently is associated with the most common drug reactions in renal allografts. However, the frequent use of heterologous antibody preparations for prophylaxis or antirejection therapy can also lead to distinctive glomerulopathy as a result of serum sickness–type reactions following host antibody production to the heterologous antibody. The most common antibody preparations now in use are mouse monoclonal antibodies (mAb) such as anti-CD3 (OKT3), horse antithymocyte globulin (ATG), and rabbit antithymocyte or anti-lymphocyte sera (ATS, ALS). Host reactions to mouse mAb most frequently are associated with minor symptoms such as fever and chills but occasionally result in dyspnea, rash, diarrhea, or seizures [207]. In addition to serum sickness–type immune complex diseases, host responses often involve the production of neutralizing antibodies against the active binding site (idiotype) of the mAb, blocking its efficacy and reuse [208]. Serum sickness reactions to heterologous polyclonal antibody preparations, especially of horse origin, are also not uncommon, and cases of immune-complex GN following ATG/ALS treatment have been reported [147]. Immunohistologic labeling for heterologous immunoglobulin deposition can clearly define the presence of such reactions (Fig. 3.12), which may confound the evaluation of host response to antirejection therapy.

Infections are the most common cause of morbidity and death following renal transplantation and are usually the direct consequence of immunosuppression [46,47]. They may be acquired by transmission in the donor organ (see above), from wound infections [209] or urinary tract infections [210], and from primary environmental exposure [211]. Although uncommon, wound infections may require cessation of immunosuppression with subsequent graft loss due to uncontrolled rejection. In contrast, urinary tract infections are relatively common, especially in the early post-transplant period, but they seldom lead to pyelonephritis [211], which normally can be

Figure 3.12
Serum sickness to horse anti-thymocyte globulin (ATG). A. Localization of horse IgG within glomeruli (×250). B. Epimembranous immune-complex deposit (×23,000).

A

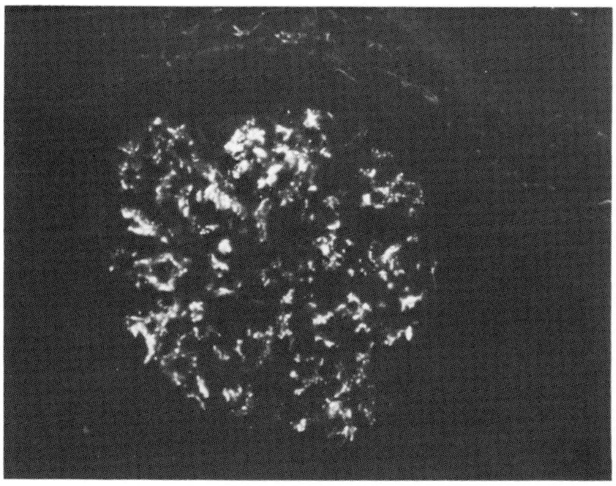

B

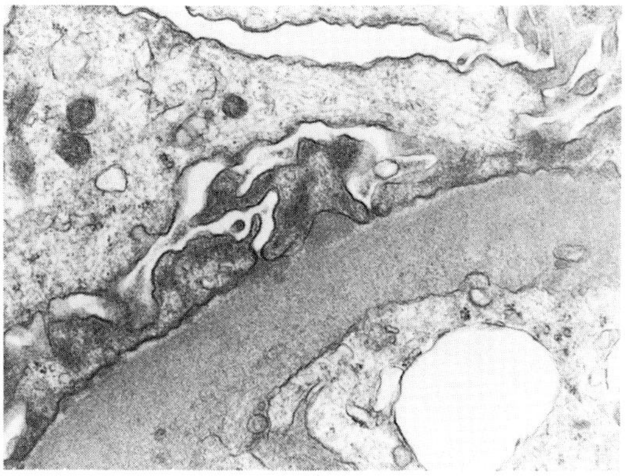

identified by the presence of leukocytes and white blood cell casts in tubules. However, in some heavily immunosuppressed patients with significant leukopenia, especially granulocytopenia, this expected picture of pyelonephritis may be altered. Renal transplant recipients are also commonly exposed to CMV either before transplantation or by receiving an organ from an infected donor [212], resulting in the majority of kidney allograft recipients being CMV seropositive [213]. However, CMV in renal allografts is usually latent and has become a less common complication with the use of CsA [214]. Nevertheless, antirejection therapy, especially with bolus steroids or antilymphocyte antibodies, increases the risk of lethal CMV infection [47]. The identification of viral infection by immunohistology, or in situ hybridization [215], is of occasional use in diagnosing serious CMV infection, although the typical morphologic features of tubular epithelial cell inclusions are usually sufficient to render a diagnosis.

As discussed above, obstructive lesions of the renal artery, vein, or ureter in the immediate post-transplant period generally provoke severe, rapid allograft injury. However, milder lesions at the anastomosis site that lead to scarring with progressive stenosis and occlusion can present with a delayed picture of allograft dysfunction. Diagnosis is usually made radiographically, but allograft biopsy can also provide histologic evidence of arterial, venous, or ureteral obstruction. Vesicoureteral reflux, although infrequent, may occur after transplantation and lead to dysfunction, usually with proteinuria [216]. Lymphocele formation can cause ureteral obstruction and infectious complications, while perirenal inflammation resulting from lymphocele, wound infection, or simple "healing-in" of the allograft can result in subcapsular inflammation that may mimic rejection on superficial biopsy specimens.

The appearance of de novo GN, even though less common than recurrent disease, is most commonly associated with proteinuria. This may be manifested as minimal change disease [217] but may also be the result of de novo membranous GN [217–219] or de novo FSGS [219,220]. We have also identified a case of de novo postinfectious-type GN, which exhibited symptoms of proteinuria and hematuria [221]. Distinction of de novo GN from recurrent or transmitted disease is essentially by exclusion, based on well-documented evaluation of the patient's native renal disease and the donor kidney before expression of the GN.

References

1. Dammin GJ. Renal transplant—correlation of histologic pattern with function. In: The Kidney (International Academy of Pathology Monograph 6). Baltimore: Williams & Wilkins, 1966;21:445–68.
2. Kincaid-Smith P. Histological diagnosis of rejection of renal homografts in man. Lancet 1967;2:849–951.
3. Porter KA. Rejection in treated renal allografts. J Clin Pathol 1967;20:518–34.
4. Kincaid-Smith P, Morris PJ, Saker BM, et al. Immediate renal graft biopsy and subsequent rejection. Lancet 1968;2:748–9.

5. Lindquist RR, Guttmann RD, Merrill JP, Dammin GJ. Human renal allografts—interpretation of morphologic and immunohistochemical observations. Am J Pathol 1968;53:851–81.
6. Glassock RJ, Feldman D, Reynolds ES, et al. Human renal isografts: a clinical and pathologic analysis. Medicine 1968;47:411–54.
7. Millard PR, Herbertson BM, Evans DB. Renal biopsy in clinical management of renal transplantation. Lancet 1:113–6.
8. Dempster WJ, Harrison CV, Shackman R. Rejection processes in human homotransplanted kidneys. Br Med J 1964;2:969–76.
9. Porter KA. Morphological aspects of renal homograft rejection. Br Med Bull 1965;21:171–5.
10. Porter KA, Marchioro TL, Starzl TE. Pathological changes in 37 human renal homotransplants treated with immunosuppressive drugs. Br J Urol 1965;37:250–73.
11. Kissmeyer-Nielsen F, Olsen S, Posborg PV, Fjeldborg O. Hyperacute rejection of kidney allografts, associated with preexisting humoral antibodies against donor cells. Lancet 1966;2:662–5.
12. Myburgh JA, Cohen I, Gecelter L, et al. Hyperacute rejection in human kidney allografts—Shwartzman or Arthus reaction? N Engl J Med 1969;281:131–5.
13. Deodhar SD, Benjamin SP. Pathology of human renal allograft rejection. Surg Clin North Am 1971;51:1141–59.
14. Porter KA, Dossetor JB, Marchioro TL, et al. Human renal transplants. I. Glomerular changes. Lab Invest 1967;16:153–81.
15. Porter KA, Andres GA, Calder MW, et al. Human renal transplants. II. Immunofluorescent and immunoferritin studies. Lab Invest 1968;18:159–71.
16. Mathew TH, Kincaid-Smith P, Eremin J, Marshall VC. Percutaneous needle biopsy of renal homografts. Med J Aust 1968;1:6–7.
17. Pillay VKG, Kurtzman NA. Percutaneous biopsy of the transplanted kidney. JAMA 1973;226:1561–2.
18. Buselmeier TJ, Schauer RM, Mauer SM, et al. A simplified method of percutaneous allograft biopsy. Nephron 1976;16:318–21.
19. Murphy GP. Percutaneous needle biopsy of human renal allotransplants. J Urol 1972;107:193–5.
20. Parker RA, Elliot WC, Muther RS, et al. Percutaneous aspiration biopsy of renal allografts using ultrasound localization. Urology 1980;15:534–5.
21. Appel GB, Saltzman MJ, King DL, Hardy MA. Use of ultrasound for renal allograft biopsy. Kidney Int 1981;19:471–3.
22. Horowitz MD, Russell E, Abitbol C, et al. Massive hematuria following percutaneous biopsy of renal allograft. Successful control by selective embolization. Arch Surg 1984;119:1430–3.
23. Salcedo JR, Silverstein CE. Postbiopsy bleeding in renal allograft: successful treatment with epsilon aminocaproic acid. J Urol 1982;127:783.
24. Moreau JF, Merland JJ, Deschamps JM. Postbiopsy false arterial aneurysm of a transplanted kidney: treatment by bucrylate transcatheter embolization. J Urol 1982;128:116–8.
25. Eckhauser ML, Haaga JR, Hampel N, et al. Arterial embolization of renal allograft to control hemorrhage secondary to percutaneous nephropyelostomy. J Urol 1981;126:679–80.
26. Kalash SS, Muakkassa WF, Campbell EW, et al. Persistent clot anuria complicating renal transplant biopsy. Urology 1985;25:591–5.
27. O'Brien DP III, Parrott TS, Walton KN, et al. Renal arteriovenous fistulas. Surg Gynecol Obstet 1974;139:739–43.

28. Matas AJ, Sibley R, Mauer M, et al. The value of needle renal allograft biopsy. I. A retrospective study of biopsies performed during putative rejection episodes. Ann Surg 1983;197:226–37.
29. Fennell RS, Donnelly WH, Purcell CA, et al. The use of the kidney biopsy to predict allograft loss in a pediatric transplant population. Int J Pediatr Nephrol 1986;7:21–6.
30. Matas AJ, Tellis VA, Sablay L, et al. The value of needle renal allograft biopsy. III. A prospective study. Surgery 1985;98:922–6.
31. Waltzer WC, Miller F, Arnold A, et al. Value of percutaneous core needle biopsy in the differential diagnosis of renal transplant dysfunction. J Urol 1987;127:1117–21.
32. Huraib S, Goldberg H, Katz A, et al. Percutaneous needle biopsy of the transplanted kidney: technique and complications. Am J Kid Dis 1989;14:13–17.
33. Finkelstein FO, Siegel NJ, Bastl C, et al. Kidney transplant biopsies in the diagnosis and management of acute rejection actions. Kidney Int 1976;10:171–8.
34. Banfi G, Imbasciati E, Tarantino A, Ponticelli C. Prognostic value of renal biopsy in acute rejection of kidney transplant. Nephron 1981;28:222–6.
35. Vangelista A, Frasca GM, Stefoni S, Bonomini V. Graft biopsy in renal transplantation: correlation with clinical, immunological, and virological investigations. Kidney Int 1983;23S:41–5.
36. Parfrey PS, Kuo YL, Hanley JA, et al. The diagnostic and prognostic value of renal allograft biopsy. Transplantation 1984;38:586–90.
37. Pardo-Muidan FJ, Guillen R, Virto R, et al. Kidney allograft biopsy: a valuable tool in assessing the diagnosis of acute rejection. Clin Nephrol 1985;24:37–41.
38. Kerman RH, ed. Immunological monitoring of the transplant patient. Transplant Proc 1984;16:1403–1718.
39. Häyry P, Koskimies S, eds. Proceedings of the Eleventh International Congress of the Transplantation Society. Transplant Proc 1987;19:1559–1694.
40. Genkins SM, Sanfilippo F, Carroll BA. Duplex doppler sonography of renal transplants: lack of sensitivity and specificity in establishing pathologic diagnosis. AJR, 1989;152:535–9.
41. Yap HK, Dietrich RB, Kangarloo H, et al. Acute renal allograft rejection. Comparative value of ultrasound vs. magnetic resonance imaging. Transplantation 1987;43:249–52.
42. Heil J, Sutherland DER, Fryd DS, et al. Acute tubular necrosis of cadaver renal allografts does not correlate with organ sharing or preservation time but portends a poorer prognosis for long-term graft survival. Transplant Proc 1984;16:270–2.
43. Sanfilippo F, Vaughn WK, Spees EK, Lucas BA. The detrimental effects of delayed graft function in cadaver donor renal transplantation. Transplantation 1984;38:643–8.
44. Canafax DM, Torres A, Fryd DS, et al. The effects of delayed function on recipients of cadaver renal allografts. Transplantation 1986;41:177–81.
45. Iwaki Y, Terasaki PI. Primary nonfunction in human cadaver kidney transplantation: evidence for hidden hyperacute rejection. Clin Transplant 1987;1:125–31.
46. Tilney NL, Strom TB, Vineyard GC, et al. Factors contributing to the declining mortality rate in renal transplantation. N Engl J Med 1978;299:1321–5.
47. Scroggs MW, Wolfe JA, Bollinger RR, Sanfilippo F. Clinical and post-mortem findings in deaths associated with renal transplantation. Arch Pathol Lab Med 1987;111:983–7.

48. Bossen EH, Johnston WW, Amatulli J, Rowlands DT. Exfoliative cytopathologic studies in organ transplantation. III. The cytologic profile of urine during acute renal allograft rejection. Acta Cytol 1970;14:176–81.
49. Simpson MA, Madras PN, Crosson AW, et al. Correlation of binding of human immunoglobulin, urinary cytology, and needle biopsy in the early posttransplant period. Transplant Proc 1987;19:1662–3.
50. Sandoz PF, Bielmann D, Mihatsch M, Thiel G. Value of urinary sediment in the diagnosis of interstitial rejection in renal transplants. Transplantation 1986;41:343–8.
51. Rapaport FT, Converse JM, Billingham RE. Recent advances in clinical and experimental transplantation. JAMA 1977;237:2835–40.
52. Matas AJ, Sablay L, Tellis VA, et al. The value of needle renal allograft biopsy. II. Reflection of acute rejection changes throughout the kidney by percutaneous biopsy. Transplantation 1984;38:92–3.
53. Colvin RB. Clinical applications of monoclonal antibodies in renal allograft biopsies. Am J Kidney Dis 1988;11:126–30.
54. Fuggle SV, McWhinnie DL. Immunohistology of the transplant kidney. In: Morris PJ, ed. Kidney transplantation, ed 3. Philadelphia: Saunders, 1988:473–89.
55. McCue PA, Santoianni RA. Expedited handling of transplantation biopsies. Am J Surg Pathol 1988;12:155–7.
56. Valenzuela R, Hamway SA, Deodhar SD, et al. Histologic, ultrastructural and immunomicroscopic findings in 96 one-hour human renal allograft biopsy specimens. Hum Pathol 1980;11:187–95.
57. Shemesh O, Golbetz H, Kriss JP, Myers BD. Limitations of creatinine as a filtration marker in glomerulopathic patients. Kidney Int 1985;28:830–8.
58. de la Riviere GB, van de Putte LBA. Preexisting glomerulonephritis in allografted kidneys. Arch Pathol Lab Med 1976;100:196–8.
59. Sanfilippo F, Croker BP, Bollinger RR. Fate of four cadaveric donor renal allografts with mesangial IgA deposits. Transplantation 1982;33:370–6.
60. Sanfilippo F. The transmission of disease to allograft recipients via donor organs. Curr Opinion Immunol 1989;1:1225–9.
61. Betts RF, Freeman RB, Douglas RG, et al. Transmission of cytomegalovirus infection with renal allograft. Kidney Int 1975;8:385–92.
62. Cohen J, Hopkin J, Kurtz J. Infectious complications after renal transplantation. In: Morris PJ, ed. Kidney transplantation, ed 3. Philadelphia: Saunders, 1988:533–73.
63. Ward JW, Holmberg SD, Allen JR, et al. Transmission of human immunodeficiency virus (HIV) by blood transfusion screened as negative for HIV antibody. N Engl J Med 1988;318:473–8.
64. Bowen PA II, Lobel SA, Caruana RJ, et al. Transmission of human immunodeficiency virus (HIV) by transplantation: clinical aspects and time course analysis of viral antigenemia and antibody production. Ann Intern Med 1988;108:46–8.
65. Penn I. Tumors arising in organ transplant recipients. Adv Cancer Res 1981; 28:31–61.
66. Spees EK, Lempert N, Olson JL, et al. Blue cadaver donor kidneys for transplantation. J Urol 1984;131:338A.
67. Leunissen KML, Ruers TJM, Bosman F, et al. Intravascular coagulation and kidney donation. Transplantation 1986;42:307–8.
68. Abouna GM, Kremer GD, Daddah SK, et al. Reversal of diabetic nephropathy in human cadaveric kidneys after transplantation into non-diabetic recipients. Lancet 1983;1:1274–6.

110. Sanfilippo F. The current use of immunosuppressive therapy to overcome immunologic risk factors associated with renal allograft rejection. In: Transplantation and Clinical Immunology XX. Combined Immunosuppressive Therapy in Transplantation. Amsterdam: Excerpta Medica; 1989:107–18.
111. Gell PGH, Coombs RRA. Clinical aspects of immunology, ed 3. Oxford: Blackwell Scientific, 1986.
112. Armstrong HE, Bolton EM, McMillan I, et al. Prolonged survival of actively enhanced rat renal allografts despite accelerated cellular infiltration and rapid induction of both class I and class II MHC antigens. J Exp Med 1987;164:891–907.
113. Dallman MJ, Wood KJ, Morris PJ. Specific cytotoxic T cells are found in the non-rejected kidneys of blood transfused rats. J Exp Med 1987;165:566–71.
114. Ruiz P, Coffman TM, Howell DN, et al. Pretransplant donor blood transfusion prevents rat renal allograft dysfunction but not the in situ cellular alloimmune or morphologic manifestations of rejection. Transplantation 1988;45:1–7.
115. Williams GM, Hume DM, Hudson RP, et al. "Hyperacute" renal homograft rejection in man. N Engl J Med 1968;279:611–18.
116. Patel R, Terasaki PI. Significance of a positive crossmatch test in kidney transplantation. N Engl J Med 1969;288:735–9.
117. Bannett A, Brynger H, Samuelsson B, et al., eds. ABO incompatibility and transplantation. Transplant Proc 1987;19:4401–4642.
118. Cardella CJ, Falk JA, Nicholson MJ, et al. Successful renal transplantation in patients with T cell reactivity to donor. Lancet 1982;2:1240–3.
119. Sanfilippo F, Vaughn WK, Spees EK, Bollinger RR. Cadaver renal transplantation ignoring peak-reactive sera in patients with markedly decreasing pretransplant sensitization. Transplantation 1984;38:119–24.
120. Wolfe JA, McCann RL, Sanfilippo F. Cyclosporine-associated microangiopathy in renal transplantation: a severe but potentially reversible form of early graft injury. Transplantation 1986;41:541–4.
121. Sturgill BC, Lobo PI, Bolton WK. Cold-reacting IgM antibody-induced renal allograft failure. Similarity to hyperacute rejection. Nephron 1984;125–7.
122. Ruers TJM, Buurman WA, van Boxtel CJ, et al. Immunohistological observations in rat kidney allografts after local steroid administration. J Exp Med 1987;166:1205–20.
123. Skoglund C, Scheynius A, Holmdahl R, van der Meide PH. Enhancement of DTH reaction and inhibition of the expression of class II transplantation antigens by in vivo treatment with antibodies against γ-interferon. Clin Exp Immunol 1988;71:428–32.
124. Imbasciati E, Banfi G, Egidi F, et al. Morphologic patterns of renal allograft rejection. Contr Nephrol 1987;55:105–22.
125. Kolbeck PC, Tatum AH, Sanfilippo F. Phenotypic evaluation of mononuclear cell infiltrates in renal allograft biopsies. Transplant Proc 1985;17:893–5.
126. Sanfilippo F, Kolbeck PC, Vaughn WK, Bollinger RR. Renal allograft cell infiltrates associated with irreversible rejection. Transplantation 1985;40:679–85.
127. Medawar PB. The behavior and fate of skin autografts and skin homografts in rabbits. J Anat 1944;78:176–99.
128. Kiaer H, Hansen HE, Olsen S. The predictive value of percutaneous biopsies from human renal allografts with early impaired function. Clin Nephrol 1980;13:58–63.
129. Sibley RK, Payne W. Morphologic findings in the renal allograft biopsy. Semin Nephrol 1985;5:294–306.
130. McWhinnie DL, Thompson JF, Taylor HM, et al. Morphometric analysis of

cellular infiltration assessed by monoclonal antibody labeling in sequential human renal allograft biopsies. Transplantation 1986;42:352–8.
131. Hancock WW, Thomson NM, Atkins RC. Monoclonal antibody analysis of interstitial cell infiltrate during human renal allograft rejection. Transplant Proc 1983;15:352–5.
132. Kormendi F, Amend WJC. The importance of eosinophil cells in kidney allograft rejection. Transplantation 1988;45:537–9.
133. Beshorner WE, Burdick JF, Williams GM, Solez K. The presence of Leu-7-reactive lymphocytes in renal allografts undergoing acute rejection. Transplant Proc 1985;17:618–22.
134. Tufveson G, Forsum U, Claesson K, et al. T-lymphocyte subsets and HLA-Dr expressing cells in rejected human kidney grafts. Scand J Immunol 1983;18:37–40.
135. Platt JL, LeBien TW, Michael AF. Interstitial mononuclear cell populations in renal graft rejection: identification by monoclonal antibodies in tissue sections. J Exp Med 1982;155:17–30.
136. Wood GS, Warner NL, Warnke RA. Anti-Leu 3/T4 antibodies react with cells of monocyte/macrophage and Langerhans lineage. J Immunol 1983;131:212–6.
137. Blue M-L, Daley JF, Levine H, Schlossman SF. Coexpression of T4 and T8 on peripheral blood T cells demonstrated by two-color fluorescence flow cytometry. J Immunol 1985;134:2281–6.
138. Kolbeck PC, Tatum AH, Sanfilippo F. The relationship between histologic pattern, intensity, and phenotypes of cells infiltrating renal allografts. Transplantation 1984;38:709–15.
139. Kolbeck PC, Scheinman JI, Sanfilippo F. Acute cellular rejection and cyclosporine nephrotoxicity monitored by biopsy in a renal allograft recipient: the differentiation of drug nephrotoxicity from rejection by phenotyping of cellular infiltrates. Arch Pathol Lab Med 1986;110:389–93.
140. Van Es A, Meyer CJLM, Oljans PJ, et al. Mononuclear cells in renal allografts. Transplantation 1984;37:134–9.
141. Sako H, Nakane Y, Okino K, et al. Immunohistochemical study of the cells infiltrating human renal allografts by the ABC and the IGSS method using monoclonal antibodies. Transplantation 1987;44:43–50.
142. Bishop GA, Hall BM, Duggin GG, et al. Immunopathology of renal allograft rejection analyzed with monoclonal antibodies to mononuclear cell markers. Kidney Int 1986;29:708–17.
143. Waltzer WC, Miller F, Arnold A, et al. Immunohistologic analysis of human renal allograft dysfunction. Transplantation 1987;43:100–5.
144. von Willebrand E, Pettersson E, Ahonen J, Häyry P. CMV infection, class II antigen expression, and human kidney graft rejection. Transplantation 1986; 42:364–7.
145. Axelsen RA, Seymour AE, Mathew TH, et al. Glomerular transplant rejection: a distinctive pattern of early graft damage. Clin Nephrol 1985;23:1–11.
146. Hiki Y, Leong ASY, Mathew TH, et al. Typing of intraglomerular mononuclear cells associated with transplant glomerular rejection. Clin Nephrol 1986;26:244–9.
147. Tatum AH, Bollinger RR, Sanfilippo F. Rapid serologic diagnosis of serum sickness from antithymocyte globulin therapy using enzyme immunoassay. Transplantation 1984;38:582–6.
148. Platt JL, Ferguson RM, Sibley RD, et al. Renal interstitial cell populations in cyclosporine nephrotoxicity. Transplantation 1983;36:343–6.
149. Barrett M, Milton AD, Barratt J, et al. Evaluation of class II major histocompatibility complex antigen expression for the differential diagnosis of

cyclosporine A nephrotoxicity from kidney graft rejection. Transplant Proc 1987;19:1769–71.
150. Rao KV, Rose JK. Incidence, histological pattern, and clinical outcome of rejection episodes occurring in the late posttransplant period. Transplantation 1985;39:631–7.
151. Soloman LR, Martin S, Short CD, et al. Late cellular rejection in renal transplant recipients. Transplantation 1986;41:262–4.
152. Ruiz P, Kolbeck PC, Scroggs MW, Sanfilippo F. Associations between cyclosporine therapy and interstitial fibrosis in renal allograft biopsies. Transplantation 1988;45:91–5.
153. Flechner SM, Kerman RH, Van Buren C, Kahan BD. Successful transplantation of cyclosporine-treated haploidentical living-related renal recipients without blood transfusions. Transplantation 1984;37:73–6.
154. Hess AD, Colombani PM, Esa A. Cyclosporine: immunobiologic aspects in transplantation. In: Williams GM, Burdick JF, Solez K, eds. Kidney transplant rejection: diagnosis and treatment. New York: Marcel Dekker, 1986; 17:353–82.
155. Myers BD. Cyclosporine nephrotoxicity. Kidney Int 1986;30:964–74.
156. Keown PA, Stiller CR, Wallace AC. Nephrotoxicity of cyclosporin A. In: Williams GM, Burdick JF, Solez K, eds. Kidney transplant rejection: diagnosis and treatment. New York: Marcel Dekker, 1986;20:423–57.
157. Sommer BG, Innes JT, Whitehurst RM, et al. Cyclosporine associated renal arteriopathy resulting in loss of allograft function. Am J Surg 1985;149:756–64.
158. Klintmalm G, Ringén O, Groth CG. Clinical and laboratory signs in nephrotoxicity and rejection in cyclosporine-treated renal allograft recipients. Transplant Proc 1983;15:2815–20.
159. Kolbeck PC, Wolfe JA, Burchette J, Sanfilippo F. Immunopathologic patterns of cyclosporine deposition associated with nephrotoxicity in renal allograft biopsies. Transplantation 1987;43:218–24.
160. Lewis RM, Janney RP, Van Buren CT, et al. A retrospective analysis of long-term renal allograft function associated with cyclosporine-prednisone immunosuppressive therapy. Transplant Proc 1988;20:534–9.
161. Sibley RK, Rynasiewicz J, Ferguson RM, et al. Morphology of cyclosporine nephrotoxicity and acute rejection in patients immunosuppressed with cyclosporine and prednisone. Surgery 1983;94:225–34.
162. Farnsworth A, Hall BM, Ng ABP, et al. Renal biopsy morphology in renal transplantation. A comparative study of the light-microscopic appearances of biopsies from patients treated with cyclosporin A or azathioprine prednisone and antilymphocyte globulin. Am J Surg Pathol 1984;8:243–52.
163. Mihatsch MJ, Bergstand A, Bohman SO, et al. Renal histopathology in kidney transplant recipients immunosuppressesd with cyclosporin A: results of an international workshop. Clin Nephrol 1985;24:107–19.
164. Mihatsch MJ, Thiel G, Ryffel B. Histopathology cyclosporine nephrotoxicity. Transplant Proc 1988;20:759–71.
165. Mihatsch MJ, Olivier W, Marbet U, et al. Giant mitochondria in renal tubular cells and cyclosporin A. Lancet 1981;1:1162–3.
166. Verani RR, Flechner S, Van Buren C, Kahan BD. Acute cellular rejection or cyclosporine A nephrotoxicity? A review of transplant renal biopsies. Am J Kidney Dis 1984;4:185–91.
167. d'Ardenne AJ, Dunnill MS, Thompson JF, et al. Cyclosporine and renal allograft histology. J Clin Pathol 1986;39:145–51.
168. von Willebrand E, Häyry P. Cyclosporine-A deposits in renal allografts. Lancet 1983;2:189–92.

169. Kolbeck PC, Wolfe JA, Burchette J, Sanfilippo F. Evaluation of cyclosporine induced nephrotoxicity by immunoperoxidase analysis of renal allograft biopsies. Transplant Proc 1987;19:1781–4.
170. Ruiz P, Kolbeck PC, Scroggs MW, et al. Cyclosporine therapy and the development of interstitial fibrosis in renal allografts. Transplant Proc 1988;20:807–11.
171. Hamburger J, Crosnier J, Dormont Y. Observations in patients with a well-tolerated homotransplanted kidney. Possibility of a secondary disease. Ann NY Acad Sci 1964;120:558–77.
172. Fish AJ, Herdman RC, Delly WD, Good RA. Glomerular changes in well-functioning human renal homografts. Transplantation 1967;5:1338–43.
173. Petersen VP, Olsen TS, Kissmeyer-Nielsen F, et al. Late failure of human renal transplants. Medicine 1975;54:45–71.
174. Zollinger HU, Moppert J, Thiel G, Rohr HP. Morphology and pathogenesis of glomerulopathy in cadaver kidney allografts treated with antilymphocyte globulin. Curr Top Pathol 1973;57:1–48.
175. Maryniak RK, First MR, Weiss MA. Transplant glomerulopathy: evolution of morphologically distinct changes. Kidney Int 1985;27:799–806.
176. Tuazon TV, Schneeberger EE, Bhan AK, et al. Mononuclear cells in acute allograft glomerulopathy. Am J Pathol 1987;129:119–32.
177. Richardson WP, Colvin RB, Cheeseman SH, et al. Glomerulopathy associated with cytomegalovirus viremia in renal allografts. N Engl J Med 1981;305:57–64.
178. Herrera GA, Alexander RW, Cooley CF, Luke RG, et al. Cytomegalovirus glomerulopathy: a controversial lesion. Kidney Int 1986;29:725–33.
179. Ulrich W, Schledere MP, Buxbaum P. The histopathologic identification of CMV infected cells in biopsies of human renal allografts. An evaluation of 100 transplant biopsies by in situ hybridization. Pathol Res Pract 1986;181:739–45.
180. Boyce NW, Hayes K, Gee D, Holdsworth SR, et al. Cytomegalovirus infection complicating renal transplantation and its relationship to acute transplant glomerulopathy. Transplantation 1988;45:706–9.
181. Mauer SM, Barbosa J, Vernier RL, et al. Development of diabetic vascular lesions in normal kidneys transplanted into patients with diabetes mellitus. N Engl J Med 1976;295:916–20.
182. Maryniak RK, Mendoza N, Clyne D, et al. Recurrence of diabetic nodular glomerulosclerosis in a renal transplant. Transplantation 1985;39:35–8.
183. Najarian JS, Sutherland DE, Simmons RL, et al. Ten years experience with renal transplantation in juvenile onset diabetics. Ann Surg 1979;190:487–500.
184. Cameron JS, Turner DR. Recurrent glomerulonephritis in allografted kidneys. Clin Nephrol 1977;7:47–54.
185. Honkanen E, Törnroth T, Pettersson E, Kuhlbäck B. Glomerulonephritis in renal allografts: results of 18 years of transplantations. Clin Nephrol 1984; 21:210–19.
186. Advisory Committee to the Renal Transplant Registry. Renal transplantation in congenital and metabolic diseases: a report from the ACS/NIH Renal Transplant Registry. JAMA 1975;232:148–53.
187. Amend WJC, Vincenti F, Feduska NJ, et al. Recurrent systemic lupus erythematosus involving renal allografts. Ann Intern Med 1981;94:444–8.
188. Kumano K, Sakai T, Mashimo S, Endo T, et al. A case of recurrent lupus nephritis after renal transplantation. Clin Nephrol 1987;27:94–98.
189. Nyberg G, Blohmé I, Svalander C, et al. Rejection and recurrence of SLE nephritis in cyclosporine-treated kidney transplant recipients. Transplant Proc 1987;19:1637–8.
190. Helin H, Pasternack A, Falck H, Kuhlbäck B. Recurrence of renal amyloid and

de novo membranous glomerulonephritis after transplantation. Transplantation 1981;32:6–9.
191. Leumann EP, Wegmann W, Largiader F. Prolonged survival after renal transplantation in primary hyperoxaluria of childhood. Clin Nephrol 1978;9:29–34.
192. Friedlaender MM, Kopolovic J, Rubinger D, et al. Renal biopsy in Fabry's diseases eight years after successful renal transplantation. Clin Nephrol 1987;27:206–11.
193. Malekzade HMH, Neustein HB, Schneider JA, et al. Cadaver renal transplantation in children with cystinosis. Am J Med 1977;63:525–33.
194. Bonsib SM, Ercolani L, Ngheim D, Hamilton HE. Recurrent thrombotic microangiopathy in a renal allograft. Am J Med 1985;79:520–7.
195. Hebert D, Sibley RK, Mauer SM. Recurrence of hemolytic uremic syndrome in renal transplant recipients. Kidney Int 1986;30S:51–8.
196. Rao TKS, Gupta SK, Butt KMH, et al. Relationship of renal transplantation to hypertension in end-stage renal failure. Arch Intern Med 1978;138:1236–41.
197. Steinman T, Jaffe B, Monaco A, et al. Recurrence of Wegeners granulomatosis after kidney transplantation. Successful re-induction of remission with cyclophosphamide. Am J Med 1980;68:458–60.
198. Woodhall PB, McCoy RC, Gunnells JC, Seigler HF. Apparent recurrence of progressive systemic sclerosis in a renal allograft. JAMA 1976;236:1032–4.
199. Mathew TH, Mathews DC, Hobbs JB, Kincaid-Smith P. Glomerular lesions after renal transplantation. Am J Med 1975;59:177–90.
200. Hamburger J, Crosnier J, Noël LH. Recurrent glomerulonephritis after renal transplantation. Annu Rev Med 1978;29:67–72.
201. Morzycka M, Croker BP, Seigler HF, Tisher CC. Evaluation of recurrent glomerulonephritis in kidney allografts. Am J Med 1982;72:588–98.
202. Cameron JS. Glomerulonephritis in renal transplants. Transplantation 1982; 34:237–45.
203. Korbet SM, Schwartz MM, Lewis EJ. Recurrent nephrotic syndrome in renal allografts. Am J Kidney Dis 1988;11:270–6.
204. Striegel JE, Sibley RK, Fryd DS, Mauer SM. Recurrence of focal segmental sclerosis in children following renal transplantation. Kidney Int 1986;30S:44–50.
205. Milliner DS, Pierides AM, Holley KE. Renal transplantation in Alport's syndrome. Anti-glomerular basement membrane glomerulonephritis in the allograft. Mayo Clin Proc 1982;57:35–43.
206. Quérin S, Noël LH, Grünfeld JP, et al. Linear glomerular IgG fixation in renal allografts: incidence and significance in Alport's syndrome. Clin Nephrol 1986;25:134–40.
207. Thistlethwaite JR, Stuart JK, Mayes JT, et al. Complications and monitoring of OKT3 therapy. Am J Kidney Dis 1988;11:112–9.
208. Jaffers GJ, Fuller TC, Cosimi AB, et al. Monoclonal antibody therapy. Anti-idiotypic and non-anti-idiotypic antibodies to OKT3 arising despite intense immunosuppression. Transplantation 1986;41:572–8.
209. Kyriakides GK, Simmons RL, Najarian JS. Wound infections in renal transplant wounds: pathogenic and prognostic factors. Ann Surg 1975;182:770–5.
210. Rubin RH, Wolfson JS, Cosimi AB, et al. Infection in the renal transplant recipient. Am J Med 1981;70:405–11.
211. Pearson JC, Amend WJC, Vincenti FG, et al. Post-transplantation pyelonephritis: factors producing low patient and transplant morbidity. J Urol 1980;123:153–6.
212. Chou S. Acquisition of donor strain cytomegalovirus by renal transplant recipients. N Engl J Med 1986;314:1418–23.

213. Rubin RH, Tolkoff-Rubin NE, Oliver D, et al. Multicenter seroepidemologic study of the impact of cytomegalovirus infection on renal transplantation. Transplantation 1985;40:243–9.
214. Sutherland DER, Payne WD, Fryd DS, et al. Comparison of cyclosporine and azathioprine for immunosuppression in diabetic and nondiabetic renal allograft recipients. Transplant Proc 1985;17:1204–11.
215. Kemnitz J, Haverich A, Gubernatis G, Cohnert TR. Rapid identification of viral infections in liver, heart, and kidney allograft biopsies by in situ hybridization. Am J Surg Pathol 1989;13:80–2.
216. McMorrow RG, Curtis JJ, Lucas BA, et al. Does vesicoureteric reflux result in renal allograft failure? Clin Nephrol 1980;14:89–91.
217. Gephardt GN, Tubbs RR, Braun WE, et al. Nephrotic range proteinuria with "minimal change glomerulopathy" in human renal allografts: report of four cases. Am J Kidney Dis 1988;12:51–61.
218. Cosyns JP, Kazatchkine MD, Bhakdi S, et al. Immunohistochemical analysis of C3 cleavage fragments, factor H, and the C5b-9 terminal complex of complement in de novo membranous glomerulonephritis occurring in patients with renal transplant. Clin Nephrol 1986;26:203–8.
219. Ward HJ, Koyle MA. Immunopathologic features of de novo membranous nephropathy in renal allografts. Transplantation 1988;45:524–9.
220. Cheigh JS, Mouradian J, Soliman M, et al. Focal segmental glomerulosclerosis in renal transplants. Am J Kidney Dis 1983;2:449–55.
221. Sanfilippo F, Croker BP. The possible occurrence of staphylococcal post-infectious glomerulonephritis in a renal allograft. Transplantation 1983;35:25–9.

4

Liver Transplantation

DALE C. SNOVER

Liver dysfunction following liver transplantation can result from processes such as infectious diseases, which are not unique to liver transplantation, or from processes that are unique, such as those related to preservation of the liver, surgical aspects of the transplantation, and allograft rejection. These latter problems constitute the major focus of this chapter.

Assessing Liver Dysfunction Following Transplantation

As the number of liver transplants performed has increased, so has the need for accurate methods of assessing liver status. The role of the pathologist in this assessment has increased in recent years, although frequency of biopsy, indications for biopsy, and the relative weight biopsy is given in decisions regarding therapy of a potential rejection episode still vary among centers. Although biochemical liver function tests and radiologic techniques provide valuable information, they are rarely diagnostic. Liver biopsy, though not 100% successful in determining the cause of dysfunction, remains the gold standard of diagnosis in many centers.

Biopsies are performed for three major reasons. In many centers protocol biopsies (i.e., biopsies taken at specific intervals after transplantation regardless of clinical status) are used to provide the earliest possible diagnosis of rejection, since the rejecting liver will show histologic changes before clinical manifestations [1]. Biopsy is also performed to assess changes in liver function, usually as first noted by abnormal liver function tests (LFTs). Finally, biopsy is often used to assess efficacy of therapy following treatment for rejection, since LFTs alone do not reliably measure disease activity.

To properly evaluate the pathological condition of the liver following transplantation, an understanding of the operative procedure and of post-operative care is necessary. These subjects are reviewed in detail elsewhere and are discussed only briefly here [2].

Livers to be transplanted are preserved for a variable period of time before transplantation, usually by flushing the organ with preservation fluid and packing it in ice [2]. Several factors may influence the integrity of the donated liver including status of the donor before death and the preservation process itself. If there is any doubt about the donor liver's quality, a biopsy should be obtained at the time of closure of the patient so that an accurate baseline is available to evaluate future pathologic changes [3]. The surgical procedure itself inflicts some degree of physical trauma on the liver, which may result in focal necrosis or even areas of infarction [4]. These areas of infarction may be biopsied in the post-transplant period and should not be overinterpreted as representing infarction due to problems with one of the vascular anastomoses.

The transplant procedure itself involves five anastomoses: the suprahepatic and infrahepatic inferior vena cava, portal vein, hepatic artery, and bile duct. The suprahepatic vena cava is technically the most difficult, since the recipient cuff is frequently quite short. Narrowing or thrombosis of this anastomosis may result in Budd-Chiari syndrome. Narrowing or thrombosis of the portal vein or arterial anastomosis may cause ischemic damage. Obstruction of the infrahepatic inferior vena cava will not cause hepatic difficulties.

Several approaches have been used for the biliary anastomosis. These include choledochodochostomy, cholecystoenterostomy, and choledochojejunostomy [5]. The choice is usually dictated in part by clinical circumstances (e.g., the absence of a patient recipient duct in sclerosing cholangitis obviously makes a choledochodochostomy impossible) as well as by the surgeon's preference. The biliary anastomosis may either leak or obstruct and has constituted a major technical problem [5].

Following transplantation all patients receive a wide variety of potentially hepatotoxic agents. These include immunosuppressants such as cyclosporine (CsA), azathioprine, and steroids; antibiotics; and hyperalimentation. The pathologist should always be aware of the pharmacopoeia in the patient before rendering a diagnosis.

One final factor that may cause a problem in diagnosis is the effect of multiple biopsies. We have seen scarring caused by a previous biopsy site

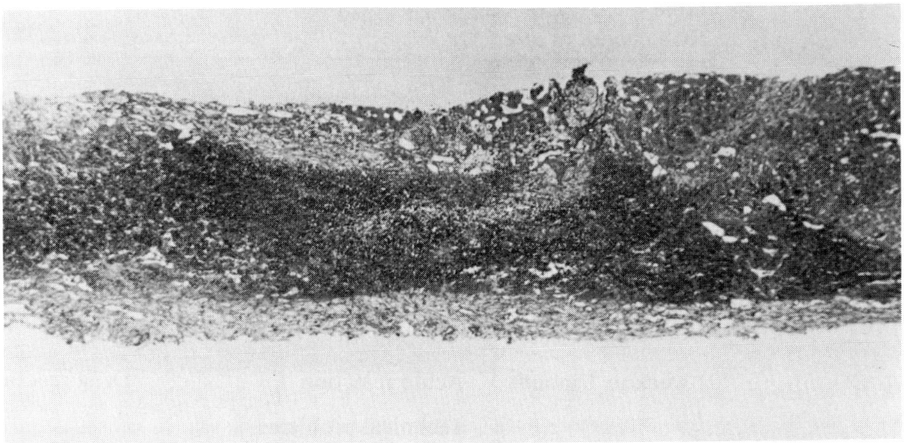

Figure 4.1
Previous biopsy site characterized by a linear area of central hemorrhage surrounded by fresh granulation tissue. Note the residual normal liver in the upper right side of the biopsy (hematoxylin-eosin ×40).

on several occasions. These areas are usually recognizable by their linear character and granulation-tissue-like quality (Fig. 4.1) and should not be mistaken for functionally significant necrosis or fibrosis.

Timing of Pathological Events Following Transplantation

The differential diagnosis of an episode of clinical liver dysfunction will be determined by the interval from transplantation (Table 4.1). For example, many technical complications will be apparent in the first few days after surgery. Similarly, acute rejection usually occurs in the first several weeks post-transplant. On the other hand, infectious diseases such as hepatitis B, which have a requisite incubation time, will arise after this incubation time. Keeping these factors in mind will help in interpretation of biopsies.

Pathology of Technical Complications

Included among technical complications following transplantation are those related to the preservation and transport of the organ and those related to problems with the various anastomoses described above.

Most livers will show histologic abnormalities at the time of transplantation. Biopsies taken at transplantation ("time-zero" biopsies) will almost invariably show rarefaction or ballooning of hepatocellular cytoplasm that may be diffuse or predominantly centrilobular (Fig. 4.2) [3]. This will sometimes be accompanied by focal accumulation of polymorphonuclear cells

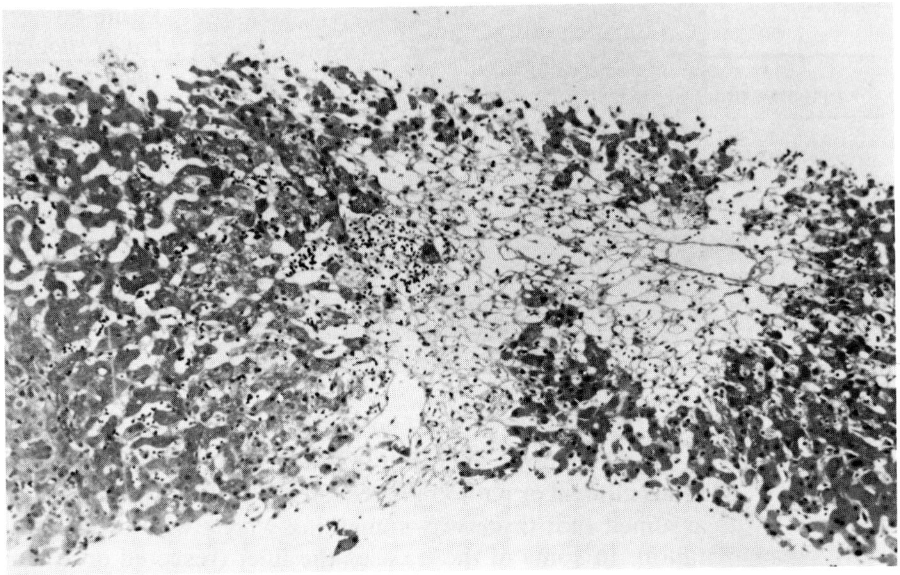

Figure 4.4
Area of centrilobular necrosis with surrounding hepatocellular atrophy and sinusoidal dilatation in a patient with portal vein obstruction (hematoxylin-eosin ×100).

lead to persistent ischemic changes in the liver. The type of extensive infarction seen with arterial stenosis is rare. Rather, the typical features are those of centrilobular hepatocellular atrophy with secondary sinusoidal dilation and areas of dropout of clusters of hepatocytes (Fig. 4.4). The type of noncirrhotic portal fibrosis seen in patients with extrahepatic portal vein thrombosis who have not undergone transplantation has not been reported to date in those who have received transplants [9].

Stenosis of the suprahepatic vena cava will lead to Budd-Chiari syndrome characterized by centrilobular congestion and atrophy (Fig. 4.5). In some cases this may be impossible to differentiate from congestion and portal vein

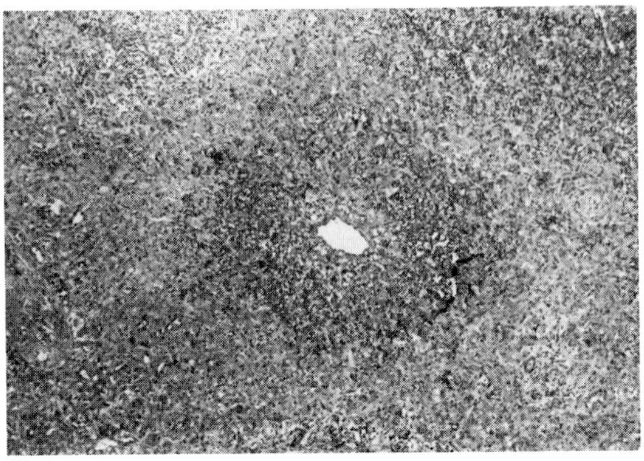

Figure 4.5
Centrilobular congestion and necrosis in a resected allograft from a patient with narrowing of the suprahepatic anatomosis of the interior vena cava and subsequent Budd-Chiari syndrome (hematoxylin-eosin ×30).

thrombosis; all cases require radiographic confirmation. These changes are the same as those of any outflow problem including veno-occlusive disease or congestive heart failure [10,11].

Biliary tract complications have decreased in frequency with improved surgical technique [5,12]. The type and frequency of complication varies with the type of surgical anastomosis employed. In general the preferred anastomoses in the United States today are the choledochochodochostomy or the choledochojejunostomy to the Roux loop. The cholecystoenterostomy is uncommonly used because of the frequency of complications, particularly obstruction.

Biliary tract complications consist primarily of leakage or obstruction [5,12]. Leakage is more common and may result from technical problems with the anastomosis, ischemia to the duct due to arterial thrombosis, or leakage around a T tube. Anastomotic leakage is more easily repaired without serious sequelae. Leakage does not generally produce liver dysfunction directly, although it may lead to sepsis and subsequent hepatic complications related to that sepsis.

Biliary obstruction may result from technical problems with the anastomosis, ischemia, formation of bile casts, or obstruction by a T tube or stent. Clinically, the patient will present with liver dysfunction that will be characteristic of obstructive liver disease. However, since these features are nonspecific, differentiation from rejection is impossible based on laboratory data alone. In addition, since biliary obstruction will interfere with the absorption of orally administered CsA, the blood CsA level may drop following obstruction, leading to rejection as a complication of obstruction. As a corollary to this, rejection in this setting may resolve after the obstruction has cleared due to an increase of blood CsA levels.

Diagnosis of obstruction relies primarily on radiologic findings. A biopsy may be characteristic of acute obstruction (portal edema, cholestasis, bile ductular proliferation, and portal polymorphonuclear infiltration), although since the type of obstruction seen in this setting is usually partial and somewhat chronic rather than acute, there is less edema, more proliferation, and an intermixture of lymphocytes with the polymorphonuclear leukocytes (PMNs). These features render the diagnosis less than straightforward. Under these circumstances there will often be a considerable degree of bile duct damage as well, although endothelialitis (a major criterion of rejection, see below) is not seen [3,13]. It is well recognized that acute rejection following partially successful treatment may manifest a histologic picture very similar if not identical to obstruction, making the task of biopsy even more difficult if the patient has been treated for rejection before biopsy [3]. In any patient with histologic findings consistent with obstruction, radiologic confirmation of the diagnosis is mandatory.

Pathology of Rejection

As in the kidney, three types of rejection can be recognized in the liver: hyperacute, acute, and chronic. The first of these, hyperacute, is mediated by preformed antidonor antibodies, whereas the latter two are presumably different manifestations of the same predominantly cell-mediated process.

Hyperacute Rejection

Although well documented in the kidney, hyperacute rejection has only recently been recognized in the liver. We have seen one case in a human, and there are now several animal models [14–17].

There is little question that hyperacute rejection has been more difficult to produce in animal models of the liver than with other organs. In addition, there also seems to be some protection against its occurrence in humans, since there appears to be little statistical decrease in survival after liver transplantation in the face of ABO incompatibility or a positive crossmatch [18,19]. An early attempt to create an animal model was interpreted as showing accelerated acute but no hyperacute rejection in presensitized rats [17]. Review of the results of this study, however, shows several animals that appear to have livers compatible with hyperacute rejection. More recent studies using slightly different strains of presensitized rats have confirmed the occurrence of antibody-mediated rejection [14]. Nine of ten grafts in sensitized rats became grossly abnormal immediately after transplantation, and death occurred in less than 4 hours. Antibodies and complement were noted in the sinusoids and vessels, and the organs showed hemorrhage and necrosis without significant lymphocytic infiltrate. No specific mention was made of arteritis, a constant component of hyperacute rejection of the human kidney, nor of a polymorphonuclear infiltrate that usually accompanies the process in humans and animal models in other organs [20,21].

We have seen one case of hyperacute rejection in a human liver transplanted into a presensitized host [16]. The liver failed to function normally from the time of transplantation, and 30 minutes after anastomosis showed histologic evidence of damage in the form of pericentral vein focal necrosis and polymorphonuclear infiltration with fibrin deposition in the central veins. By 5 days after transplantation there were extensive areas of infarction in conjunction with a predominately polymorphonuclear portal infiltrate, necrotizing arteritis, and some evidence of superimposed acute rejection in the form of endothelialitis and bile duct damage (Fig. 4.6). When the patient died 11 days after transplantation, the liver was extensively infarcted with no evidence of infection or technical vascular problems. Unfortunately, no immunofluorescence studies were available from the early biopsies to confirm the presence of immunoglobulin deposition. However, the importance of this absent data is debatable, since it is often difficult to identify the offending antibody in human renal hyperacute rejection, and there is evidence in animal models of cardiac hyperacute rejection that the antibody may be seen only for an hour or so after transplantation [21].

An important question to be raised in conjunction with human hyperacute rejection remains that of the organ's relative resistance to this process. The answer to this may lie in two factors. First, the liver has a large native reserve that allows considerable organ destruction to take place before disease begins to manifest itself. This factor accounts for the early underestimate of

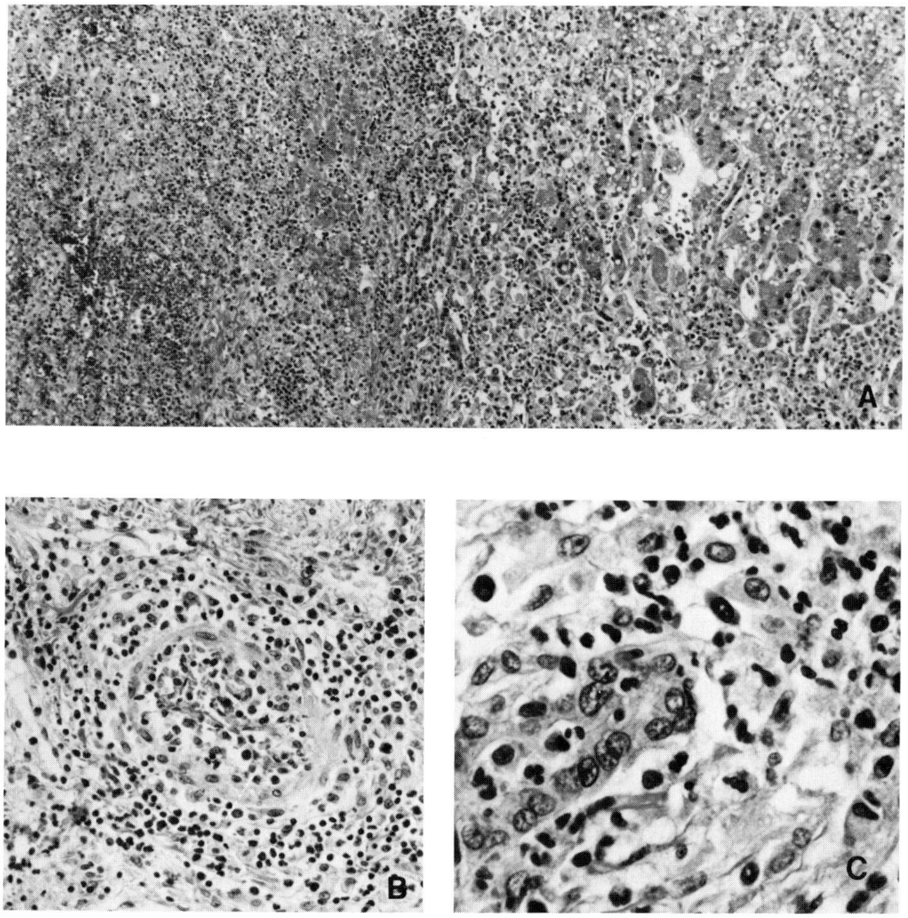

Figure 4.6
Biopsy at day 5 in a patient who underwent transplantation despite a positive crossmatch. A. Confluent ischemic necrosis is evident in the left part of the field (hematoxylin-eosin ×100). B. Portal tract showing occlusive arteritis and a dense predominately polymorphonuclear infiltrate (hematoxylin-eosin ×190). C. Bile duct showing intraepithelial lymphocytes and intraluminal PMNs. Note the surrounding polymorphonuclear infiltrate (hematoxylin-eosin ×480). (Source: From Snover DC. The pathology of acute rejection. Transplant Proc 1986;18 (Suppl 4):123–7. Reproduced with permission of the publisher, Grune & Stratton, Inc.)

the significance of acute rejection as well as the paucity of reported cases of hyperacute rejection. Second, hyperacute rejection relies on the presence of circulating preformed antibodies. In most cases of liver transplantation, there is a significant "washout" of native antibodies by large amounts of blood loss and transfusion during the transplant procedure. For example, in our patient the titer of specific antidonor antibody dropped markedly immediately after transplant only to rise again later. This may have been due in part to the transfusions and in part to absorption of antibody to the organ but in either case may have delayed the full effect of antibody-mediated damage. It may be possible, in fact, that this dilution of antibody combined with the liver's large capacity to absorb antibody may be why hyperacute liver rejection is rare.

A second question is why it has taken so long to recognize a probable case of human hyperacute rejection even if it is rare. One possible answer is that the end stage of a hyperacutely rejected organ, be it the kidney or the liver, looks like any other infarcted organ regardless of the cause of ischemia. Since for many years clinicians were hesitant to biopsy the transplanted liver, many organs were examined only after they had failed and were removed for retransplantation or at autopsy. A totally infarcted liver was likely to be designated as primary graft failure, although unrecognized hyperacute rejection may have been just as likely. It seems probable that buried in the diagnosis of primary graft failure are a number of cases of hyperacute rejection.

Acute Rejection

Acute rejection constitutes a major problem following transplantation. In some series as many as 16% of all transplanted livers fail due to chronic rejection [22]. If one assumes that chronic rejection is the end stage of unsuccessfully treated acute rejection, then the importance of early recognition of the acute process is obvious. Although early series reported acute rejection to be a relatively rare phenomenon, most centers are now reporting rejection rates of at least 75% [23].

Acute rejection in its untreated state is characterized by a diagnostic triad of findings [3,8,22,24,25]: (1) a portal infiltrate composed predominantly of lymphocytes with lesser numbers of polymorphonuclear cells and eosinophils, (2) damage to interlobular bile ducts in association with intraepithelial lymphocytes, and (3) venous endothelialitis, i.e., the attachment of lymphocytes to the endothelium of portal or central veins. These features are present in virtually all patients experiencing rejection, although their appearance may be modified somewhat by factors such as type of prophylaxis, time after transplant that rejection occurs, and type of fixative used in biopsy preparation. In addition, a number of less specific findings may be present, some having prognostic significance.

Portal Infiltrate The portal infiltrate of acute rejection is usually mixed in type, although plasma cells are uncommonly found (Fig. 4.7). Although obviously nonspecific, the presence of an infiltrate is the most sensitive sign of early rejection. The only time an infiltrate is not present in rejection is in the "vanishing bile duct syndrome," described below. The infiltrate varies from being focal in early mild rejection to being diffuse and obliterating portal structures in severe disease. The mix of cell types varies somewhat with the prophylactic regimen in our experience, with patients receiving "triple drug therapy" (CsA, prednisone, and azathioprine) showing an increase in the prominence of PMNs relative to patients receiving CsA and prednisone only [8].

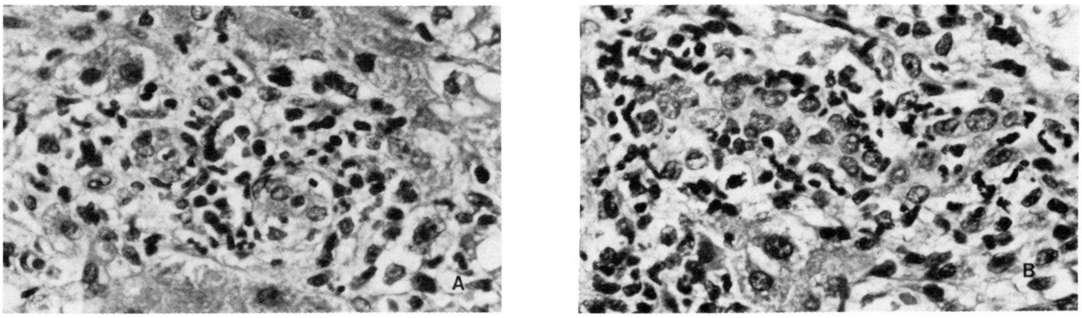

Figure 4.7
Portal areas from two biopsies with rejection. Both show a mixed portal inflammatory infiltrate. A. The bile duct in this tract has undergone loss of individual cells, luminal loss, and vacuolation of the cytoplasm in association with several intraepithelial inflammatory cells (hematoxylin-eosin ×480). B. The bile duct in this tract differs from that in (A) in that there is nuclear atypia and overlapping but no actual loss of individual cells (hematoxylin-eosin ×480).

Of the cell types seen in acute rejection, the significance of the eosinophil is the most intriguing. The role of this cell in the pathogenesis of liver damage is unknown, but its presence in an infiltrate is a useful sign of rejection if the possibility of a drug reaction can be ruled out.

Damage to Bile Ducts The presence of bile duct damage is a prerequisite for the diagnosis of rejection. The role of the bile duct as a target of rejection may be due to its expression of major histocompatibility complex (MHC) antigens, particularly of class I [26]. The damage takes several forms including vacuolation of cytoplasm, pleomorphism, anisocytosis and overlapping of nuclei, and actual loss of individual cells or entire ducts (see Fig. 4.7). At times the density of the portal infiltrate will obscure the ducts, making evaluation difficult on hematoxylin-eosin stain. In such cases we have found the trichrome stain invaluable for visualizing the structures. Immunoperoxidase staining for keratin is also useful to identify bile ducts. The interlobular bile ducts (i.e., those accompanying arterioles in the center of portal tracts) rather than the proliferating bile ductules should be evaluated, since the latter frequently show changes of the type described above regardless of the cause of the proliferation. Also, the simple absence of an occasional epithelial cell or "telescoping" of epithelial cells should not be misconstrued as true damage, since these changes may occasionally be seen in healthy livers.

As with the infiltrate, bile duct damage may be focal in early disease. The damage is usually identified in conjunction with an infiltrate, and careful examination will almost always disclose lymphocytes within the damaged duct. In addition, PMNs are a frequent finding both in the wall and the lumen of the ducts and do not imply a biliary tract infection or obstruction.

Although bile duct damage is characteristic of rejection and limits the differential diagnosis, it is not absolutely diagnostic, since several other agents including some drugs and viral infections will produce similar changes [27,28]. In addition, recurrent primary biliary cirrhosis may manifest similar changes. In most conditions other than rejection that manifest bile duct damage, the damage is limited to fewer than 50% of the ducts.

Venous Endothelialitis Endothelialitis is the most specific change seen in rejection (Fig. 4.8). If carefully searched for in untreated rejection specimens, it will be identified in at least 90% of cases [8]. However, several factors may obscure this finding.

1. Endothelialitis is the first feature of rejection to disappear following treatment for rejection. Hence, the chance of finding it drops to less than 40% following therapy.
2. It is almost always focal, so that it may not be seen in small biopsies, particularly if central veins are not present in the biopsy. In general, endothelialitis is easier to identify in the central vein, since a dense portal infiltrate makes portal veins difficult to identify.
3. Some fixatives seem to obscure this finding by coagulating plasma in the veins. It is most easily identified in 10% buffered formalin–fixed tissue and is most obscured with fixatives such as B5.

Another problem with endothelialitis is defining the process. Although previously defined simply as the attachment of lymphocytes to the endothelium of vessels, there are many liver biopsies in which a few lymphocytes are seen adjacent to but not clearly attached to the endothelium (Fig. 4.9). Depending on the magnitude, this finding may be overinterpreted as endothelialitis and result in an overdiagnosis of rejection. We now prefer to define endothelialitis not only by the proximity of lymphocytes to the endothelium, but also by evidence of damage to the endothelium, usually in the form of

Figure 4.8
Central vein (A) and portal vein (B) showing florid endothelialitis. Note the accumulation of lymphocytes adherent to the endothelium with resultant damage to the endothelium in the form of lifting of the endothelium from its underlying basement membrane (hematoxylin-eosin ×480).

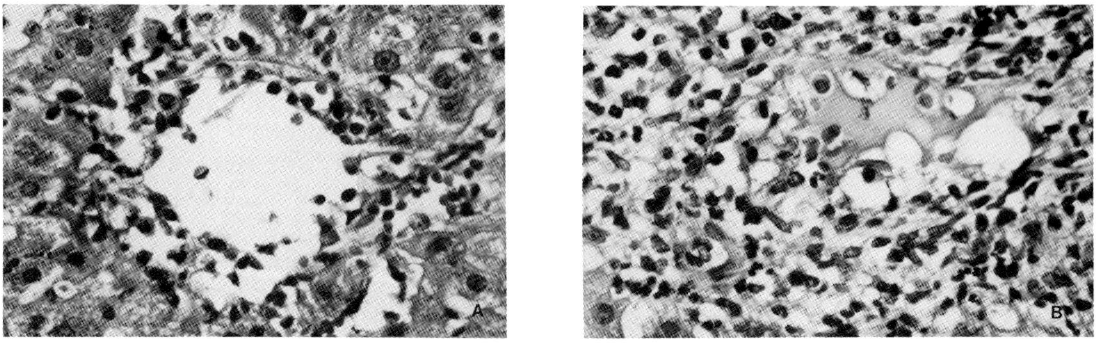

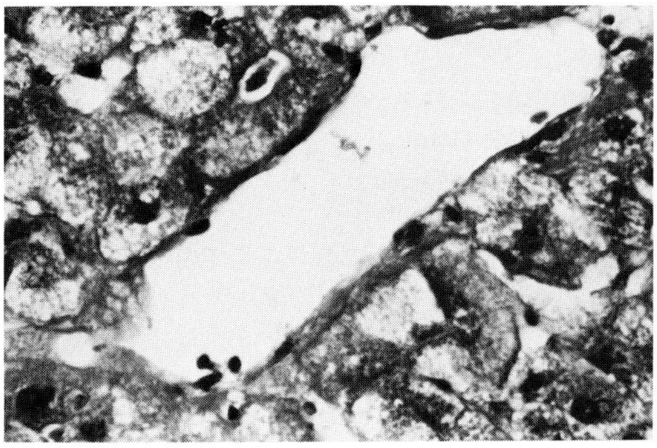

Figure 4.9
Central vein from a nontransplant liver biopsy showing apparent attachment of three lymphocytes to the endothelial surface. There is no evidence of damage to the endothelium, however, and therefore this does not constitute significant endothelialitis (hematoxylin-eosin ×480).

lifting of the endothelium from the underlying basement membrane (see Fig. 4.8). There should be a clear attachment of the lymphocytes to the endothelium as evidenced by a "tenting" of the endothelium or by a cytoplasmic bridge between the lymphocyte and endothelium.

Although almost specific, there are some circumstances in which the finding of endothelialitis should be interpreted with caution. Apparent attachment of lymphocytes may be noted in areas of confluent central hepatocellular necrosis, such as may be caused by pretransplant ischemia, and in this situation endothelialitis should be ignored. In addition, in areas of artifactual disruption of the specimen (e.g., a tear caused by the microtome knife during sectioning) there may be structures resembling veins with endothelialitis (Fig. 4.10). However, the absence of endothelium in these areas should be a clue that the spaces are really not veins and hence endothelialitis is not present.

Although it is our general practice to make an absolute diagnosis of rejection only in the presence of the complete triad, we will diagnose rejection without identifying endothelialitis under certain circumstances. If more than 50% of the bile ducts are damaged and there is an appropriate infiltrate, then we will diagnose rejection. This circumstance will occur in only a handful of cases. More common is to find less than 50% bile duct damage with an in-

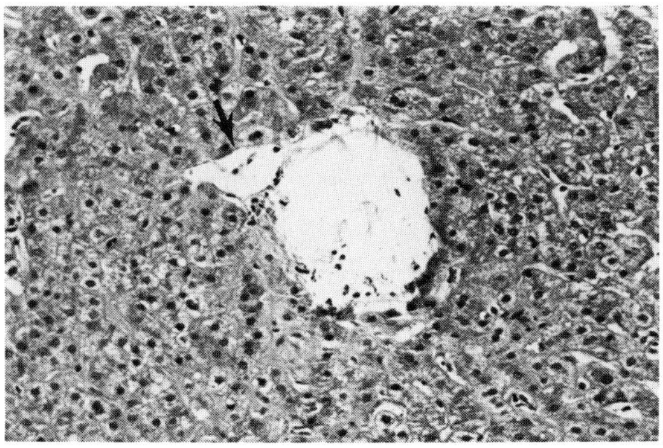

Figure 4.10
Artifactual disruption of the liver adjacent to a central vein simulating endothelialitis. Note that there is no endothelium lining the artifactual space. The true central vein is located adjacent to the tear (arrow) and does not show endothelialitis (hematoxylin-eosin ×192).

filtrate. In this latter circumstance, rejection should be diagnosed *only* if endothelialitis is present. In approximately 33% of such cases without endothelialitis, the infiltrate and all signs of rejection will disappear without any increase in therapy [8]. Therefore, we use the diagnosis of "consistent with but not diagnostic of" rejection for biopsies with no endothelialitis and less than 50% bile duct damage.

In an occasional case, endothelialitis willl be easily identified in conjunction with an infiltrate, but bile duct damage will be difficult to find. Such cases should be diagnosed as rejection, since it is our experience that careful search will identify some bile duct damage. It is possible that some of these cases are a predominately vascular type of rejection in which the bile ducts are not a major target of attack.

Nonspecific Findings in Rejection A number of nonspecific findings may be seen in conjunction with rejection but have no diagnostic or prognostic value. Most common of these is canalicular cholestasis. This finding is almost ubiquitous in the early post-transplant biopsy regardless of the presence of rejection. There has been speculation that it may be related to CsA toxicity. However, it is also commonly seen in patients receiving only azathioprine-prednisone prophylaxis. Hepatocellular damage either in the form of ballooning or focal necrosis may be seen. Ballooning in conjunction with confluent necrosis may be caused by vascular rejection and as such is related to a bad prognosis (see below). However, ballooning is a nonspecific finding in that it may be due to any cause of vascular insufficiency and is particularly common in the first several weeks after transplantation. During this early period it is assumed that such ballooning is due to so-called preservation damage and as such should resolve spontaneously with time. In this case repeat biopsies show gradual resolution of the process in the first 2 weeks. Other causes of ballooning include vascular insufficiency for technical reasons, drug toxicities, and viral infections.

Focal hepatocellular necrosis or the presence of acidophil bodies may also be seen in the early post-transplant period, although either is more common in biopsies several weeks to months post transplant, especially in patients with a previous diagnosis of rejection [8]. The significance of this necrosis is unclear, but in the late cases it may relate to a cell-mediated reaction to increased expression of class I antigens, found on hepatocytes following rejection (see below) [29,30].

Implications for Management Several systems of grading of acute rejection have been proposed in the literature, although most have not been tested. We use a system based on the three factors found to have prognostic significance: arteritis, ischemic centrilobular damage (probably secondary to arteritis), or paucity of bile ducts (Fig. 4.11) (Table 4.2) [8]. Any biopsy with these features has severe rejection. These changes may not be seen in the initial rejection biopsy. Their development in follow-up biopsies taken in the course of treatment of a rejection episode should be taken as an indication that increased immunosuppression is needed. Biopsies without these bad features are diagnosed as mild or moderate rejection based on bile duct damage of less than or greater than 50%.

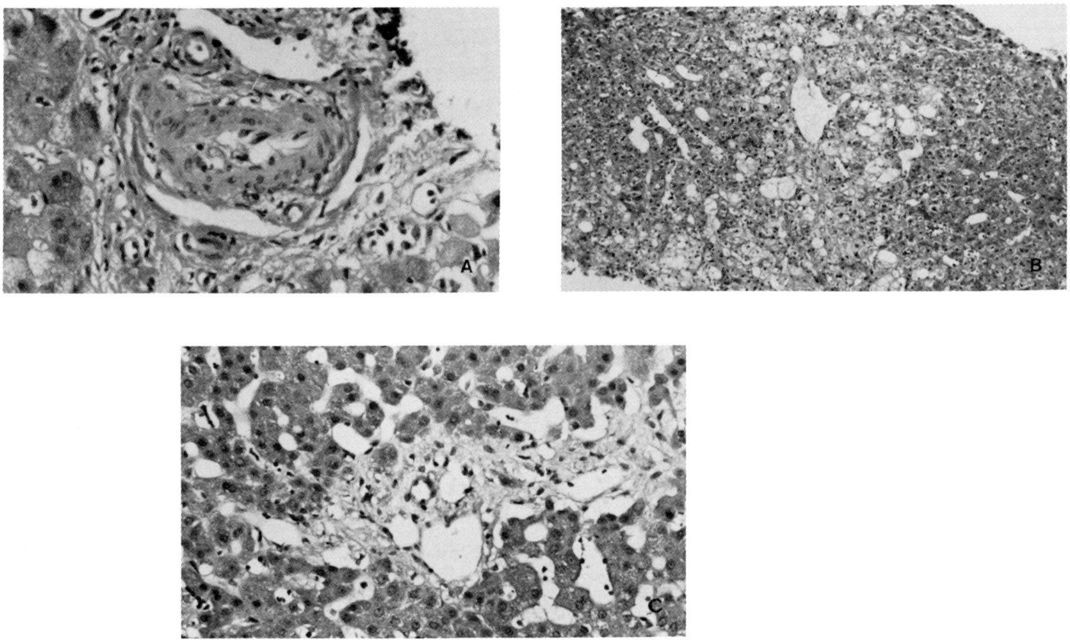

Figure 4.11
Histologic features portending a bad prognosis when found in association with the diagnostic features of rejection. A. Mild lymphocytic arteritis (hematoxylin-eosin ×480). B. Centrilobular ballooning degeneration and dropout of clusters of hepatocytes (hematoxylin-eosin ×100). C. Paucity of bile ducts in one portal tract. Note the absence of inflammation in addition to the absence of an interlobular bile duct (hematoxylin-eosin ×192).

Table 4.2
Grading of acute rejection

Diagnosis	*Description*
Consistent with rejection (nondiagnostic)	Mixed portal infiltrate with <50% bile duct damage, no endothelialitis
Acute rejection, grade I (mild)	As above, with endothelialitis
Acute rejection, grade II (moderate)	Mixed portal infiltrate, >50% bile duct damage, with or without endothelialitis
Acute rejection, grade III (severe)	Grade I or II plus arteritis, paucity of bile ducts, or central ballooning with confluence dropout of hepatocytes

Source: From Snover DC. The pathology of acute rejection. Transplant Proc 1986;18(Suppl 4):123–7. Reprinted by permission of the publisher, Grune & Stratton, Inc.

Acute rejection may show several responses to therapy with prednisone, antilymphocyte globulin, or monoclonal antibody OKT3. The best response is total resolution of all signs of rejection within a week of treatment. This is, in our experience, a rather uncommon response. More common is for the liver to remain abnormal but to show improvement. The first feature of rejection to disappear is the endothelialitis, followed by bile duct inflammation and damage, with the portal infiltrate being last to go [8]. Whether the patient should continue to receive medication and on what regimen depends on the pathologist's and clinician's judgment of the patient's status and the degree of ongoing damage to the liver. In general, if the bile duct damage is markedly diminished and intraepithelial lymphocytes are difficult to find, treatment may be discontinued despite some persistence of portal inflammation. Repeat biopsy is suggested until all bile duct damage and most inflammation is gone, however.

Although it is clear that percutaneous biopsy is now the gold standard for the diagnosis of rejection, the role of fine needle aspiration biopsy (FNAB) has yet to be defined [31,32]. In the kidney this technique has been used with great success to identify rejection [33]. However, the situation in the liver is quite different.

1. The process of rejection in the liver is predominately confined to the portal areas, as opposed to the relatively diffuse infiltrate found in renal rejection. Therefore, sampling error may be more of a problem in the liver than in the kidney.
2. The diagnosis of rejection in the liver relies heavily on notation of the distribution of the inflammation in regard to vessels and bile ducts, a distribution that cannot be identified by FNAB.
3. Finally, the differential diagnosis of liver dysfunction is somewhat greater than that of renal dysfunction following kidney transplant, and several of the differential diagnostic items (e.g., drug reactions and viral infections) are characterized by an infiltrate very similar to that of rejection.

Several preliminary studies have indicated that FNAB is safe in the liver and that it can identify an inflammatory process [31,32]. This in itself may be of value in limiting the differential diagnosis in a particular case of dysfunction. However, determination of its absolute diagnostic accuracy will await a prospective study comparing FNAB with standard needle biopsy.

Chronic Rejection

Chronic rejection is defined, for working purposes, as irreversible cell-mediated rejection resulting in loss of liver function and death if the organ is not replaced. Recent attempts to define chronic rejection as a function of an arbitrary time cutoff of 100 days as are used in graft-vs-host disease (GVHD) are unacceptable [34]. Although the use of a 100-day definition of chronic GVHD has been a useful tool in defining that process, the situation in bone marrow transplanation differs considerably from that of solid organ transplantation, and in fact the pathogenesis of acute and chronic GVHD is such that acute GVHD almost never occurs after day 100 [35]. On the other hand, in solid organ transplantation, as best exemplified by the kidney experience, acute rejection may occur as a superimposed process on a backdrop of chronic rejection, a situation that could not occur if the arbitrary 100-day definition is used. This fact is important because use of the term *acute rejection* to mean a potentially reversible process tells the clinician something crucial about treatment; in a similar way, use of the term *chronic* to imply irreversible prevents overimmunosuppressing the patient with an irreversible process.

Diagnostic Features It is presumed, as stated above, that chronic rejection represents the end result of insufficiently treated acute rejection. The precise reason that an episode of acute rejection may not be controlled remains to be elucidated. The diagnosis of chronic rejection by biopsy is much more difficult than that of acute rejection and, in our experience, requires both pathologic and clinical input.

As seen in resected transplant specimens or at autopsy, chronic rejection is usually manifest by obliterative endarteritis and resultant ischemic damage (Fig. 4.12). It may be accompanied by fibrosis, cirrhosis, or the "vanishing bile duct syndrome" [8,22,36]. The vessels involved are generally larger-order arteries. The lumen is narrowed by subintimal accumulation of fat-laden histiocytes or fibrous tissue (see Fig. 4.12A). The vessels with histiocytes may appear yellow to the naked eye, as in atherosclerosis. Frequently the endarteritis will be quite focal, being present in only a few of many sections of liver examined.

Unfortunately, because of this focality and the size of the involved arteries, the vessels showing endarteritis are rarely present in needle biopsies.

Figure 4.12
Chronic rejection in a resected liver. A. Portal area showing near-total obliteration of arteries by subendothelial accumulation of foamy histiocytes (hematoxylin-eosin ×100). B. Central area of the same biopsy showing areas of hepatocellular swelling and fibrosis (hematoxylin-eosin ×75).

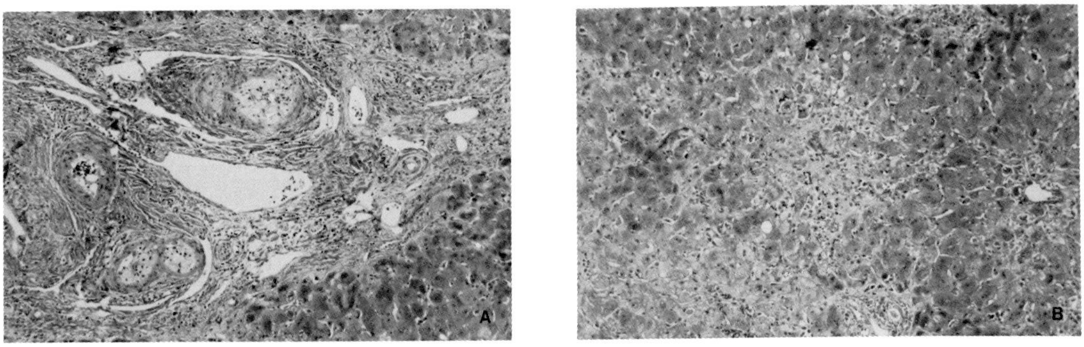

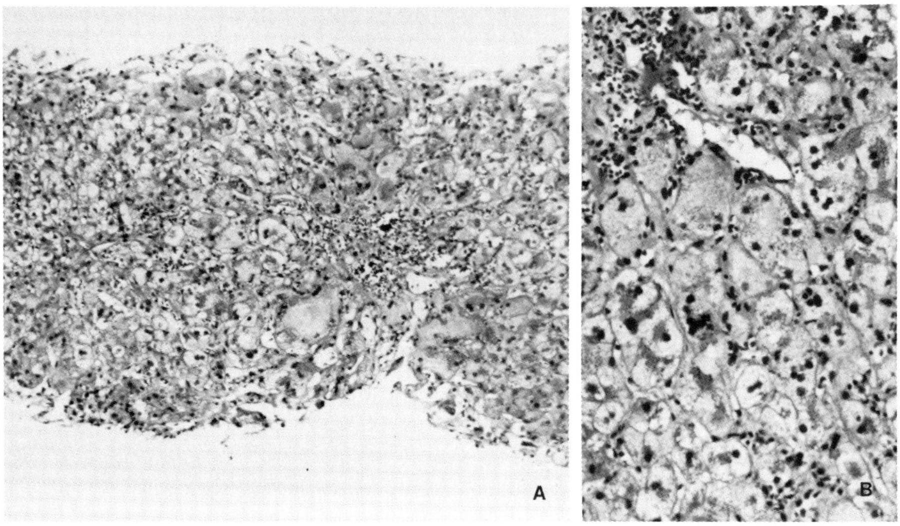

Figure 4.13
Needle biopsy of chronic rejection. A. Central area showing generalized hepatocellular ballooning and focal infiltration by lymphocytes (hematoxylin-eosin ×100). B. Same area showing giant cell transformation of hepatocytes adjacent to the central vein. Many of these cells contain abundant lipofuscin (hematoxylin-eosin ×192).

Therefore, we must rely on more subtle, less diagnostic changes. Most commonly one will see central ischemic damage (ballooning degeneration with hepatocellular dropout), fibrosis, and loss of bile ducts. The hepatocellular damage will frequently dominate the picture. Because it is a chronic ischemic process, there frequently will be an extensive accumulation of lipofuscin pigment in the hepatocytes, and giant cell transformation indicative of regenerative activity may be present, especially in the centrilobular regions (Fig. 4.13). The fibrosis will also frequently manifest a central pericellular

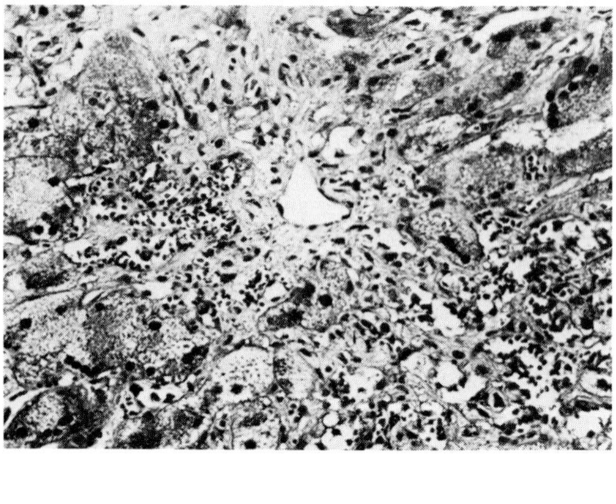

Figure 4.14
Trichrome stain of the biopsy in Figure 4.13 demonstrating fibrosis around the central vein with extension into surrounding sinusoids (hematoxylin-eosin ×192).

character indicating its origin in these ischemic areas (Fig. 4.14). Occasionally a true micronodular cirrhosis will develop, although this appears to be the exception. It is our experience that none of these findings, except possibly cirrhosis, is absolutely irreversible or diagnostic. However, when seen in a patient with continued deterioration of liver function who fails to show evidence of response to repeated therapeutic efforts, a diagnosis can be made. Another finding of chronic rejection felt to be helpful by some is the presence of clusters of foamy histiocytes in the sinusoids [37]. This finding often accompanies long-standing cholestasis and is common in such diseases as primary biliary cirrhosis [38]. We have seen it early after transplantation in patients with severe cholestasis. Therefore, its diagnostic potential remains to be proved. Other causes of ischemia, including narrowing of the arterial anastomosis, must be considered in the differential diagnosis of ischemic lesions even in the face of rejection. Occasionally a correctable arterial stenosis will be superimposed on a rejection episode, leading to features suggesting chronic irreversible rejection.

Vanishing Bile Duct Syndrome A possible form of irreversible rejection is the vanishing bile duct syndrome (VBDS), characterized by loss of ducts in the absence of vascular rejection [34,36]. Such a form of rejection may be analogous to chronic tubulointerstitial rejection of the kidney [20]. However, the specificity of loss of bile ducts for chronic rejection remains to be defined. It has been suggested that persistent total absence of bile ducts in repeated biopsies is a bad prognostic sign requiring consideration of retransplantation. The occasional absence of a duct is considered to be of less import [8,34]. However, it has become apparent that many cases of VBDS are reversible, despite the usual designation of this process as irreversible or chronic. Of five patients with pure VBDS (i.e., VBDS without ischemic change suggesting vascular rejection) at the University of Minnesota, three have shown complete clinical and biochemical recovery, all after more than 1 year following the diagnosis. The fourth patient is showing improvement but not complete recovery at 13 months, and the fifth is stable at 4 months.* In addition, one patient at the Mayo Clinic has recovered, again at greater than 12 months from onset.† All these patients have shown acute rejection followed by total loss of ducts at the time of greatest bilirubin elevation. Subsequent biopsies have shown presence of ducts accompanied or even preceded by ductular proliferation. This latter feature has persisted despite normal liver function in several patients. Thus, we no longer consider the histologic diagnosis of VBDS to represent chronic rejection. Rather, we suggest that such biopsies be designated simply by the descriptive term of VBDS. Patients with such histologic findings should not undergo retransplantation unless they develop evidence of significant synthetic or degradative dysfunction in addition to jaundice.

*Freese et al., unpublished data.

†Weisner RH, personal communication.

tion will by necessity be left untreated until an infectious episode has been successfully treated. Monitoring the progress of the rejection by frequent biopsy during this time will allow optimal decision making in regard to therapy.

The specific hepatotropic viral infections such as hepatitis B have particular relevance to transplantation, since they may recur in the transplanted liver and the infectious agent might theoretically simulate rejection.

It is clear that hepatitis B will recur frequently in patients who have undergone transplantation because of cirrhosis due to chronic infection [50,51]. The frequency of recurrence following transplantation for fulminant hepatitis B infection is less well characterized. The fact that the virus will infect the new liver does not necessarily mean that the liver will develop clinical hepatitis or eventual failure, however, and therefore the role for transplantation in these patients is not clear. The immunosuppression may convert these patients into permanent carriers of the virus, although in such patients withdrawal of immunosuppression could prove disastrous [52]. At least one liver transplant patient appears to have suffered massive hepatic necrosis as a result of reduction of immunosuppression [51]. Recurrent hepatitis B does not cause difficulties in the diagnosis of acute rejection [51]. There is recent indication that hepatitis delta may recur in conjunction with hepatitis B [53].

The problem of recurrence of non-A–non-B (NANB) hepatitis is one that is impossible to address directly in view of the lack of serologic or immunohistochemical tests to define this agent. To date, however, reports of recurrence of chronic active hepatitis and cirrhosis in patients transplanted for cryptogenic or possible NANB-induced cirrhosis have not occurred. A more significant potential problem with NANB hepatitis is the role that primary infections may play in the post-transplant period, since the major source of infection with this (or these) virus(es) is transfusion. With a usual incubation time of 5 to 10 weeks, confusion of NANB hepatitis with acute rejection is not likely in the first month after transplantation. However, cases of late rejection may be difficult to distinguish accurately from chronic NANB, especially in view of the reported frequency of bile duct damage in NANB [54]. It has been our experience that some patients with successfully treated early acute rejection will develop low-grade liver function abnormalities 6 months or more after transplantation. Biopsy of these patients will show a picture of focal portal lymphocytic infiltrate with mild bile duct damage, no endothelialitis, and little or no hepatocellular necrosis. Whether these cases represent low-grade "smoldering" rejection or chronic persistent NANB hepatitis is impossible to determine at present.

Other viruses such as cytomegalovirus (CMV), herpes, and adenovirus may occur following transplantation. Diagnosis of the first two can usually be made by the finding of typical inclusions or by culture [55]. Immunohistochemical staining may also provide a specific diagnosis. Adenovirus infection also has a characteristic if not diagnostic histologic appearance and may be stained with commercially available antisera [56]. Although bile duct involvement can occur with these viruses, such involvement has not caused problems in the diagnosis of rejection.

Drug Reactions Following Transplantation

The patient in the post-transplant period receives many potentially hepatotoxic agents including CsA, azathioprine, multiple antibiotics, and hyperalimentation. The evaluation of biopsies under these circumstances requires knowledge of the forms of potential damage from these agents, although for some such as CsA, the morphology of toxicity in the human has not been clearly defined. As a general rule, hypersensitivity reactions are marked by eosinophilic infiltration of the liver. Since eosinophilia is a very common component of rejection, however, this feature is of little value in differential diagnosis. On the other hand, hepatocellular damage is a prominent component of many drug reactions of both the idiosyncratic and toxic varieties and therefore is a useful feature distinguishing possible drug or viral reactions from rejection.

There is no doubt that CsA is hepatotoxic, although the seriousness of the toxicity is much less than that of renal toxicity. Abnormalities of liver function tests have been reported in from 20% to 50% of renal transplant patients receiving CsA immunosuppression [57]. Bilirubin, the aminotransferases, and alkaline phosphatase appear to be elevated in roughly equal frequencies. In over 80% of cases the abnormalities are self-limited, although in some patients they recur. Cholelithiasis has also been reported in 2.4% patients receiving CsA immunosuppression; a concurrent series of azathioprine-treated patients had no cholelithiasis [57].

Despite the high incidence of liver abnormalities, the histology of CsA toxicity in the human has not been adequately described. In animal experiments there is some degree of species variability in terms of liver damage. Dogs seem to be resistant to the effect of the drug, whereas rats and monkeys do develop liver toxicity with chronic administration [58]. In rats receiving oral CsA for 13 weeks, the livers showed centrilobular hepatocellular ballooning degeneration. In monkeys, 4 weeks of intravenous administration led to cholestasis, fatty change, and focal hepatocellular necrosis. We have noted marked canalicular cholestasis in some of our patients with very high blood levels of CsA, but in view of the high frequency of cholestasis in the transplanted liver regardless of other pathologic findings, the significance of this finding is debatable. In fact, patients receiving only azathioprine as immunosuppression have an incidence of cholestasis roughly equal in frequency to CsA-treated patients.* Nothing in the literature or in our experience suggests that CsA toxicity may mimic the features of rejection.

Azathioprine has been associated with cholestatic hepatitis in renal transplant patients [59]. Histologically, some of these cases show centrilobular ballooning degeneration with cholestasis and a mild, nonspecific portal infiltrate. As with CsA, differential problems with rejection have not been encountered, since bile duct damage and endothelialitis are not features of azathioprine toxicity.

Steroids have been associated with the development of nodular regenerative hyperplasia (NRH) as well as mild fatty change in the liver [60]. This

*Gouw A, personal communication.

drug may be responsible for some of the reported cases of NRH occurring in renal and bone marrow transplant patients [61]. There is very little significance to this diagnosis except that it explains hepatomegaly or occasionally ascites or mild jaundice.

Antibiotics have the greatest potential of any of the aforementioned drugs to cause differential problems in the diagnosis of rejection. Some of these drugs cause bile duct damage and a portal infiltrate that may suggest rejection. Although endothelialitis has not been reported to be a feature of drug reactions, it is certainly possible (if not probable) that careful search will someday reveal that even this finding can be simulated by drugs. We have seen a reaction to sulfamethoxizole-trimethoprim that simulated GVHD quite well, although it would probably have been distinguishable from rejection by its more prominent hepatocellular reaction.

Figure 4.15
A. Liver biopsy 3 weeks after transplantation showing marked discrete centrilobular hepatocellular ballooning. This change had been present in two previous weekly biopsies (hematoxylin-eosin ×40). B. Biopsy from the same patient as (A) 1 week after stopping total parenteral alimentation (hematoxylin-eosin ×40).

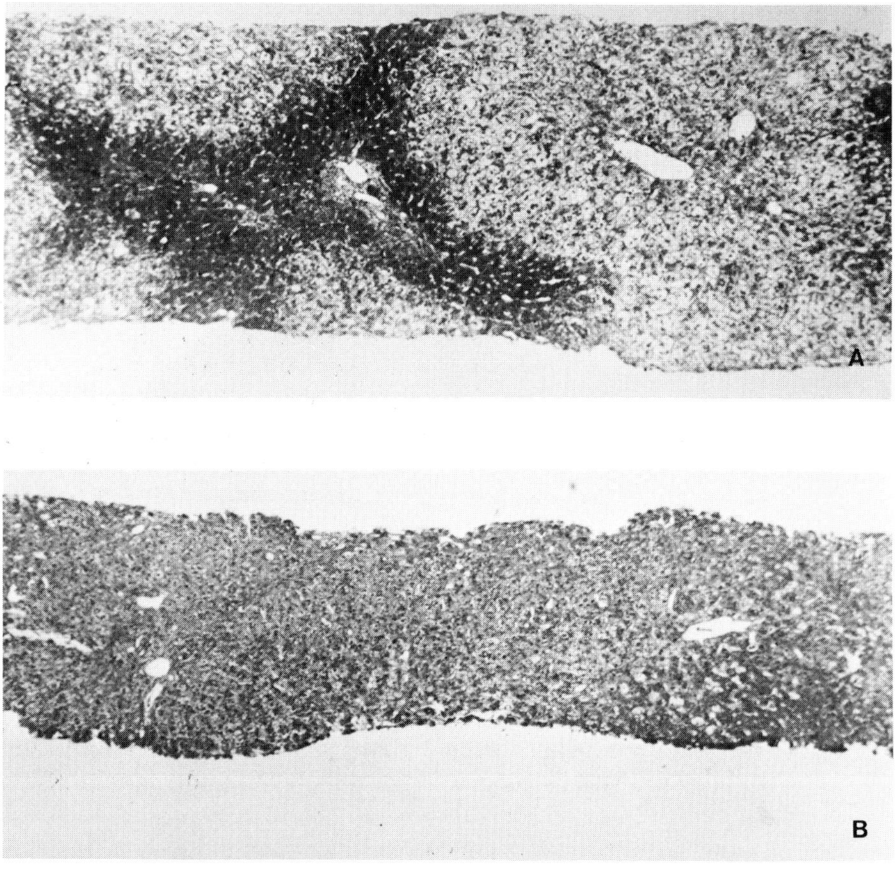

The role of hyperalimentation in producing significant liver damage in the post-transplant period is controversial. There is no doubt that significant liver damage, including the development of cirrhosis, can occur, particularly in neonates [62]. In these cases the toxicity is manifest by fatty change, cholestasis, bile duct proliferation, and a portal polymorphonuclear infiltrate simulating large duct obstruction. In addition, periodic acid–Schiff (PAS)-positive material is commonly present in Kupffer cells. In the adult the situation appears to be somewhat different in that the reaction is less frequent and usually less severe. It has been our experience in several patients with post-transplant jaundice to find a histologic picture of a notably discrete centrilobular ballooning with cholestasis that has responded both clinically and histologically to withdrawal of parenteral nutrition (Fig. 4.15). Although the specificity of this histologic picture has not been tested, the possibility of this type of reaction should be considered in these patients. This histologic picture is quite similar to one reported by Williams et al. as a nonimmunologic form of post-transplant cholestasis [63]. Some authors have suggested that these findings are possibly due to CsA toxicity [57].

Recurrence of Original Disease Following Transplantation

Recurrence of the disease process for which a patient originally underwent transplantation is a potential problem facing the transplant team. Although some diseases such as extrahepatic biliary atresia or alpha-1-antitrypsin deficiency seem unlikely to recur, others, such as malignancies, can be expected to recur quite often.

Documentation of recurrence varies with different diseases. There is no question that most primary liver malignancies, including both hepatocellular and cholangiocarcinoma, will recur at a high frequency [50]. Certain tumors, such as hepatoblastoma and fibrolamellar hepatoma, may have a lower recurrence rate, although some of these will recur as well [64]. In many centers, therefore, these diseases are considered a contraindication to transplantation. This is not the case universally, however, since occasional long-term survivors have been reported.

As mentioned previously, hepatitis B infection almost invariably recurs, except in those patients with fulminant hepatitis B [51]. Since many of these patients will develop a carrier state rather than have clinical manifestations of significant disease, most centers will consider these patients as transplantation candidates. The long-term outcome of reinfected patients remains to be determined, however [51,65].

Recurrence of other diseases has been more difficult to assess. As discussed above, primary biliary cirrhosis has been reported to recur, although documentation of such recurrence is difficult [49,66]. In addition, whether recurrence leads to liver failure, and at what rate, remains to be shown. Recurrence of autoimmune chronic active hepatitis and Budd-Chiari syndrome has also been reported [50]. In none of these diseases does the frequency of recurrence provide sufficient cause to reject a candidate for transplantation.

Future Developments

Although much has been learned regarding the basic pathology of liver transplantation, many questions remain. For example, should patients with normal liver function but rejection by biopsy be treated with increased immunosuppression, or should treatment be withheld until signs of dysfunction develop? As a corollary to this, will protocol biopsies reduce the incidence of liver failure from chronic rejection while at the same time preventing undue immunosuppression and increased infectious complications? Since these questions form the basis for the use of protocol biopsies, their answers are crucial. Providing the data for those answers may be difficult, however, since it would require randomizing patients to two treatment protocols. Since it has been our experience that patients with biopsy evidence of rejection even in the face of normal liver function require therapy, it would be difficult to refuse treatment to anyone with these biopsy findings. Therefore, the less than perfect data provided by retrospective or interinstitutional comparison of results of centers acting on protocol biopsies may be the best that can be expected.

Another crucial question is that of the potential toxicity of CsA. Since this drug clearly has some short-term effect on liver function, it would be crucial to determine its pathologic effect(s) and long-term significance. Unfortunately, liver transplant patients are not a good group to study for liver toxicity, and data in this regard would more likely come from recipients of other transplants.

From a histopathologic perspective, it remains probable that other histologic forms of rejection will be discovered. This possibility stems from occasional patients who manifest liver dysfunction and have biopsies that do not show the classic features of rejection but who respond to immunosuppression given when all other known possible causes of liver dysfunction have been eliminated. Answering this question, of course, requires definition of rejection without using histologic findings as a basis for the diagnosis and will require accumulation of a number of such cases to define this "aberrant" histologic state.

The role of immunologic studies in the diagnosis of rejection also provides an area of future potential. Although there has been some data generated in regard to the role of subsetting of infiltrating cells in the diagnosis of rejection, the specificity and prognostic value of the data remain to be determined [44]. The same can be said for the use of monitoring of immunologic parameters in the peripheral blood, a technique that has not proved of great value with other organs. In addition, the role of new immunologic diagnostic techniques such as in situ hybridization in the evaluation of infectious disease is in the early phase of study and may provide an additional tool toward the management of these patients.

Obviously, the answer to any of these questions requires the cooperation of surgeons, hepatologists, pediatricians, radiologists, and pathologists who deal daily with these patients. Only through this continued cooperation will the data and tissue be accumulated to answer many questions.

References

1. Stock PG, Snover DC, Payne W, et al. Biopsy guided immunosuppressive therapy in the treatment of liver transplant rejection: an individualized approach. Clin Transplant 1987;1:179–86.
2. Starzl TE, Iwatsuki S, Van Thiel DH, et al. Evolution of liver transplantation. Hepatology 1982;2:614–36.
3. Snover DC, Sibley RK, Freese DK, et al. Orthotopic liver transplantation: a pathological study of 63 serial liver biopsies from 17 patients with specific reference to the diagnostic features and natural history of rejection. Hepatology 1984;4:1212–22.
4. Russo PA, Yunis EJ. Subcapsular hepatic necrosis in orthotopic liver allograft. Hepatology 1986;6:708–13.
5. Lerut J, Gordon RD, Iwatsuki S, et al. Biliary tract complications in human orthotopic liver transplantation. Transplantation 1987;43:47–51.
6. Cardella JF, Castaneda-Zuniga WR, Hunter D, et al. Angiographic and interventional radiological considerations in liver transplantation. AJR 1986;146:143–53.
7. Wozney P, Zajko AB, Bron KM, et al. Vascular complications after liver transplantation: a 5-year experience. AJR 1986;147:657–63.
8. Snover DC, Freese DK, Sharp HL, et al. Liver allograft rejection: an analysis of the use of biopsy in determining outcome of rejection. Am J Surg Pathol 1987;11:1–10.
9. Mikkelsen WP, Edmundson HA, Peters RL, et al. Extra- and intrahepatic portal hypertension without cirrhosis (hepatoportal sclerosis). Ann Surg 1965;162:602–20.
10. Leopold JG, Parry TE, Storring FK. A change in the sinusoidal-trabecular structure of the liver with hepatic venous outflow block. J Pathol 1970;100:87–98.
11. Shulman HM, McDonald GB, Matthews D, et al. An analysis of hepatic veno-occlusive disease and centrilobular hepatocyte degeneration following bone marrow transplantation. Gastroenterology 1980;79:1178–91.
12. Starzl TE, Ishikawa M, Putnam CW, et al. Progress in and deterrents to orthotopic liver transplantation, with special reference to survival, resistance to hyperacute rejection and bile duct reconstruction. Transplant Proc 1974;6:129–39.
13. Poulson H, Christofferson P. Histological changes in liver biopsies from patients with surgical bile duct disorders. Acta Pathol Microbiol Scand 1970;78A:571–9.
14. Knechtle SJ, Kolbeck PC, Tsuchimoto S, et al. Hepatic transplantation into sensitized recipients: demonstration of hyperacute rejection. Transplantation 1987;43:8–12.
15. Gubernatis G, Lauchart W, Jonker M, et al. Signs of hyperacute rejection of liver grafts in Rhesus monkeys after donor-specific presensitization. Transplant Proc 1987;19:1082–3.
16. Hanto DW, Snover DC, Noreen HJ, et al. Hyperacute rejection of a human orthotopic liver allograft in a presensitized recipient. Clin Transplant 1987;1:304–10.
17. Houssin D, Gugenheim J, Brunaud MD, et al. Accelerated but not hyperacute rejection of liver allografts in hypersensitized rats. In: Thiede A, Deltz E, Engemann R, Hamelmann H, eds. Microsurgical models in rats for transplantation research. Heidelberg: Springer-Verlag, 1985;227–31.
18. Gordon RD, Esquivel CO, Iwatsuki S, Starzl TE. Liver transplantation across ABO blood groups. Surgery 1986;100:342–8.

19. Iwatsuki S, Iwaki Y, Kano T, et al. Successful liver transplantation from cross-match-positive donors. Transplant Proc 1981;13:286–8.
20. Corson JM, The pathologist and the kidney transplant. Pathol Annu 1972;8:251–92.
21. Forbes RDC, Guttman RD. Pathogenetic studies of cardiac allograft rejection using inbred rat models. Immunol Rev 1984;77:5–29.
22. Demetris AJ, Lasky S, Van Thiel DH, et al. Pathology of hepatic transplantation: a review of 62 adult allograft recipients immunosuppressed with a cyclosporine/steroid regimen. Am J Pathol 1985;118:151–61.
23. Discussion. The first international workshop and colloquium on the pathology of liver transplantation. Transplant Proc 1986:18(Suppl 4):144–5.
24. Wight DGD. Pathology of rejection. In: Calne RV, ed. Liver transplantation. New York: Grune & Stratton, 1983;247–77.
25. Williams JW, Peters TG, Vera SP, et al. Biopsy directed immunosuppression following hepatic transplantation in man. Transplantation 1985;39:589–96.
26. Daar SA, Fuggle SV, Fabre JW, et al. The detailed distribution of HLA-A,B,C, antigens in normal human organs. Transplantation 1984;38:289–92.
27. Snover DC, Weisdorf SA, Ramsay NKC, et al. Hepatic graft-versus-host disease: a study of the predictive value of biopsy in diagnosis. Hepatology 1987;4:123–30.
28. Review by an international group. Histopathology of the intrahepatic biliary tree. Liver 1983;3:161–75.
29. So SKS, Platt JL, Ascher NL, Snover DC. Increased expression of class I antigens on hepatocytes in rejecting liver allografts. Transplantation 1987;43:79–85.
30. Steinhoff G, Wonigeit K, Ringe B, et al. Modified patterns of major histocompatibility antigen expression in human liver grafts during rejection. Transplant Proc 1987;19:2466–9.
31. Lautenschlager I, Hockerstedt K, von Willebrand TM, et al. Aspiration cytology of a human liver allograft. Transplant Proc 1984;16:1243–6.
32. Hockerstedt K, Lautenschlager I, Scheinin TM, et al. Diagnosis of rejection in liver transplantation. Transplant Proc 1987;19:2483–4.
33. Häyry P, von Willebrand E. Monitoring of human renal allograft rejection with fine needle aspiration cytology. Scand J Immunol 1981;13:87–97.
34. Ludwig J, Weisner RH, Butts KP, et al. The acute vanishing bile duct syndrome (acute irreversible rejection) after orthotopic liver transplantation. Hepatology 1987;7:476–83.
35. Snover DC. Acute and chronic graft-versus-host disease: histopathological evidence for two pathogenetic mechanisms. Hum Pathol 1984;15:202–5.
36. Portmann B, Neuberger JM, Williams R. Intrahepatic bile duct lesions. In: Calne RV, ed. Liver transplantation. New York: Grune & Stratton, 1983;279–87.
37. Grond J, Gouw ASH, Poppema S, et al. Chronic rejection in liver transplants: a histopathologic analysis of failed grafts and antecedent serial biopsies. Transplant Proc 1986;18(Suppl 4):128–35.
38. Desmet VJ. Cholestasis: extrahepatic obstruction and secondary biliary cirrhosis. In: MacSween RNM, Anthony PP, Scheuer PJ, eds. Pathology of the liver. Edinburgh: Churchill-Livingstone, 1979;272–305.
39. Daar AS, Fuggle SV, Fabre JW, et al. The detailed distribution of MHC class II antigens in normal human organs. Transplantation 1984;38:293–8.
40. Barbatis C, Woods J, Morton JA, et al. Immunohistochemical analysis of HLA (A,B,C) antigens in liver disease using a monoclonal antibody. Gut 1981;22:985–91.

41. Demetris AJ, Lasky S, Van Thiel DH, et al. Induction of DR/Ia antigens in human liver allografts: an immunohistochemical and clinicopathologic analysis of 20 failed grafts. Transplantation 1985;40:504–9.
42. Dilly SA, Sloane JP. An immunohistological study of human hepatic graft-versus-host disease. Clin Exp Immunol 1985;62:545–53.
43. Si L, Whiteside TL, Van Thiel DH, Rabin BS. Lymphocyte subpopulations at the site of "piecemeal" necrosis in end stage chronic liver diseases and rejecting liver allografts in cyclosporine-treated patients. Lab Invest 1984;50: 341–7.
44. Perkins JD, Weisner RH, Banks PM, et al. Immunohistologic labeling as an indicator of liver allograft rejection. Transplantation 1987;43:105–8.
45. Eggink HF, Houthoff HJ, Huitema S, et al. Cellular and humoral immune reactions in chronic active liver disease. I. Lymphocyte subsets in liver biopsies of patients with untreated idiopathic autoimmune hepatitis, chronic active hepatitis B and primary biliary cirrhosis. Clin Exp Immunol 1982;50:17–24.
46. Si L, Whiteside TL, Schade RR, Van Thiel DH. Studies of lymphocyte subpopulations in the liver tissue and blood of patients with chronic active hepatitis (CAH). J Clin Immunol 1983;3:408–19.
47. Shulman HM, McDonald GB. Liver disease after marrow transplantation. In: Sale GE, Shulman HM, eds. The pathology of bone marrow transplantation. New York: Masson, 1984;104–35.
48. Fennel RH Jr. Cellular damage in liver transplantation rejection: its similarity to that of primary biliary cirrhosis and graft-versus-host disease. Pathol Annu 1981;16:289–94.
49. Neuberger J, Portmann B, Macdougall BR, et al. Recurrence of primary biliary cirrhosis after liver transplantation. N Engl J Med 1982;306:1–4.
50. Portmann B, O'Grady J, Williams R. Disease recurrence following orthotopic liver transplantation. Transplant Proc 1986;18(Suppl 4):136–43.
51. Demetris AJ, Jaffe R, Sheahan DG, et al. Recurrent hepatitis B in liver allograft recipients: differentiation between viral hepatitis B and rejection. Am J Pathol 1986;125:161–72.
52. Hanson CA, Sutherland DE, Snover DC. Fulminant hepatic failure in an HBsAg carrier renal transplant patient following cessation of immunosuppressive therapy. Transplantation 1985;39:311–12.
53. Marinucci G, Valeri L, Alfani D, et al. Delta infection and liver disease recurrence in hepatic allografts. Transplant Proc 1986;18:1402–4.
54. Schmid M, Pirovino M, Altorfer J, et al. Acute hepatitis non-A, non-B: are there any specific light microscopic features? Liver 1982;2:61–7.
55. Snover DC, Hutton S, Balfour HH, Bloomer JR. Cytomegalovirus infection of the liver in transplant recipients. J Clin Gastroenterol 1987;9:659–65.
56. Koneru B, Jaffe R, Esquivel CO, et al. Adenoviral infections in pediatric liver transplant recipients. JAMA 1987;258:489–92.
57. Lorber MI, Van Buren CT, Flescher SM, et al. Hepatobiliary and pancreatic complications of cyclosporine therapy in 466 renal transplant recipients. Transplantation 1987;43:35–40.
58. Ryffel B, Donatsch P, Madorin M, et al. Toxicological evaluation of cyclosporine A. Arch Toxicol 1983;53:107–41.
59. Sparberg M, Simon N, Del Greco F. Intrahepatic cholestasis due to azathioprine. Gastroenterology 1969;57:439–41.
60. Stromeyer FW, Ishak KG. Nodular transformation (nodular "regenerative" hyperplasia) of the liver. Hum Pathol 1981;12:60–71.

61. Snover DC, Weisdorf S, Bloomer J, et al. Nodular regenerative hyperplasia of the liver following bone marrow transplantation. Hepatology 1989;9:443–8.
62. Cohen C, Olsen MM. Pediatric total parenteral nutrition. Liver histopathology. Arch Pathol Lab Med 1981;105:152–6.
63. Williams JW, Vera S, Peters TG, et al. Cholestatic jaundice after hepatic transplantation: a nonimmunologically mediated event. Am J Surg 1986;151:65–70.
64. Starzl TE, Iwatsuki S, Shaw BW, et al. Treatment of fibrolamellar hepatoma with partial or total hepatectomy and transplantation of the liver. Surg Gynecol Obstet 1986;162:145–8.
65. Snover DC. Hepatitis B virus infection and liver transplantation. Hepatology 1987;7:973–9.
66. Demetris AJ, Marcus BH, Esquivel C, et al. Pathological analysis of liver transplantation for primary biliary cirrhosis. Hepatology 1988;8:939–47.

5

Cardiac Transplantation

MARGARET E. BILLINGHAM

It is now generally accepted that heart transplantation is no longer an experimental procedure but rather a highly effective therapy for the treatment of patients with end-stage heart disease. The Registry of the International Society for Heart Transplantation recorded 78 centers in the United States and 37 centers from other sites around the world performing cardiac transplantation in 1987 [1]. The database of the Registry now consists of more than 10,300 patients. The average age for patients undergoing heart transplantation is 41.68 years with a range from newborn to 66 years. The majority of patients in the heart transplant group have been male, with only 15% of heart transplant patients being female. My experience of cardiac transplantation pathology is based on the Stanford University Medical Center experience where cardiac transplantation has been steadily ongoing since 1968 and where more than 500 cardiac transplants have been performed. The oldest survivor in this cohort is now 19 years past cardiac transplantation. Overall survival as calculated from actuarial tables continues to improve. For those patients treated with cyclosporine, the 1-year actuarial survival is now 79% and the 5-year actuarial survival is increased to 78.3%. Many centers have a first-year survival of almost 90%.

a day are being performed, as in our center, electron microscopy becomes impracticable.

Pathology of Acute Rejection

Early postoperative cardiac pathologic findings can be considered under the headings of immediate graft failure, hyperacute cardiac rejection, ischemic or reperfusion changes in the myocardium, and acute cardiac rejection, which is uncommon but can occur in the first week following transplantation.

Immediate Graft Failure

On rare occasions the donor heart will fail to function satisfactorily before the patient has left the operating room following cardiac transplantation. This can be due to a number of surgical problems as well as to damage to the donor heart, either by prolonged ischemic time (if the heart has been distantly procured) or by actual trauma to the heart if the donor was an accident victim. If the recipient has severe pulmonary hypertension, the right ventricle may become discolored, dilate, and fail to contract adequately at reperfusion. In this case, the donor heart's nonhypertrophied normal right ventricle is unable to overcome the increased pulmonary pressure and fails. Recipients are generally not accepted for cardiac transplantation if they have a pulmonary artery wedge pressure over 10 Wood units. Patients with increased pulmonary hypertension will do better with a combined heart-lung transplant or a heart from a donor with pulmonary hypertension who is receiving a heart-lung transplant ("domino transplant"). Pathologically, the heart that fails immediately may be unremarkable, although it is usual to find some degree of dilatation; some diffuse hemorrhage in the right ventricle is also occasionally seen. Ischemic damage from poor reperfusion is usually not morphologically evident because it has not had time to develop. Careful inspection of the heart may reveal fibrin thrombi in small vessels.

Hyperacute Rejection

Hyperacute rejection is also very rare, since it results from inaccurate cross-matching of the blood and major histoincompatibility differences of the donor and recipient. Usually, the heart dilates, becomes darker, and begins to fibrillate or does not contract well before the patient leaves the operating room. The patient will not survive in this condition unless another donor is obtained immediately or a mechanical "bridge-to-transplant" is applied until another donor is found. Histopathologic changes of hyperacute rejection consist of marked interstitial hemorrhage seen diffusely throughout the heart in contrast to the focal hemorrhage seen in the right ventricle of the failing right ventricle (see above) or the localized hemorrhage in a myocardial infarct. There may be evidence of marked interstitial edema as well. If the heart is supported with a mechanical "bridge" for a while before retransplantation, then neutrophils may be seen marginating in vessels or even in the interstitium. These changes are similar to those seen in animal models in which deliberate histocompatibility mismatch is used between donor and recipient. Small vessels often contain "sludging" of red cells, which may block the capillaries, and fibrin thrombi.

Reperfusion and Ischemic Injury

Many of the transplanted donor hearts will show some evidence of ischemic and reperfusion injury during the first week and up to 3 weeks following cardiac transplantation. This may be seen even in hearts that are not distantly procured and that have minimum ischemic time. The myocardium at this time may show patchy areas of myocyte shrinkage with either hypereosinophilia or nuclear pyknosis. These changes are highlighted by a Masson's trichrome stain, which will show a distinct tinctorial difference between the gray damaged myocytes and the bright red normal myocytes (Fig. 5.1). Inflammatory infiltrate is absent at this stage, a marked distinction between necrosis due to acute rejection and that due to ischemia. Ul-

Figure 5.1
Endomyocardial biopsy 1 week after cardiac transplantation showing focal ischemia (arrows) (Masson's trichrome ×400).

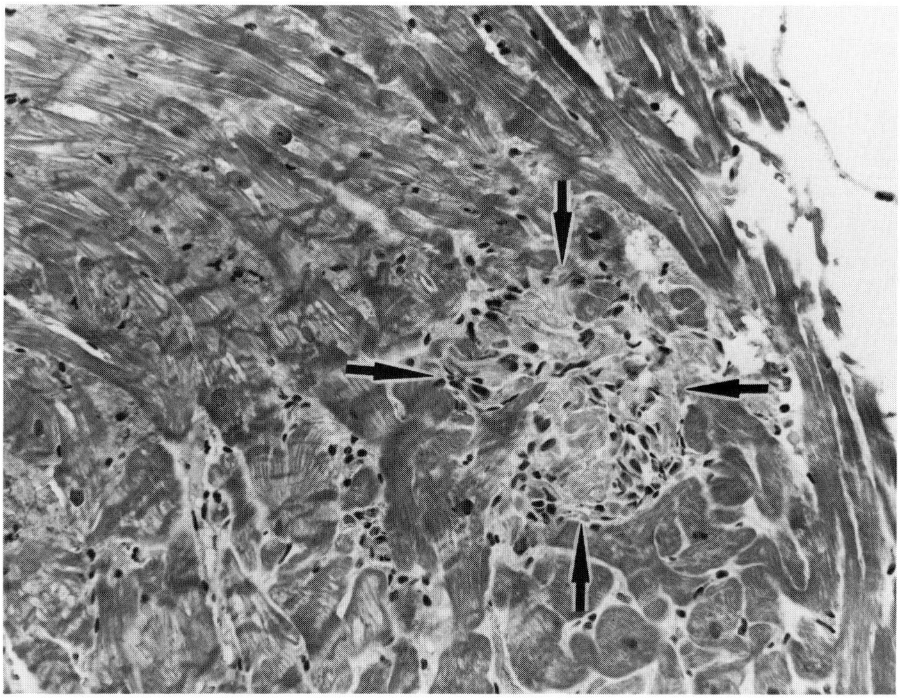

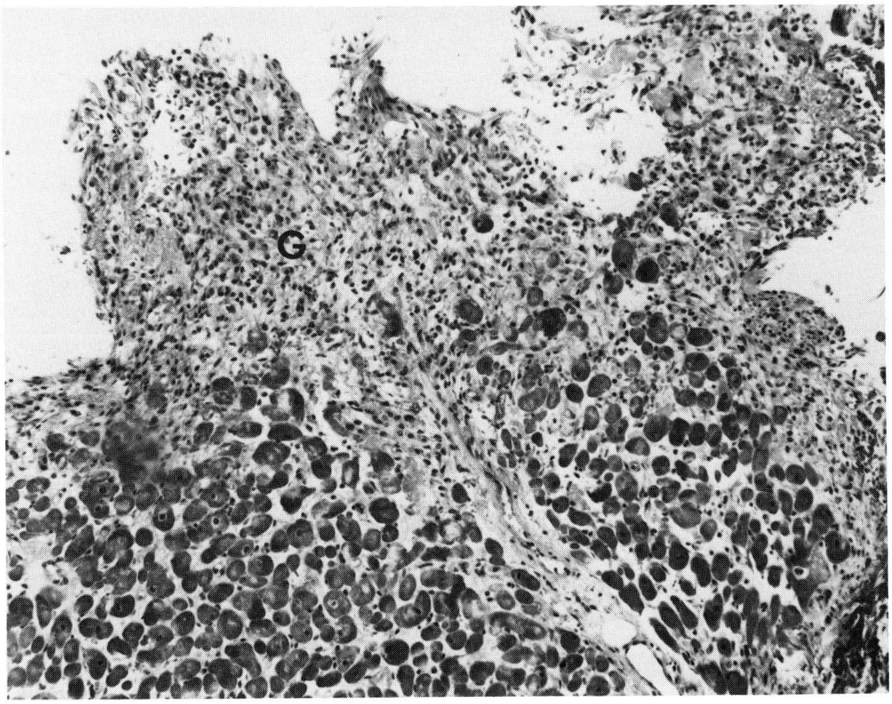

Figure 5.2
Biopsy 2 weeks after cardiac transplantation showing granulation tissue G (hematoxylin-eosin ×200).

trastructurally, the capillaries show marked endothelial swelling and rupture as well as microscopic hemorrhage [9]. Ultrastructurally, mitochondria also show swelling and matrix lucency in the affected areas. Ten days to 2 weeks following ischemia and reperfusion damage, focal granulation tissue may be seen in the previously damaged areas of myocardium. The granulation tissue is also unlike the inflammatory infiltrate seen in acute rejection, since it is mixed infiltrate and not monomorphous lymphocytes (Fig. 5.2).

Other Changes Seen in the Early Postoperative Period

High-dose pressor agents may be used liberally during early postoperative resuscitation of the patient and also may have been used in resuscitation and support of the donor before the transplantation. The results of this may lead to the typical focal "catecholamine effect" described below. This usually results in small focal lesions where two or three myocytes are damaged and there is a mixed inflammatory infiltrate. These "microinfarcts" are thought to result from spasm of small end vessels in the myocardium due to the pressor agents (Fig. 5.3).

Microinfarcts may also be due to trapped air bubbles that have not been

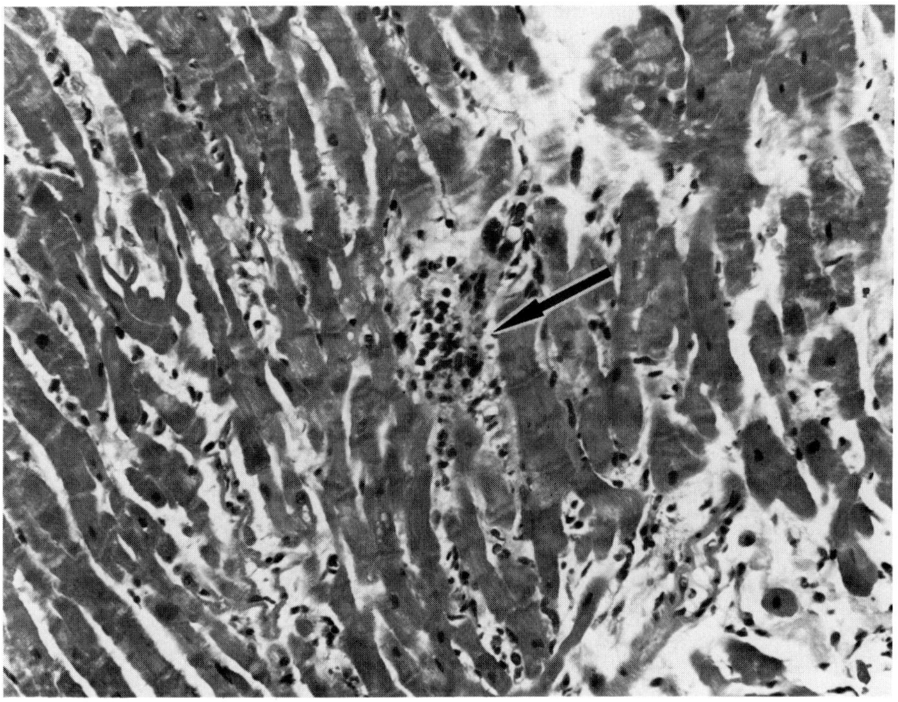

Figure 5.3
Focal myocyte damage and infiltrate (arrow) due to "pressor" effect (hematoxylin-eosin ×200).

adequately removed from the coronary circulation during closure of the transplanted heart. These changes may be seen toward the end of the first week or within 10 days of cardiac transplantation. Although small, these infarcts are larger than those caused by the pressor agents described above. These microinfarcts are usually seen on the endocardial surface. After 10 days, reparative changes may be present, with histiocytes marginating around the edge of the previously damaged myocardium or an early neutrophilic infiltrate. These changes are quite unlike the perimyocytic mononuclear infiltrate that occurs in acute rejection and should not be confused with it. We emphasize that these small areas of myocyte damage will be highlighted by a connective tissue stain, particularly Masson's trichrome, before the inflammatory infiltrate has developed.

It is also possible, of course, to have acute rejection within the first week following cardiac transplantation. In this case, the changes of acute rejection may be mixed with those of ischemia, but differentiation is not difficult: In ischemia, necrosis of the myocyte occurs first and an acute inflammatory infiltrate follows, whereas in acute rejection, the mononuclear infiltrate occurs first and the myocyte necrosis follows. In all diagnostic endomyocardial biopsies, this rule is helpful in distinguishing ischemia from rejection.

Histopathologic Changes in Cardiac Transplants During the First Year Following Transplantation

During the first year following cardiac transplantation, particularly the first 3 months, the most common changes are those of acute rejection and infection affecting the myocardium.

Acute Cardiac Rejection

Most patients who undergo cardiac transplantation will have an episode of acute rejection within the first 3 months following transplantation depending on the type of treatment and the histoincompatibility of the donor heart. In a few cases the cardiac recipient will not reject noticeably for the duration of the graft. On the other hand, some recipients will reject in a low-grade, but persistent, way for the first 2 or 3 months, often necessitating a retransplantation. Acute cardiac rejection may occur later due to poor absorption of immunosuppressive drugs or may be precipitated by weight gain in the patient, thereby effectively diluting the amount of immunosuppression.

Grading of Acute Rejection There are now several different grading systems for acute rejection [10,11]. We have found that the simplest form of grading is best for reproducibility and understanding by clinicians. Transplantation centers should use whatever grading systems they prefer, but a particular transplant program must use a system consistently, and each participating pathologist and each clinician must be familiar with the particular grading system in use. For the purpose of this chapter, we will use the simple grading system of mild, moderate, severe, and resolved acute rejection. Although there is a spectrum of changes within each of these categories, we have found it more useful to use this simplified version, since each grade requires a definitive modification of immunosuppression or some other definite treatment. Intermediate grades do not require any actions and are more useful for computerization or research purposes. A summary of the different grading systems is given in Table 5.2.

Mild Acute Rejection Mild acute rejection is characterized by a perivascular or an endocardial infiltrate of large, plump, mononuclear cells with prominent nucleoli and pyroniophilic cytoplasm. These cells are sometimes sparsely distributed within the interstitium but are more commonly perivascular in location (Fig. 5.4). Myocyte necrosis is not usually present at this stage. However, very focal myocyte necrosis should not preclude a diagnosis of mild acute rejection. The infiltrates of mild acute rejection are usually patchy and focal. The infiltrating plump mononuclear cells are T cells and, depending on the type of immunosuppressive treatment, have a preponderance of cytotoxic suppressor T cells, although a few helper T cells may also be present [12]. The diagnosis of mild acute rejection is twofold: to alert the clinician of an impending cardiac rejection episode, confirmation of which is required by a rebiopsy within 5 days for cyclosporine-treated patients; and

Table 5.2
Summary of some published biopsy grading systems in cardiac allografts

Stanford (Billingham) Heart Transplant 1:25, 1987	*Hannover (Kemnitz) Am J Surg Pathol 11:503, 1987*	*Texas (McAllister) Tex Heart Instit J 13:1, 1986*
No rejection	A0	0–1
Mild	A1, A2	0–4
Moderate	A3	4–9
Severe	A4	10
Resolving	A5a	—
Resolved	A5b	—
	C1 (chronic rejection)	

to treat immediately in the case of azathioprine-treated patients. The patient who has a mild acute rejection and is being treated with cyclosporine may develop a moderate acute rejection within 5 days. It has been shown that approximately 30% to 40% of patients with biopsies showing mild acute rejection proceed to a moderate acute rejection that requires treatment, while

Figure 5.4
Endomyocardial biopsy showing mild acute rejection (focal infiltrates, arrows) without myocyte damage (hematoxylin-eosin ×200).

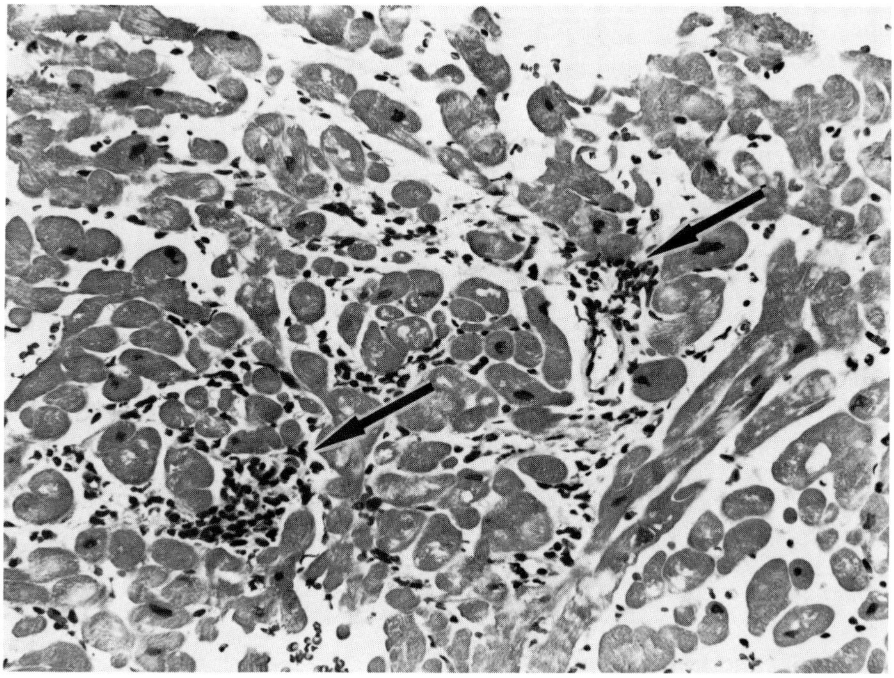

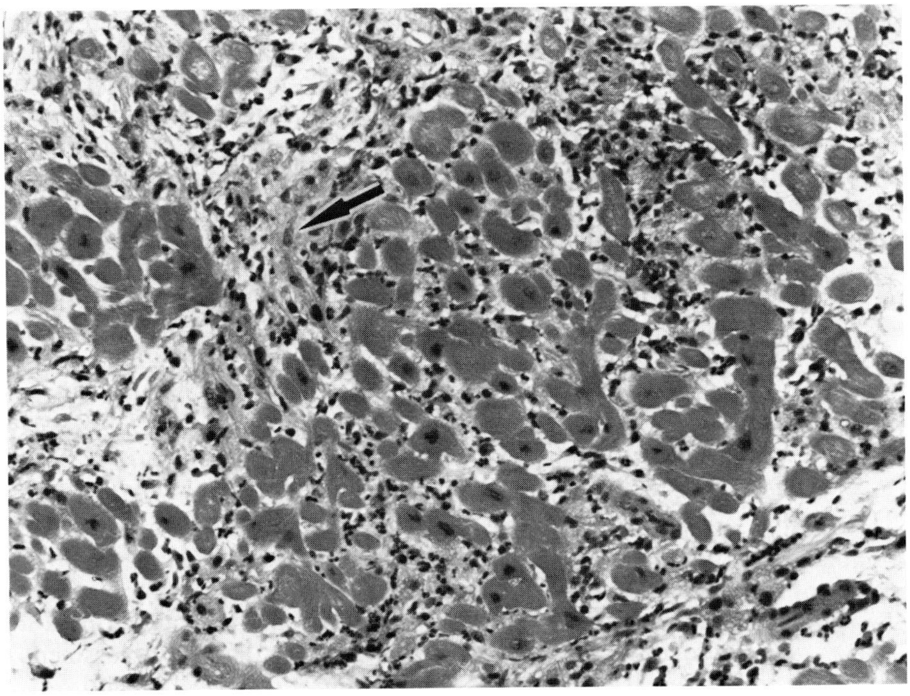

Figure 5.6
Severe acute rejection with mixed infiltrates (lymphocytes, neutrophils, and eosinophils) and myocyte damage (arrow) (hematoxylin-eosin ×200).

or 40 biopsy procedures overall, at which three or four pieces of tissue are taken at any one time, the presence of previous biopsy sites is almost inevitable. Recent biopsy sites (1 or 2 weeks) are usually marked by a fibrinous exudate as well as granulation tissue, and a useful marker is the myocyte disarray at the base of the biopsy crater. Myocyte disarray is not usually seen as a result of acute rejection alone. Older biopsy sites can be distinguished by fibrous tissue but also by the myocyte disarray at the base of the biopsy site (Fig. 5.7). The mixed infiltrate in granulation tissue is quite different from that of acute rejection.

2. The inflammatory infiltrate caused by infectious organisms in the cardiac recipient can be mistakenly diagnosed as acute rejection. This problem does not appear to arise too frequently. The most common infectious organisms causing a myocarditis in immunosuppressed-cardiac recipients are cytomegalovirus (CMV) and *T. gondii*. In the case of CMV, usually the virus does not evoke an inflammatory infiltrate. However, we have seen a mixed infiltrate associated with it, and therefore confusion with acute rejection is not a problem. Unfortunately, it is possible to have acute rejection and CMV infection at the same time; this presents a diagnostic and treatment dilemma. Often the infection is treated first unless the rejection is severe. In the case of toxoplasmosis causing a myocarditis, the inflammatory infiltrate is usually mixed and contains neutrophils and eosinophils. The inflammatory in-

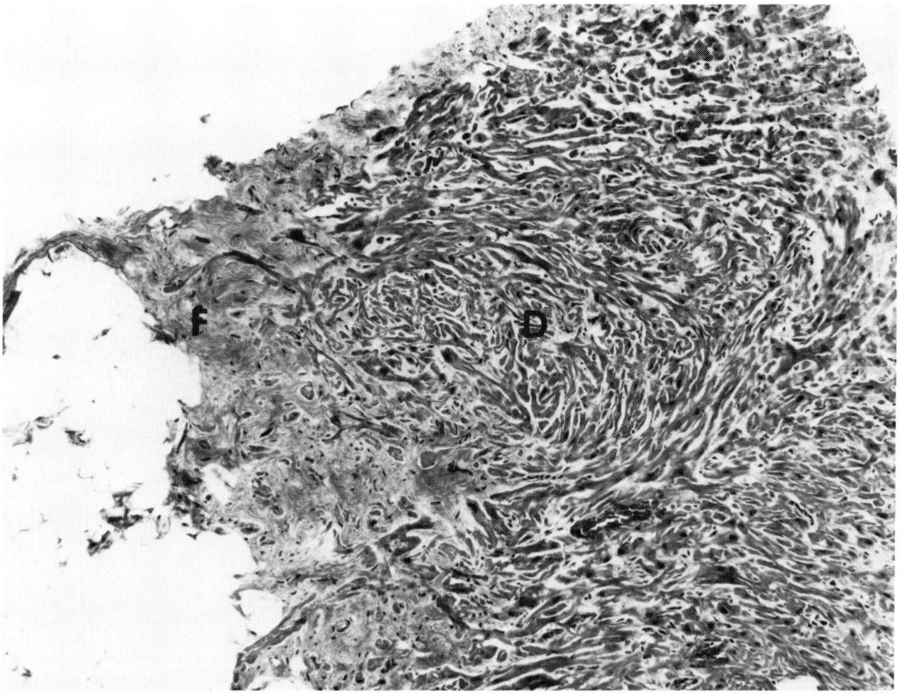

Figure 5.7
Endomyocardial biopsy showing biopsy site with peripheral fibrin, F, and myocyte disarray, D (hematoxylin-eosin ×200).

filtrate tends to be focal, and there is no accompanying vasculitis or hemorrhage that could be confused with severe acute rejection. The *T. gondii* cysts should be looked for away from the inflammatory infiltrate, since the intact cysts usually do not evoke an infiltrate. We have not had trouble distinguishing viral myocarditis from an acute rejection morphologically.

3. The presence of the "quilty" effect may sometimes be a problem in the diagnosis of acute rejection. The quilty effect refers to a predominantly endocardial infiltrate of lymphocytes that are pyroninophilic. This infiltrate, although usually confined to the endocardial surface, may "spill over" into the subjacent myocardium (Fig. 5.8). It has been shown that the infiltrate in the subendocardium can also cause focal myocyte necrosis. At Stanford, the policy is not to treat the quilty effect, even if spillover exists, if it can be shown that the intramyocyte infiltrate is definitely an extension of the endocardial one. If the infiltrates are separated and are in other moieties of the biopsy, we assume that acute rejection is also present and treat the patient in the usual way. The quilty effect usually disappears spontaneously in subsequent biopsies. It is most likely a rejection phenomenon of some kind, since it can be seen in rat models, especially those treated with cyclosporine. The quilty effect is seen in approximately 9% of endomyocardial biopsies of patients treated with cyclosporine at Stanford. To date, we have not seen any evidence of the quilty effect in patients treated with OKT3 up to the first

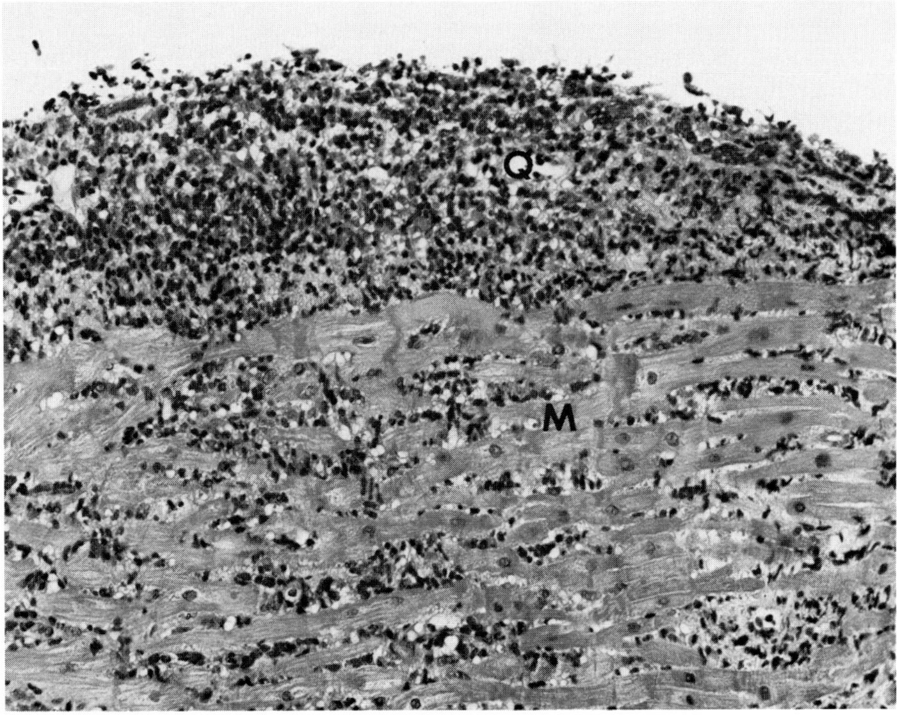

Figure 5.8
Endocardial infiltrate or "quilty" effect with some "spillover" into the adjacent myocyte, M (hematoxylin-eosin ×200).

6 months following transplantation. The etiology of the quilty effect is not clear, and several studies have tried to address this problem* [13].

It is appropriate to warn pathologists that because of the side effects of cyclosporine, there is a trend in many centers to give less cyclosporine and more azathioprine so that a clear distinction between these two forms of treatment is becoming more blunt. Therefore, the pathologist should be aware of the changes for both sets of treatment. Table 5.3 summarizes the difference in the two forms of therapy. Other ways (particularly noninvasive methods) for identifying acute rejection are nonmorphologic and therefore will not be discussed in this chapter.

Infection in the Cardiac Recipient

Acute infection is known to be the most important cause of morbidity and death in the cardiac recipient. Acute infection has caused the death of 37.8%

*Unpublished results, Stanford University, 1989.

Table 5.3
Differences in morphologic responses to cyclosporine vs conventional treatment

Response	*Cyclosporine*	*Conventional*
Rejection	Slow onset (5–7 days)	Rapid onset (24–36 hours)
Reversal of rejection	Slow	Rapid
Clinical signs	Often absent	Usually present
Rejection infiltrate	Eosinophils present	Eosinophils only in infection
Endocardial infiltrates ("quilty" effect)	9% of all biopsies	Very rare

cardiac transplant recipients, out of a total of 10,334 patients in the International Society of Heart Transplant Registry. The overall number of infections occurring in patients treated with cyclosporine versus those treated with azathioprine is approximately the same, although the probability of death from infection is less in the cyclosporine-treated cohort.† This is because there are approximately 10% fewer viral infections in cyclosporine-treated patients in the early postoperative years and approximately 20% fewer fungal infections (which are less easily reversed) in cyclosporine-treated patients over a 5-year period. The gap with bacterial infections is less pronounced between the two groups (approximately 5% fewer bacterial infections in the cyclosporine-treated group over 5 years in the Stanford study). The most common acute infections during the early postoperative period, as stated previously, are *T. gondii* and CMV. It is well known that placing a donor heart from a CMV-seropositive donor into a seronegative recipient almost always results in a CMV infection. It is also now well known that CMV infection predisposes to acute rejection, and the pathologist should be alert to this. The range of organisms responsible for infectious disease in cardiac recipients is extensive and exotic (Table 5.4). Infections in this group of patients may be seen in other organs of the body, since they

Table 5.4
Infections in cyclosporine-treated cardiac recipients (Stanford, December 1980 to September 1988)

1. Bacterial	242
2. Viral	187
Titer rise only	40
3. Fungal	52
4. Protozoal	28
5. *Nocardia*	15

†Unpublished results, Stanford University, 1989.

become disseminated, including to the brain and skin, and will not be detailed in this chapter.

Pathology of Long-Term Cardiac Transplantation Survival

In the late postoperative period, a number of potential complications can limit long-term survival.

Acute Rejection

Although occurring mainly in the early postoperative period, acute rejection can occur in the late postoperative period. Episodes of acute rejection in the late postoperative period may follow an infection with CMV or may be due to a reduction in immunosuppressives due to cushingoid features, osteoporosis, hirsuteness, hypertension, or nephrotoxicity. Occasionally, an inadvertent marked increase in the recipient's weight effectively reduces the amount of immunosuppression and can precipitate a rejection episode. It has been noticed in the Stanford series that a mild acute rejection in a long-term cardiac survival patient is less likely to proceed to a moderate acute rejection.

Accelerated Graft Coronary Disease in Long-Term Survivors

This condition is sometimes referred to as "chronic" rejection, but this is a confusing term and preferably should not be used. The coronary circulation in the transplanted organ is subject to the development of a rapidly progressive form of concentric intimal proliferation, often extending along the length of the vessel and including the small branches. In the heart, the small penetrating branches of the epicardial coronaries may be occluded totally while the main vessel is only partially occluded. This is why myocardial infarcts can occur in cardiac recipients, even though the angiographic changes of the epicardial coronaries are apparently not occluded. These changes can occur as rapidly as 3 months following cardiac transplantation, and death from infarcts has been reported as early as 9 months after cardiac transplantation. Accelerated graft coronary disease can be detected on coronary arteriogram in 40% of cardiac recipients by 2.5 years following cardiac transplantation [3].

The incidence of graft coronary disease does not appear to differ significantly in patients who were treated with cyclosporine and those who were treated with the conventional (azathioprine and steroids) regimen. In two separate studies, one an autopsy and another a clinical study at Stanford, there was no definite correlation of incidence of graft coronary disease with the number of acute rejection episodes or HLA mismatches, age or sex of the donor heart, or whether the cardiac recipient previously had cardiomyopathy or coronary disease [14]. There may be a correlation with CMV in-

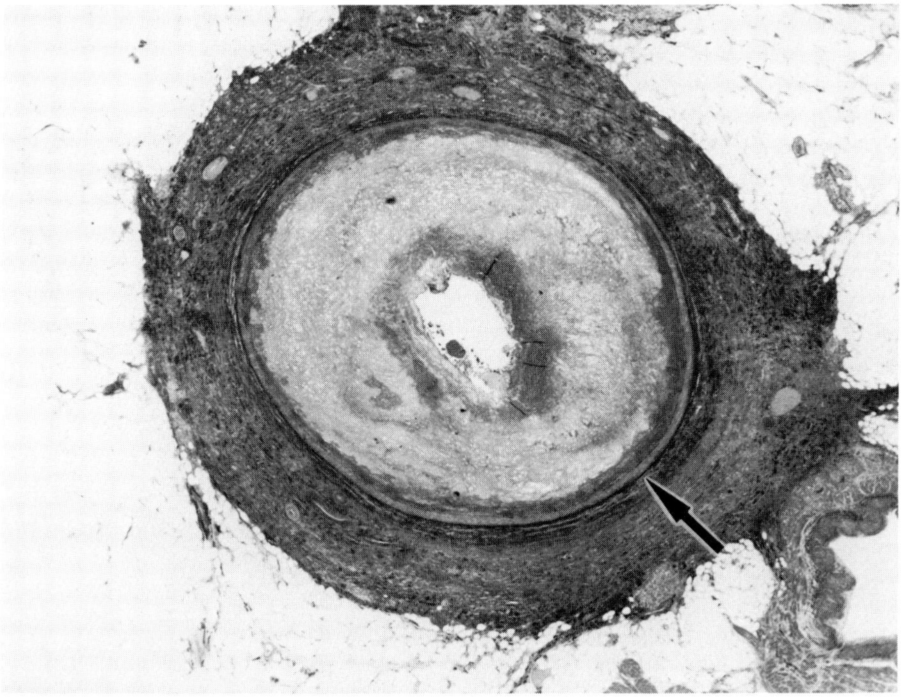

Figure 5.9
Section of coronary artery 1 year following cardiac transplantation showing concentric intimal proliferation and almost intact elastic lamina (arrow) (elastic van Giesen ×12.5).

fection, although this is unlikely to be the whole cause of this complication [15].

The pathologic findings take the form of a concentric intimal proliferation that is unlike naturally occurring atherosclerosis in that it is not focal or asymmetric (Fig. 5.9). Also, the internal elastic lamina is frequently intact, in contrast to the fragmentation and partial disappearance seen in naturally occurring atherosclerosis. Although occasional plaques with cholesterol clefts and very focal calcification can be seen in graft recipients, it is not clear whether these are legacies of the donor heart. The intimal proliferation appears to consist mainly of modified smooth muscle cells and lipid-filled macrophages. The lining endothelium is usually intact.

It is of interest that graft coronary disease may also occur in combined heart-lung transplants, both in the heart and in the lungs, even though in some cases actual rejection episodes are not documented in the heart. Graft coronary disease can occur in children who have undergone transplantation as well as in adult recipients. Accelerated graft coronary disease is one of the most discouraging aspects of cardiac transplantation at this time, and it accounts for the greatest number of retransplantation procedures [1].

Chronic Hypertrophy and Fibrosis of the Graft

It has been observed that all transplanted hearts become larger within weeks of transplantation. In addition, 1 year after transplantation, most transplanted hearts show myocyte hypertrophy as well as an increase in interstitial fibrosis. Early on it was demonstrated that the longer the donor ischemic time, the worse the reperfusion changes in small vessels at an ultrastructural level [9]. It is thought that this may result in some of the fibrosis, and this is supported by the fact that patients with longer ischemic time and distantly procured donor hearts have more fibrosis and compensatory hypertrophy than those who have on-site donor hearts. Several morphometric studies have been performed to support this [16]. It is also well known that restrictive and constrictive functional changes occur in long-term survivors of heart transplantation. It is thought that these changes may be related. Some evidence shows that high cyclosporine levels result in an increase in fine perimyocytic fibrosis in the heart [17,18]. With the reduced cyclosporine levels currently in use, this type of fibrosis is not often seen now.

The Effects of Denervation of the Transplanted Heart

At least in the early stages following cardiac transplantation, the heart remains denervated and is not under the usual control of the autonomic nervous system. The heart rate, in response to dynamic exercise, tends to be slower and not to achieve peak levels during maximum exercise when compared with age-matched normal controls. As judged by pharmacologic electrophysiologic studies on cardiac recipients, the transplanted heart remains denervated in long-term survivors. Serial cardiac biopsies studied by electron microscopy after transplantation show ongoing degeneration of the sympathetic and sensory nerves in the first few months following transplantation. Long-term studies, however, show that the postganglionic nerves remain intact, since their ganglia remain viable in the atrioventricular groove. Serial studies up to 11 years after cardiac transplantation have failed to reveal reinnervation from the morphologic standpoint [19]. However, these studies are done in biopsies, which in turn obtain tissue from the apex of the right ventricle. More recently, it has been reported [20] that there is some physiologic evidence of the reinnervation. In the sinoatrial and atrioventricular nodes there is about a 50% chance of surgical damage during procurement of the heart to both the recipient and donor tissue.

Transplantation Malignancies

It has been known since the advent of organ transplantation that malignancies have an increased rate of development in the immunosuppressed recipient [21,22]. This is thought to be the result of immunosuppression or chronic alloantigen stimulation. Unfortunately, this complication also occurs in cardiac allograft recipients. The distribution of malignancies is similar to that described in renal transplant recipients. The lymphoproliferative malignancies have been of particular concern. However, in some cases, these can be reduced or even abolished by lowering immunosuppression, particularly cyclosporine, and also by treating the patient with acyclovir. Patients with other lymphoproliferative malignancies have responded well to radiation. Extranodal lymphomas have been found in the gastrointestinal tract in cyclosporine-treated patients and at the site of injection of antithymoycte globulin in the thighs of cardiac recipients. The etiology of these malignancies has been a source of controversy, and several good publications express the various views on this subject [23,24].

Summary

Cardiac transplantation is now an accepted form of treatment for end-stage heart disease in all age groups. Long-term cardiac recipient survivors still require ongoing immunosuppression and, as a result, suffer from the side effects of these drugs. Coronary artery graft disease is one side effect that may necessitate retransplantation. Despite this, cardiac recipients may live productive lives for up to 19 years after transplantation.

The early pathologic findings of cardiac transplantation are mainly those of acute rejection episodes and acute infectious episodes. Although both can occur in long-term survivors, they are less frequent. The particular problems of long-term survivors are those of accelerated graft coronary disease and other complications related to immunosuppression, including malignancies. Malignancies have become much less common with widespread use of lower doses of immunosuppression. The pathologic findings of cardiac transplantation are similar in children except that children with acute rejection appear to be more labile and are sometimes difficult to treat. Children with cardiac transplants have done well, however, and there are many survivors at 5 and 6 years after transplantation.

References

1. Fragomeni LS, Kay MP. The Registry of the International Society for Heart Transplantation: fifth official report—1988. J Heart Transplant 1988;7:249–53.
2. Billingham ME. Some recent advances in cardiac pathology. Hum Pathol 1979;10:367–86.
3. Schroeder JS, Hunt SA. Cardiac transplantation: where are we? N Engl J Med 1986;315:961–2. (Editorial.)
4. Mason JW. Techniques for right and left ventricular endomyocardial biopsy. Am J Cardiol 1978;41:887–92.
5. Tilkian AG, Daily EK. Endomyocardial biopsy. In: Tilkian AG, Daily EK, eds. Cardiovascular procedures. St. Louis: Mosby, 1986;180–203.
6. Billingham ME. The post-surgical heart: the pathology of cardiac transplantation. Am J Cardiovasc Pathol 1988;1:319–34.

7. Spiegelhalter DJ, Stovin PGI. An analysis of repeated biopsies following cardiac transplantation. Stat Med 1983;2:33–40.
8. Myles JL, Ratliff NB, McMahon JT, et al. Reversibility of myocyte injury in moderate and severe acute rejection in cyclosporine-treated cardiac transplant patients. Arch Pathol Lab Med 1987;111:947–52.
9. Billingham ME, Baumgartner WA, Watson DC, et al. Distant heart procurement for human transplantation: ultrastructural studies. Circulation 1980;1:11–19.
10. Kemnitz J, Cohnert T, Schafers H-J, et al. A classification of cardiac allograft rejection. Am J Surg Pathol 1987;11:503–15.
11. McAllister HA, Schnee MJ, Radovancevic B, Frazier H. A system for grading cardiac allograft rejection. Texas Heart Inst J 1986;13:1–2.
12. Weintraub D, Masek M, Billingham ME. The lymphocyte subpopulations in cyclosporine-treated human heart rejection. Heart Transplant 1985;4:213–6.
13. Radio SJ, McManus BM, Winters G, et al. Preferential endocardial residence of B cells in "quilty" effect of human heart allografts: immunohistochemical distinction from rejection. Presented at the International Symposium on Inflammatory Heart Disease. Snowmass, CO: July 1988, p. 467.
14. Billingham ME. Cardiac transplant atherosclerosis. Transplant Proc 1987;5:19–25.
15. Oyer P. Heart, heart/lung transplantation. (Abstr.) Presented at the Twelfth International Congress of the Transplantation Society, book II. Sydney, Australia: Aug. 14–19, 1988.
16. Imakita M, Tazelaar H, Rowan R, et al. Hypertrophy of the transplanted heart: a morphometric analysis. Transplantation 1987;43:839–42.
17. Billingham ME. Diagnosis of cardiac rejection by endomyocardial biopsy. Heart Transplant 1981;1:25–30.
18. Karch SB, Billingham ME. Cyclosporine-induced myocardial fibrosis: a unique controlled case report. Heart Transplant 1985;4:210–12.
19. Rowan RA, Billingham ME. Myocardial innervation in long-term cardiac transplant survivors: a quantitative ultrastructural survey. J Heart Transplant, 1988;7:448–52.
20. Stovin PGI, Hewitt S. Conduction tissue in the transplanted human heart. J Pathol 1986;149:183–9.
21. Penn I. Malignant lymphoma in organ transplantation recipients. Transplant Proc 1981;13:736–8.
22. Starzl TE, Porter KA, Iwatsuki S, et al. Reversibility of lymphomas and lymphoproliferative lesions developing under cyclosporine steroid therapy. Lancet 1984;1:583–7.
23. Cleary ML, Sklar J. Lymphoproliferative disorders in cardiac transplant recipients are multiclonal lymphomas. Lancet 1982;2:489–93.
24. Cleary ML, Warnke R, Sklar J. Monoclonality of lymphoproliferative lesions in cardiac transplant recipients: clonal analysis based on immunoglobulin-gene rearrangements. N Engl J Med 1984;310:477–82.

6

Combined Heart-Lung Transplantation

SAMUEL A. YOUSEM
HENRY D. TAZELAAR

The first unilateral human lung transplant was performed in 1963, and since then many investigators, particularly Veith and colleagues, have explored this therapeutic option in patients with terminal vascular, interstitial, or obstructive lung disease [1–6]. Their germinal work in experimental animals and humans provided the first glimpses into the surgical complications, immunosuppressive complications, and rejection phenomena, associated with this procedure [3,7]. Between 1963 and 1980 over 40 solitary lung transplants were performed for end-stage lung disease, and no long-term clinical successes were observed, with only two patients surviving (6 and 10 months, respectively) [7]. In 1981, coinciding with the introduction of cyclosporine, investigators at Stanford University performed the first heart-lung transplantation under the leadership of Reitz and Shumway [8–10]. Since then, over 200 combined heart-lung transplant operations have been performed, primarily for patients with pulmonary hypertension due to Eisenmenger's complex and for primary plexogenic ateriopathy [11].

Surgical complications resulted in the death of 8 of 28 patients postoper-

Acknowledgment: This work is supported by the Pathology Education and Research Foundation.

The Reimplantation Response

Early work with unilateral human lung transplants, heart-lung transplantation, and autotransplantation of lungs in dogs and monkeys demonstrated an immediate transient disruption in lung function. The morphologic, roentgenographic, and functional changes that occur in a lung transplant as a result of surgical trauma, ischemia, denervation, and lymphatic interruption, *exclusive of pulmonary rejection,* have been labeled the reimplantation response [9,16]. This phenomenon is manifested by alveolar infiltrates and perihilar shadows on chest radiographs that resemble pulmonary edema. These changes peak at 3 days after surgery and slowly regress over the following 1 to 2 weeks. This finding is associated with independent disturbances of ventilation and perfusion of the lung grafts with decreased compliance. This process is worsened by hilar stripping, stenosis of vascular and bronchial anastomoses, and prolonged graft ischemia [16]. Histologically, the lungs demonstrate interstitial and alveolar edema, which is reflected in edematous clear zones cuffing the bronchovascular bundles and lymphatic routes within the interlobular septa. This reaction is seen primarily in the central or perihilar lung parenchyma. Small numbers of neutrophils within alveolar septa and alveoli may also be seen, probably due to ischemic damage. The edema is resolved with dehydrating therapy. Presumably, regrowth of lymphatics or redistribution of lymphatic flow over weeks results in intrinsic elimination of edema fluid. Although the histologic findings of this process are easy to identify, clinical presentation may mimic pulmonary rejection and precipitate a diagnostic biopsy.

Acute Pulmonary Rejection

If a lung is allotransplanted without the patient's receiving immunosuppressive therapy, it undergoes a series of clinical, radiographic, functional, and morphologic disturbances that we recognize as manifestations of acute pulmonary rejection [3,12,17]. These findings appear to be uniform, whether occurring in rats, mongrel dogs, baboons, rhesus monkeys, or unilateral lung or heart-lung transplants in humans (Table 6.1). In the latter group, it was initially thought that lung and heart rejection occurred simultaneously. However, both clinical and experimental studies have shown that although heart rejection is almost uniformly associated with pulmonary abnormalities, lung rejection can occur with a normal endomyocardial biopsy [18–21]. These findings may be a result of quantitative differences in expression of HLA antigens in the two organs [22–24]. Furthermore, the addition of cyclosporine to the immunosuppressive protocol has blunted the clinical and histologic manifestations of lung rejection but has allowed more expeditious reversal of the rejection crisis [15].

The precise incidence of early pulmonary rejection in transplant recipients is unknown, although the Pittsburgh group has indicated that more than half the recipients were felt to have had a rejection episode within the first 2 to 3 weeks [13]. For the most part, patients present with pyrexia, dyspnea, and cough without serologic, culture, or histologic evidence of pulmonary infection. Other patients may be asymptomatic. Chest roentgenograms reveal a progression of *bilateral,* predominantly lower lobe infiltrates unresponsive to antibiotic therapy [2]. This progressive opacification occurs over a 1- to 2-day period and has a diffuse homogeneous appearance. Blood gas studies show progressive hypoxemia, which coincides with an increase in pulmonary vascular resistance and the presence of transformed lymphocytes in peripheral blood smears. Bronchoalveolar lavage has revealed a lymphocytosis, and the lymphocytes have shown high levels of cell-mediated lympholysis during episodes of acute rejection [25,26]. Because the transplanted lungs have their full complement of bronchial-associated lymphoid tissue, they undergo repetitive interactions with the immunocompetent host lymphocytes [27,28]. An in vivo mixed lymphocyte reaction results, and lavage studies have revealed that during the first 6 weeks after transplantation, the vast majority of donor lymphocytes and macrophages are replaced by those of the recipient. This phenomenon may be an integral part of the early rejection period.

Veith and colleagues have described the manifestations of the early rejection period—classic rejection, atypical or alveolar rejection, and vascular rejection [7,29]. We believe these three "distinct" patterns represent a continuum in the spectrum of early lung rejection. The classic form was initially described in dogs, monkeys, and human recipients of solitary lung allografts [3]. At Pittsburgh and Stanford, we have had experience with six patients who had open lung biopsies during clinical acute rejection episodes, and their histologies [12] have closely resembled those of experimental models (see Table 6.1) [21]. Initially, there is an intensive perivascular, particularly perivenular, cuff of small round and transformed large lymphoid cells (Figs.

Table 6.1
*Acute pulmonary rejection**

Mild: edema of interstitium and mild perivenular and later periarterial cuffing by small round and transformed lymphocytes; endothelial cell hyperplasia with subendothelial infiltration by lymphocytes (endothelialitis); occasional eosinophilia
Moderate: intense perivenular, peribronchiolar, and periarterial cuffing by lymphocytes and immunoblasts with endothelialitis; round cells in alveolar septa and pleura with intra-alveolar edema; active bronchioliltis; neutrophils may be seen late in this stage
Severe: fibrinoid necrosis and thrombosis of veins and arteries with hemorrhage and necrosis of parenchyma; marked acute suppurative bronchiolitis, with sloughing of epithelial cells; alveolar pneumocyte hyperplasia and atypia with neutrophilic infiltrate; prominent airspace macrophages

*The stage at which treatment for acute pulmonary rejection is necessary is unclear at present.

tation of rejection, especially since many of the animals and human recipients were superinfected or had experienced ischemic episodes. These two conditions are common causes of diffuse alveolar damage in any normal adult, and we doubt that it represents a rejection reaction unless associated with tight perivascular mononuclear infiltrates.

How do these histopathologic findings influence the diagnosis of lung allograft rejection? We believe, first and foremost, that clinical evaluation is the most important method of diagnosing acute rejection. The presentation of a transplant recipient with fever, leukocytosis, bilateral lung infiltrates, and no change in the type of sputum bacteria predicts lung rejection [13,14,19]. Bronchoscopy and lavage should be used primarily to isolate infectious agents, since at present cell differential counts show no consistent correlations with rejection episodes [13,34–36]. Recent studies at Pittsburgh have shown that increased lymphocyte cytotoxicity in lavage and peripheral blood lymphocytes is associated with early rejection and may be a helpful adjunct to its diagnosis (A. Zeevi, personal communication). Finally, we have found the tissue diagnosis of acute rejection by either transbronchial or open biopsy to be extremely difficult because many viral and idiopathic reactions are accompanied by perivascular infiltrates. The features described previously in acute rejection combined with negative special stains and cultures for microorganisms and clinical information are necessary for definitive diagnosis. Reversal of radiographic, clinical, and functional abnormalities by intravenous boluses of methylprednisolone provide the ultimate confirmation. One myth that should be discarded is that lung rejection cannot occur without simultaneous cardiac rejection.

Long-Term Pathologic Alterations and Chronic Rejection

Progressive pulmonary dysfunction has occurred in half the long-term survivors of heart-lung transplantation at Stanford University and the University of Pittsburgh [11,12,14,30]. Table 6.2 represents a composite study of patients on whom autopsy or retransplantation material was obtained at Stanford [30]. Open lung biopsy findings on 5 of 6 patients were confirmed at autopsy in patients 14 through 19. As indicated, several pathologic alterations have occurred within the recipient lungs, the most striking finding being OB. The major pathologic abnormalities will be discussed sequentially.

Bronchiolitis Obliterans In 14 of the 28 long-term survivors at Stanford, a uniform pattern of clinical signs and symptoms appeared [30]. Bronchitic disturbances such as cough, mucopurulent sputum, and recurrent upper respiratory tract infections with persistent postnasal drainage and sinusitis were noted [12,37]. Radiologic abnormalities included bronchiectasis and reticulonodular or alveolar opacities found especially in the lower lobes [38]. Pulmonary function studies revealed an obstructive ventilatory defect with progressive global reductions of air flow to very low values (decreased forced expiratory volume at one second [FEV1], and decreased ratio of

FEV1 to forced vital capacity [FEV1/FVC], unlike classic chronic obstructive lung disease [14]. Total lung capacity was reduced, and restrictive lung disease coexisted. These abnormalities were noted as early as 2 months after transplant but became fully developed after 1 to 2 years. Average length of time to onset of obstructive disease was 11.2 months with a range of 2 to 35 months postoperatively. In eight of the ten patients the clinical course was progressive, while two were treated with high-dose corticosteroids at first detection of lung disease. Both showed recovery of lung function [11,39,40].

These functional abnormalities coincided with the pathologic changes of OB. OB is a clinical syndrome characterized by progressive dyspnea and obstructive lung disease at function testing, which is associated with a dynamic process of bronchiolar injury that at some point demonstrates exuberant intraluminal granulation tissue [41]. The functional effect of OB is primarily related to the severity of bronchiolar injury and to its diffuseness throughout all lobes of lung, i.e., the number of bronchioles affected [12].

OB develops through a consistent sequence of epithelial injury [12,30]. It is initiated by an active cellular phase of acute lymphocytic bronchiolitis with ulceration and denuding of the mucosa (Fig. 6.3). Lumenal ingrowth of stellate wispy fibroblasts from the submucosa ensues with intralumenal organization (proliferative phase) and the formation of a polypoid mass of granulation tissue (Masson body) (Fig. 6.4). A submucosal infiltrate of lymphocytes and histiocytes is usually observed. One-third of cases are accompanied by a perivascular infiltrate of lymphocytes. Depending on the severity of injury and its chronicity, several outcomes are possible.

1. The injury may resolve and the submucosa reepithelialize, leaving an intact bronchiole of normal diameter.
2. An eccentric or concentric submucosal scar may form with reepithelialization of the mucosa and lumenal narrowing (cicatricial phase). This sequel may only be obvious with elastic tissue stains that highlight the scar and the disrupted bronchiolar elastica (Fig. 6.5).
3. The entire bronchiole may be "obliterated," i.e., completely replaced by dense scar tissue and obvious only by its location next to pulmonary arterioles, its residual smooth muscle layer, and elastic tissue stains (Fig. 6.6). Peribronchiolar fibrosis with loss of the smooth muscle wall may occur, resulting in "extrinsic" compression of the lumen, the so-called constrictive form of OB.

In six of the transplant patients the constellation of histologic findings typical of OB was identified. Although patchy in distribution, the injury was panlobar, bilateral, and extensive.

OB, which causes destruction or constriction of small airways, was associated with an unusual finding in the major airways: cylindrical bronchiectasis and mucostasis. Large bronchi showed acute and chronic inflammation with extensive squamous metaplasia (Fig. 6.7). The submucosa was densely fibrotic and scarred, and the smooth muscle layer was focally absent, replaced by fibrovascular connective tissue. This loss of bronchial smooth muscle and supporting matrix resulted in the fusiform dilatation of the large

Table 6.2
Summary of autopsy findings in heart-lung transplant recipients

Patient	*Age*	*Sex*	*Preoperative diagnosis*	*Survival (mo.)*	*Cause of death*[a]	*Primary pathology*[b]	*Proximal bronchi-ectasis*	*OB*	*Arterio-sclerosis*	*Phlebo-sclerosis*	*Acute rejection*	*Additional findings*
Postoperative deaths												
1	26	F	PPH	21 d	Broncho-pneumonia	Broncho-pneumonia	—	—	—	—	—	*Candida*
2	21	M	CHD	1 d	Hemorrhage	Pleural hemorrhage	—	—	—	—	—	—
3	29	F	PPH	4	ARDS	ARDS	—	—	—	—	—	*Candida* tracheitis and gastritis
4	42	M	CHD	1	Multiorgan failure	ARDS; herpes pneumonia	—	—	—	—	—	Herpes esophagitis; acute pancreatitis
5	28	F	CHD	4 d	Hemorrhage	Pleural hemorrhage	—	—	—	—	—	—
6	37	M	CHD	4	Hemorrhage	ARDS	—	—	—	—	—	—
7	34	F	CHD	4	Hemorrhage	—	—	—	—	—	—	—
8	29	M	PPH	4	*Candida* sepsis	ARDS; broncho-pneumonia	—	—	—	—	—	—
9	37	M	PPH	1	Acute broncho-pneumonia ? etiology	Acute broncho-pneumonia	—	—	—	—	—	—
10	30	F	CHD	4	*Candida* sepsis	*Candida* pneumonia	—	—	—	+1	+1	Splenic infarcts
11	26	F	PPH	1	Herpes pneumonia	ARDS; Herpes pneumonia	—	—	—	—	—	—

Long-term survivors without OB												
12	37	F	PPH	52	ARDS	ARDS ? etiology	—	—	—	1+	—	—
13	45	F	PPH	63	Iatrogenic	ARDS	—	—	—	1+	—	Smoker's bronchiolitis
Long-term survivors with OB												
14	40	M	CHD	44	Complications after appendectomy	ARDS	+1	3+	1+	2+	+1	Lacerated liver
15	22	M	CHD	37	OB	Acute broncho-pneumonia	+2	3+	—	1+	—	—
16	27	M	CHD	15	Myocardial infarct	*Aspergillus* pneumonia	+1	3+	1+	2+	—	Acute aspiration
17	40	M	CHD	9	OB	*Pneumocystis* pneumonia	+1	3+	2+	2+	—	—
18	24	F	PPH	14	OB	Acute broncho-pneumonia ? etiology	+1	3+	—	—	+1	Iatrogenic pneumothorax
19	32	M	CHD	15	OB	*Coccidioides* pneumonia	+2	3+	2+	2+	—	Disseminated coccidio-domycosis

M, male; F, female; PPH, primary pulmonary hypertension; CHD, congenital heart disease with secondary pulmonary hypertension; ARDS, adult respiratory distress syndrome; OB, obliterative bronchiolitis.

Grading: –, negative; 1 to 3+, intensity of finding; [a], underlying cause of death; [b], acute (terminal) cause of death.

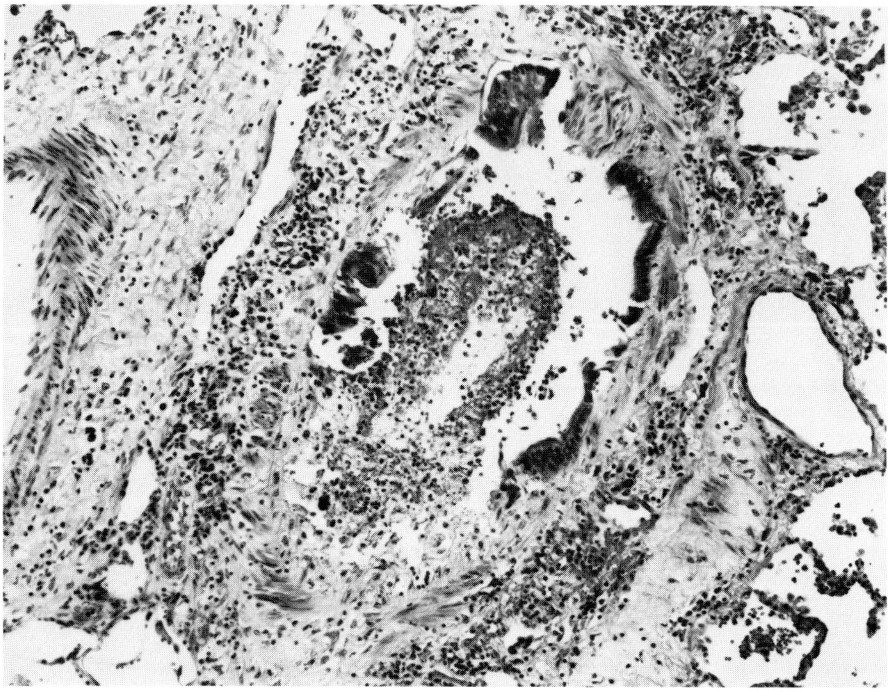

Figure 6.3
Acute bronchiolitis. Small distal bronchiole with an acute and chronic inflammatory infiltrate traversing its wall. The epithelium is denuded, and there is a fibrinous exudate within the lumen (hematoxylin-eosin ×250).

Figure 6.4
Acute bronchiolitis obliterans. A. Longitudinal section of bronchiole with its muscularis infiltrated by acute and chronic inflammatory cells. The lumen is occluded by an inflamed polypoid plug of granulation tissue. The epithelium is focally intact but in some areas has undergone squamous metaplasia (left) (hematoxylin-eosin ×100). B. Transverse section showing similar features (×500).

A

B

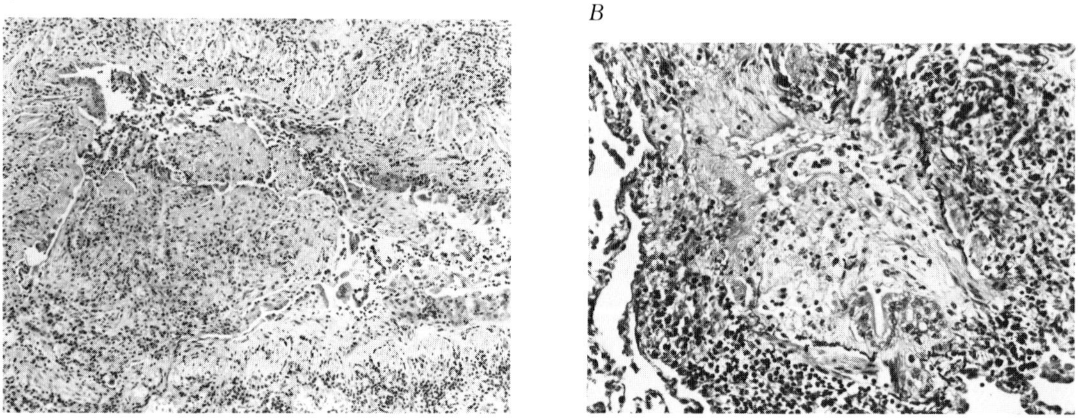

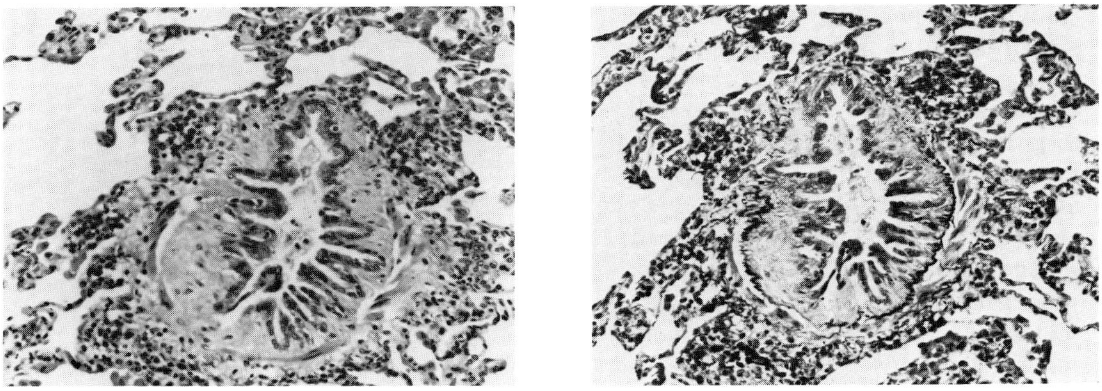

A *B*

Figure 6.5
Bronchiolitis obliterans, cicatricial phase. A. The bronchiolar lumenal diameter has been compromised by submucosal scar tissue containing a chronic inflammatory cell infiltrate. (hematoxylin-eosin ×200.) B. The elastic van Giesen stain highlights the original luminal diameter by staining the residual elastic lamella just internal to the smooth muscle (×200).

cartilaginous airways on specimen bronchograms (Fig. 6.8) [12]. The acute peripheral tapering and pruning of the bronchi contrasted with the paradoxical obliteration and luminal constriction of the terminal respiratory bronchioles. Recent studies have suggested that large airway inflammation may be a good marker for small airway disease in this patient cohort.

Figure 6.6
Bronchiolitis obliterans, cicatricial phase. A. Completely scarred bronchiole without a residual lumen (hematoxylin-eosin ×200). B. The elastic van Giesen stain highlights the presence of its elastic lamina and shows its companion arteriole (×200).

A *B*

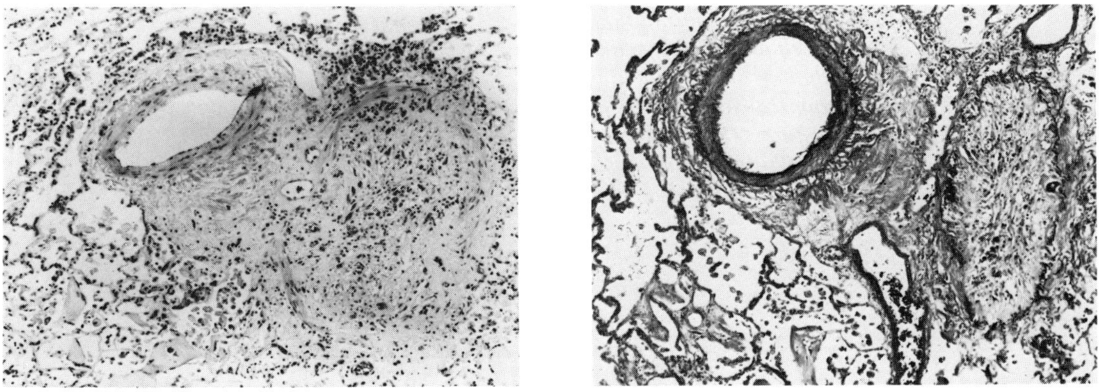

Visceral Pleura Although one would expect extensive pleural fibrosis due to implantation of a massive heart-lung bloc, pleural adhesions were not prominent. They occurred in 19% of patients, and a dense uniform adherence, similar to fibrothorax, was seen in only two patients, who are not functionally incapacitated. These adhesions usually formed over the posterior-basal portions of the lung and seemed to correlate with the degree of operative hemorrhage. Pleural scars frequently extended down the interlobular septa, giving the lung a latticework-like pattern of coarse scarring at low magnification.

Interstitium Initial studies, particularly by Veith et al. [2], suggested that diffuse interstitial fibrosis and honeycombing were a consequence of pulmonary rejection. This has not been our experience. The parenchymal scarring that was identified in our cases was focal and usually associated with bronchiectasis or overlying pleural adhesions. A mild interstitial chronic inflammatory infiltrate was rarely seen and we believe it is probably associated with a resolving viral or bacterial pneumonia which occurred during the clinical course.

Infections Both the Stanford and Pittsburgh groups have reported an incidence of infectious complications in over 85% of heart-lung recipients [35,46]. Between 67% and 89% of them involved the lung or thoracic cavity, and they were overwhelmingly bacterial (71%) [35]. Gram-negative bacilli, particularly *Serratia, Pseudomonas, Bacteroides,* and *Hemophilus* sp., comprised 66% of these pulmonary infections [35]. These episodes usually occurred within the first 6 weeks after surgery. Forty-two percent of patients with transplants also developed cytomegalovirus (CMV) infection, while 8% had episodes of cutaneous herpes simplex infection [46]. In the Pittsburgh experience, a much higher incidence of *Pneumocystis pneumonia* was observed [13,47], and all recipients not receiving antibiotic prophylaxis apparently developed pneumocystosis. Two-thirds of infections were also diagnosed unexpectedly during routine bronchoalveolar lavage. This incidence is in marked contrast to the Stanford experience, in which pneumocystosis was a rare infestation in this patient cohort [35].

In our autopsy study of heart-lung recipients, *Candida* pneumonia and tracheitis (Fig. 6.10) was noted in three patients and herpes tracheobronchitis was found in two others [30]. One patient each died of aspergillosis, coccidiodomycosis, and pneumocystotis. Except for two patients, long-term survivors died of progressive unrelenting bronchiolitis obliterans.

Other Findings In addition to the pulmonary findings, cardiac abnormalities have been observed. In contrast to those patients dying in the immediate postoperative period or without bronchiolitis obliterans, patients with bronchiolitis obliterans are predisposed to develop accelerated coronary arteriosclerosis [42]. Although two of thirteen patients without OB had mild disease, all six patients with OB at autopsy had marked coronary abnormalities, including one patient who died of a massive left ventricular myocardial infarction. This vascular disease was manifested by a concentric fibroelastosis occurring on the inner aspect of an intact internal elastica. In

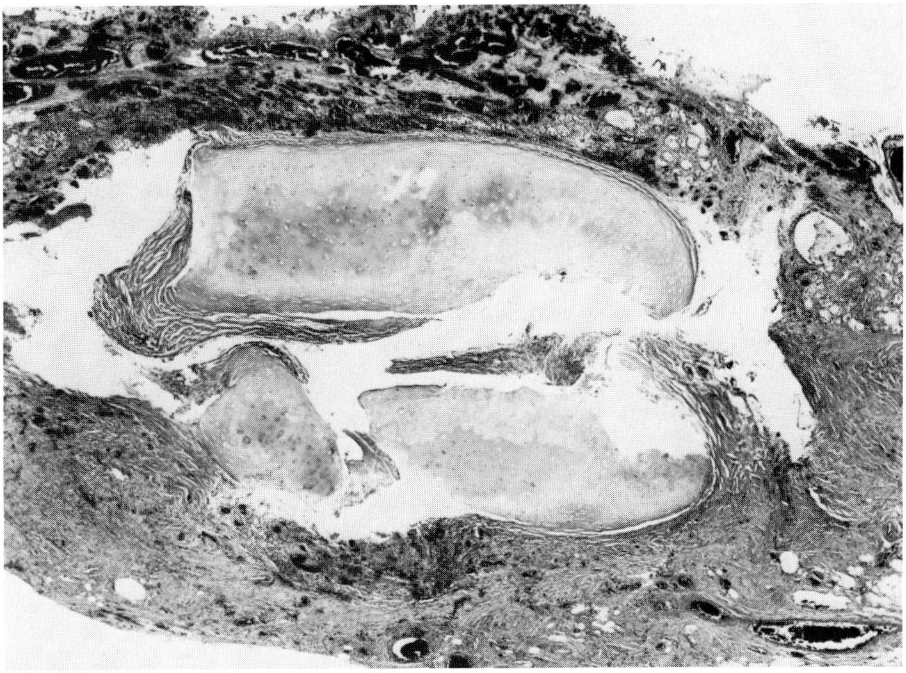

A

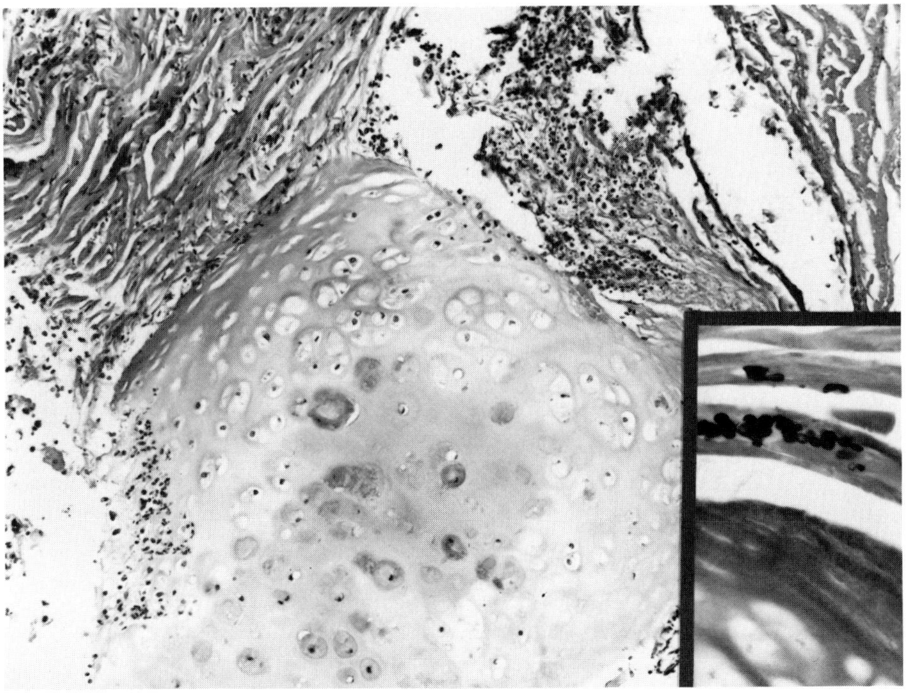

B

Figure 6.10

Acute tracheitis with Candida. *The low-power photomicrograph (A) shows the tracheal anastomosis surrounded by granulation tissue containing dilated vessels. There is an acute chondritis (B) with a Gomori's methenamine silver stain showing the presence of yeast forms consistent with* Candida *organisms (insert). (A. hematoxylin-eosin ×20; B. hematoxylin-eosin ×200; insert: gram stain ×400.)*

one case an active endovasculitis was observed. Two of six patients with OB had myocardial infarcts at autopsy; the remainder showed patchy fibrosis of uncertain etiology. The coronary arterial changes were closely related to vascular disease of the pulmonary arteries and veins and, as in renal and cardiac transplantation, have been attributed to chronic graft rejection. The vascular changes in the heart and lungs did not correlate with the number of acute rejection episodes in either organ.

Renal abnormalities attributed to cyclosporine A therapy were noted in all long-term survivors. This consisted of focal glomerular sclerosis, tubular atrophy, and interstitial fibrosis with rare mononuclear inflammatory cell infiltrates.

Heart-lung recipients also appear to be at increased risk for Epstein-Barr virus–induced lymphoproliferations [48,49]. At Pittsburgh we have also seen four patients develop pseudoaneurysms of the aorta at the anastomotic site, which has led to rupture and rapid exsanguination.

Clinical Implications

The development of an animal model and the initiation of cyclosporine immunosuppression has contributed significantly to the success of heart-lung transplantation. Cardiopulmonary transplantation has proved to be the most successful therapy for patients with primary and secondary pulmonary hypertension and has also been used in select cases of end-stage interstitial lung disease, which comprises 15% of all lung disease in the United States. After initial failures due to surgical complications (primarily hemorrhage), heart-lung transplantation has resulted in a return to normal life-style in more than two thirds of patients. Experience with this procedure has resulted in numerous clinical and pathologic lessons.

The most important factor in survival is patient selection. Individuals who have had median sternotomies, extensive operations for congenital heart disease, and bilateral thoracotomies are at high risk for intraoperative and perioperative hemorrhage from adhesions and collaterals and are now considered poor candidates for transplantation. Similarly, those potential recipients with extensive pleural adhesions should be carefully evaluated. An additional surgical factor that has been especially espoused by the Pittsburgh group is the need for wrapping the tracheal anastomosis with an omental pedicle to prevent tracheal dehiscence [13]. This complication, which was noted in the precyclosporine, high-steroid-dose era, has ceased to be a major complication in recent years but should be considered as longer graft ischemic times are recorded with distant procurement of organs.

Diagnosis and Management

The diagnosis of acute pulmonary rejection has remained a clinical enigma. Although a usual clinical presentation of dyspnea, shortness of breath, and pyrexia with progressive lung opacification despite antibiotic therapy has been recognized, the histologic diagnosis is extremely difficult [12]. Perivascular lymphocytic infiltrates are not specific for acute pulmonary rejection but can be seen in a variety of hypersensitivity and infectious processes. Similarly, the use of bronchoalveolar lavage, lymphocyte cytotoxicity studies, and nuclear scans, particularly ventilation-perfusion studies, have not individually resolved this diagnostic dilemma. Endomyocardial biopsy has not been reliable in predicting pulmonary rejection. Consequently, the diagnosis of acute graft rejection requires close and continued interaction and consultation between cardiopulmonary surgeons, pulmonologists, and pathologists, and for the most part the diagnosis is one which requires exclusion of infectious processes. Empiric therapy with intravenous glucocorticoids will confirm the clinicopathologic diagnosis.

Bronchiolitis Obliterans OB has presented a major problem in the development of post-transplant airway disease [12,30]. Its emergence in half the patients at Stanford University and the University of Pittsburgh has raised questions about its pathogenesis. Potential causes are listed in Table 6.3 and will be discussesd sequentially.

Our favored hypothesis is that OB represents a manifestation of chronic pulmonary rejection, despite a lack of absolute correlation of its development with the number of clinical acute pulmonary or cardiac rejection episodes [11,12]. OB has been frequently documented in patients with immunologic lung disease, e.g., collagen vascular diseases, and Geddes et al. [50] and Epler et al. [51] have shown an association with rheumatoid arthritis, Sjøgren's syndrome, eosinophilic fasciitis, and systemic lupus erythematosus. An immunologic mechanism has been proposed as the underlying reaction. Although this provides background evidence that immunologic phenomena can cause bronchiolar disease, recent studies by Ralph et al. [52] and Wyatt et al. [53] indicate that a minority of bone marrow transplant recipients have developed rapidly progressive and severe obstructive lung disease associated with sinusitis, bronchitis, and esophagitis. Beschorner et al. have described a similar airway process, lymphocytic bronchiolitis, which they propose as a direct graft-vs-host attack on bronchial epithelium [54].

OB in heart-lung recipients is probably due to recipients' lymphocytes attacking the foreign bronchiolar epithelium [55,56]. Evidence shows that

Table 6.3
Potential causes of bronchiolitis obliterans

Chronic rejection
Recurrent or persistent infection
Impaired mucociliary clearance—abnormal ciliary function and mucous chemistry
Inadequate vascular supply to trachea and bronchi
Drugs: cyclosporine
Chronic aspiration

the donor bronchiolar epithelium expresses larger amounts and different classes of type I and II major histocompatibility complex (MHC) antigens, perhaps due to viral infections, and that this phenomenon is closely tied to OB [34,57]. Animal studies have also demonstrated the increased expression of class II antigens as part of the rejection process [58]. Further evidence that the bronchiolar epithelium may be a target of the rejection process and that this is related to OB comes from the following: (1) recent animal studies [59] have shown that the extent of bronchiolar damage is related to the degree of histocompatibility mismatch and (2) the longest surviving heart-lung transplant patient who did not develop OB also had the closest HLA match when compared with other recipients [60]. Evidence also comes from lavage lymphocyte cytotoxicity studies which show that the presence and titers of a positive primed lymphocyte test correlates with histologic and functional obstructive airway disease.

We have alluded to the influence of infectious agents in the development of OB. Certainly the most common cause of OB in the normal population is bacterial and viral infestation [61–64]. Respiratory syncytial virus, adenovirus, and parainfluenza virus are frequent causes of bronchiolitis in children, while *Hemophilus influenzae*, *Legionella* sp., *Mycoplasma* sp., and *Chlamydia* sp. are usual adult pathogens. Many OB patients experienced repeated upper and lower respiratory tract infections, and chronic and persistent epithelial injury could result in bronchiolitis obliterans. They also may induce immunogenic antigens on the respiratory epithelium or nonspecifically upregulate the alloreactive response of resting, primed lymphocytes. Infectious episodes may be worsened by these hosts' greater susceptibility and impaired defense mechanisms. Bronchiolar injury may subsequently initiate a cycle of progressive dysfunction in that chronic inflammation results in squamous metaplasia, loss of mucociliary clearance, mucus stasis and plugging, and therefore a propensity for secondary infection. CMV has been a particularly suspect agent, especially since an association between CMV infection and OB has been noted in bone marrow transplant recipients. In general, however, OB has been a rare pathologic manifestation of CMV infection. Nevertheless, an analysis of the Stanford experience [65] showed that patients with CMV pneumonitis appeared to be at risk for developing OB, although patients who seroconverted were not. At Pittsburgh, previous pneumocystis and EBV infection are harbingers of OB. It is possible that, as has been shown in animals [66], the additional antigenic stimulation caused by infectious agents might provoke or worsen the rejection response and lead to OB.

Another less likely cause of OB includes impaired healing of the bronchial tree due to ligation of the bronchial circulation. With their vascular supply compromised, injured bronchi and bronchioles may develop smoldering reparative responses to injurous agents. The young plugs of granulation tissue that destroy the cartilage and smooth muscle walls of large airways (resulting in bronchiectasis) and obliterate the lumens of terminal bronchioles (bronchiolitis obliterans) may be a manifestation of this delayed and inadequate healing process, although such changes have not been observed in isolated nonimmunosuppressed, noninfected animals [60]. This is supported by the marked degenerative changes seen in the cartilage plates of large bronchi—calcification, ossification, and shaggy irregular perichondrial surfaces.

Drugs, especially penicillamine [67,68], are also well-known causes of OB. Cyclosporine has a well-recognized fibroproliferative effect that, if inflicted on bronchioles, would cause progressive narrowing and obliteration [69]. We doubt this possibility, however, since airway disease has not been reported in renal or cardiac transplant recipients receiving this drug.

Finally, OB could result from denervation of the bronchial tree. The cough reflex beyond the tracheal anastomosis is lost, and self-initiated pulmonary toilet is limited. Inadequate clearance of secretions, along with impaired action of the ciliary escalator, may result in mucostasis, a fertile soil for colonization by infectious agents. Again, such changes have not been observed in animal models [59].

Although probably a manifestation of rejection (either the result of multiple unrecognized acute rejection episodes or a form of "chronic rejection"), OB may appear anywhere in the clinical course of heart-lung recipients, from 2 to 35 months postoperatively. Airway toilet programs and antibiotic, bronchodilator, and physiotherapy have not resulted in a sustained clinical remission. Only one fifth of patients responded to augmented steroid therapy [11]. Therefore, when OB develops, an immediate therapeutic trial of high-dose corticosteroids or antilymphocyte globulin is indicated, once infection has been adequately excluded. Patients with OB can also be effectively monitored by transbronchial biopsy, allowing early diagnosis [17].

Other Pathologic Findings One additional morphologic finding noted in cardiopulmonary transplants, which does not appear to relate to the occurrence of OB, is accelerated intimal fibroelastosis of pulmonary arteries and veins [12,42]. In addition, concentric intimal fibrosis of the coronary arteries of all patients has been observed [34,69]. In both heart and renal transplant patients, this vascular disease, sometimes associated with an endovasculitis, has been attributed to chronic graft rejection [70–74]. The perivascular nature of infiltrates and evidence of endothelial injury in acute rejection supports this theory and suggests that the fibrotic lesions may be due to repetitive bouts of rejection. Still, only one patient has developed increased pulmonary vascular resistance. Nonetheless, careful monitoring of pulmonary pressures may be necessary as the length of recipient survival increases.

Course and Prognosis Despite the bronchiolar and vascular changes noted above, over half the patients at Stanford University and the University of Pittsburgh have returned to normal life-styles from a preoperative state of end-stage respiratory failure [11,13]. Function studies in this group have shown relatively normal pulmonary mechanics and gas exchange with only a slight restrictive deficit [11,37]. A continuing problem, however, is renal toxicity due to cyclosporine (100% of the patients). The need to reduce dosage, carefully monitor drug levels, and find alternative therapies cannot be overemphasized.

Future Directions

The surgical and therapeutic success with heart-lung transplantation has reinitiated work with single lung transplantation begun in the 1960s but terminated in the early 1970s. Veith and colleagues [7], along with Toronto Lung Transplant Group, have recently reported new successes in this field [75–77]. For patients without severe heart disease secondary to persistent pulmonary dysfunction, unilateral lung transplants have several advantages. One lung is sufficient for satisfactory pulmonary function, and because of the paucity of donors, the second could be used for an additional recipient (and the heart used for a third). Avoidance of heart transplantation eliminates cardiac-related complications, including advanced coronary artery disease associated with chronic rejection. Finally, transplantation from donors with only one diseased lung should be possible. To our knowledge, the pathologic disturbances in unilateral lung transplants are similar to heart-lung transplants, except for infrequent reports of OB.

In summary, heart-lung transplantation has proved to be the most beneficial therapy for individuals with primary or secondary pulmonary hypertension. Unfortunately, a significant proportion have developed severe obstructive changes on ventilatory studies corresponding to OB pathologically. In addition, accelerated atherosclerosis has been observed. These two sequelae are probably a manifestation of chronic pulmonary graft rejection, and their occurrence may be a severe limitation in the future success of heart-lung transplantation. Future efforts should be directed at identifying more sensitive means of diagnosing rejection, elucidating the mechanism of post-transplant OB, developing alternative immunosuppressants to cyclosporine, and finding suitable methods to preserve donor organs in vitro.

References

1. Veith F, Sinha S, Blumcke S, et al. Nature and evolution of lung allograft rejection with and without immunosuppression. J Thorac Cardiovasc Surg 1972;63:509–20.
2. Veith F, Koerner S, Siegelman S, et al. Diagnosis and reversal of rejection in experimental and clinical lung allografts. Ann Thorac Surg 1973;16:172–81.
3. Joseph W, Morton D. Morphologic alterations in the transplanted primate lung. Surg Gynecol Obstet 1971;133:821–5.
4. Baker R, Sabanayagan P, Zarins C, et al. Functional and morphologic changes after lung allografting in baboons. Surg Gynecol Obstet 1973;137:650–4.
5. Byers J, Sabanayagan P, Zarins C, et al. Pathologic changes in baboon lung allografts. Ann Surg 1973;178:754–60.
6. Halasz N, Catanzaro A, Trummer M, et al. Transplantation of the lung: correlation of physiologic, immunologic and histologic findings. J Thorac Cardiovasc Surg 1973;66:581–7.

7. Veith F, Kamholz S, Mollenkoph F, Montefusco C. Lung transplantation 1983. Transplantation 1983;34:271–8.
8. Reitz B, Burton N, Jamieson S, et al. Heart and lung transplantation: autotransplantation and allotransplantation in primates with extended survival. J Thorac Cardiovasc Surg 1980;80:360–72.
9. Reitz B. Heart-lung transplantation: a review. Heart Transplant 1982;1:291–7.
10. Jamieson S, Baldwin J, Stinson E, et al. Clinical heart-lung transplantation. Transplantation 1984;37:81–4.
11. Burke CM, Theodore J, Baldwin JC, et al. Twenty-eight cases of human heart-lung transplantation. Lancet 1986;1:517–9.
12. Yousem S, Burke C, Billingham M. Pathologic pulmonary alterations in long-term human heart-lung transplantation. Hum Pathol 1985;16:911–23.
13. Griffith BP, Hardesty RL, Trento A, et al. Heart-lung transplantation: lessons learned and future hopes. Ann Thorac Surg 1987;43:6.
14. Burke C, Theodore J, Dawkins K, et al. Post-transplant obliterative bronchiolitis and other late lung sequelae in human heart-lung transplantation. Chest 1984;86:824–9.
15. Veith FJ, Norin AJ, Montefusco CM, et al. Cyclosporine A in experimental lung transplantation. Transplantation 1981;32:474–81.
16. Prop JM, Ehrie MG, Crapo JD, et al. Reimplantation response in isografted rat lungs. J Thorac Cardiovasc Surg 1984;87:702–11.
17. Yousem SA, Paradis IL, Dauber JH, Griffith BP. Efficacy of transbronchial lung biopsy in the diagnosis of bronchiolitis obliterans in heart-lung transplant recipients. Transplantation, 1989;47:893–5.
18. Novitsky D, Cooper DKC, Rose AG, Reichart B. Acute isolated pulmonary rejection following transplantation of the heart and both lungs. Ann Thorac Surg 1986;42:180–4.
19. McGregor CB, Baldwin JG, Jamieson SW, et al. Isolated pulmonary rejection after combined heart-lung transplantation. J Thorac Cardiovasc Surg 1985;90:623–30.
20. Glanville AR, Imoto E, Baldwin JC, et al. The role of right ventricular endomyocardial biopsy in the long term management of heart-lung transplant recipients. Heart Transplant 1987;6:357–61.
21. Prop JM, Tazelaar HD, Billingham ME. Rejection of combined heart-lung transplants in rats: function and pathology. Am J Pathol 1987;127:97–105.
22. Prop JM, Wildevuur CRH, Nieuwenhuis P. Lung allograft rejection in the rat. III. Corresponding morphological rejection phases in various rat strain combinations. Transplantation 1985;40:132–8.
23. Prop JM, Wildevuur CRH, Nieuwenhuis P. Lung allograft rejection in the rat. II. Specific immunological properties of lung grafts. Transplantation 1985;40:126–31.
24. Halloran PF, Wadgymar A, Anteuried P. The regulation of expression of major histocompatibility complex products. Transplantation 1986;41:413–20.
25. Zeevi A, Fung JJ, Paradis IL, et al. Lymphocytes of bronchoalveolar lavages from heart-lung transplant recipients. Heart Transplant 1985;4:417–21.
26. Gryzan S, Paradis IL, Hardesty RL, et al. Bronchoalveolar lavage in heart-lung transplantation. Heart Transplant 1985;4:414–6.
27. Prop JM, Nieuwenhuis P, Wildevuur CRH. Lung allograft rejection in the rat. I. Accelerated rejection caused by graft lymphocytes. Transplantation 1985;40: 25–40.
28. Prop JM, Kuijpers K, Peterson AH, et al. Why are lung allografts more vigorously rejected than hearts? Heart Transplant 1985;4:433–6.

29. Veith F, Hagstrom J. Alveolar manifestations of rejection: an important cause of the poor results with human lung transplantation. Ann Surg 1972;175:336–48.
30. Tazelaar HD, Yousem S. Pathologic findings in heart-lung transplantation: an autopsy study. Hum Pathol 1988;19:1403–16.
31. Marck KW, Prop JM, Wildevuur CRH, Nieuwenhuis P. Lung transplantation in the rat. Histopathology of left lung isolated allografts. Heart Transplant 1985;4:263–6.
32. Bieber C, Hunt S, Schwinn D, et al. Complications in long-term survivors of cardiac transplantation. Transplant Proc 1981;13:207–14.
33. Billingham ME. Some recent advances in cardiac pathology. Hum Pathol 1979;10:367–86.
34. Paradis IL, Marrari M, Zeevi A, et al. HLA phenotype of lung lavage cells following heart-lung transplantation. Heart Transplant 1985;4:422–9.
35. Brooks RG, Hofflin JM, Jamieson SW, et al. Infectious complications in heart-lung transplant recipients. Am J Med 1985;79:412–22.
36. Dummer JS, Bahnson HT, Griffith BP, et al. Infections in patients on cyclosporine and prednisone following cardiac transplantation. Transplant Proc 1983;15:2779–83.
37. Theodore J, Jamieson SW, Burke CM, et al. Physiologic aspect of human heart-lung transplantation. Chest 1984;86:349–57.
38. Skeens J, Furham C, Yousem SA. Bronchiectasis and bronchiolitis obliterans in heart-lung transplant recipients: radiologic and pathologic correlation. Am J Radiol, 1989;153:253–6.
39. Allen MD, Burke CM, McGregor CGA, et al. Steroid responsive bronchiolitis after human heart-lung transplantation. J Thorac Cardiovasc Surg 1986;92: 449–51.
40. Glanville AR, Baldwin JC, Burke CM, et al. Obliterative bronchiolitis after heart-lung transplantation: apparent arrest by augmented immunosuppression. Ann Intern Med 1987;107:300–4.
41. Gosink B, Friedman P, Liebow A. Bronchiolitis obliterans. AJR 1973;117: 816–32.
42. Yousem SA, Paradis IL, Dauber J, et al. Vascular abnormalities in long term heart-lung transplant recipients. Transplantation 1989;47:564–9.
43. Heath D, Edwards JE. The pathology of hypertensive pulmonary vascular disease. A description of six grades of structural changes in the pulmonary arteries with special reference to congenital septal defects. Circulation 1958;18:533–62.
44. Wagenvoort CA, Wagenvoort N. Pathology of pulmonary hypertension. New York: Wiley, 1977;1–80.
45. Harris P, Heath D. The human pulmonary circulation. Its form and function in health and disease, ed 2. New York: Churchill Livingstone, 1977;62–78.
46. Dummer JS, White LT, Ho M, et al. Morbidity of cytomegalovirus infection in recipients of heart or heart-lung transplant who received cyclosporine. J Infect Dis 1985;152:1182–91.
47. Gryzan S, Paradis IL, Zeevi A, et al. Unexpectedly high incidence of *Pneumocystis carinii* infection after lung-heart transplantation. Am Rev Respir Dis 1988;137:1268–74.
48. Yousem SA, Randhawa PS, Paradis IL, et al. Post-transplant lymphoproliferative disorders in heart-lung transplant recipients: primary presentation in the allograft. Hum Pathol 1989;20:361–9.
49. Randhawa PS, Yousem SA, Paradis IL, et al. The clinical spectrum, pathology and clonal analysis of Epstein-Barr virus associated lymphoproliferative disorders in heart-lung transplant recipients. Am J Clin Pathol, 1989;92:177–85.

50. Geddes D, Corrin B, Brewerton D, et al. Progressive airway obliteration in adults and its association with rheumatoid disease. Q J Med 1977;46:427–44.
51. Epler G, Snider G, Gaensler E, et al. Bronchiolitis and bronchitis in connective tissue disease. JAMA 1979;24:528–32.
52. Ralph D, Springmeyer S, Sullivan K, et al. Rapid progressive airflow obstruction in marrow transplant recipients. Am Rev Respir Dis 1984;129:641–4.
53. Wyatt S, Nunn J, Yin J, et al. Airways obstruction associated with graft-versus-host disease after bone marrow transplantation. Thorax 1984;39:887–94.
54. Beschorner W, Saral R, Hutchins G, et al. Lymphocytic bronchitis associated with graft-versus-host disease in recipients of bone marrow transplants. N Engl J Med 1978;299:1030–41.
55. Stein-Streilein J, Lipscomb M, Hart D, Darden A. Graft-versus-host reaction in the lung. Transplantation 1981;32:38–46.
56. Grebe S, Streilein J. Graft-versus-host reactions: a review. Adv Immunol 1976;22:119–42.
57. Glanville AR, Tazelaar HD, Theodore J, et al. The distribution of MHC class I and class II antigens on bronchial epithelium. Am Rev Respir Dis 1989; 139:330–4.
58. Romaniuk A, Prop J, Petersen AH, et al. Increased expression of class II MHC-antigens in rejecting and cyclosporine-treated rat lung allografts. Transplantation 1989;44:209–20.
59. Tazelaar HD, Prop J, Nieuwenhuis P, et al. Airway pathology in the transplanted rat lung. Am J Clin Pathol 1986;86:384. (Abstr.)
60. Harjula A, Baldwin JC, Glanville AR, et al. HLA compatibility in heart-lung transplantation. Heart Transplant 1986;5:375. (Abstr.)
61. Wohl M, Chernick V. Bronchiolitis. Am Rev Respir Dis 1978;118:759–81.
62. Becroft D. Bronchiolitis obliterans, bronchioectasis and other sequelae of adenovirus type 21 infection in younger children. J Clin Pathol 1971;24:72–6.
63. Epler G, Colby T. The spectrum of bronchiolitis obliterans. Chest 1983;83: 161–2.
64. Moran T, Hellstrom H. Bronchiolitis obliterans. Arch Pathol 1958;66:691–707.
65. Burke CM, Glanville AR, Macoviak JA, et al. The spectrum of cytomegalovirus infection following human heart-lung transplantation. Heart Transplant 1986;5:267–72.
66. Prop J, Janset HM, Wildevuur CRH, Nieuwenhuis P. Lung allograft rejection in the rat. V. Inhaled stimuli aggravate the rejection response. Am Rev Respir Dis 1985;132:168–72.
67. Murphy K, Alkins C, Offer R, et al. Obliterative bronchiolitis in two rheumatoid arthritis patients treated with penicillamine. Arthritis Rheum 1981;24:557–60.
68. Herzog C, Miller R, Hoidal J. Bronchiolitis and rheumatoid arthritis. Am Rev Respir Dis 1981;124:636–9.
69. Myers B, Ross J, Newton L, et al. Cyclosporine A associated with chronic nephropathy: a potential irreversible renal injury. N Engl J Med 1984;311:699–721.
70. Griepp R, Stinson E, Bieber C, et al. Control of graft arteriosclerosis in human heart transplant recipients. Surgery 1977;81:262–70.
71. Crosnier B. The transplanted kidney. Contrib Nephrol 1977;7:177–346.
72. Busch G, Galvanek EG, Reynolds ES. Human renal allografts: analysis of lesions in long term survivals. Hum Pathol 1971;2:253–62.
73. Corson J. The pathologist and the kidney transplant. Pathol Annu 1972; 7:251–71.
74. Porter K. Renal transplantation. In: Heptinstall RH, ed. Pathology of the kidney. Boston: Little, Brown, 1974;171–252.

deemed necessary to obtain a biopsy. Thus our understanding of the causes of graft dysfunction and failure is limited and relies heavily on the clinical impression. The discussion in this chapter is based primarily on the transplantation experience at the University of Minnesota Hospital and Clinic [5–9], where 195 transplants were performed between July 1978 and July 1987; we will refer also to data from institutions with broad experience with neoprene [10–14] and prolamine [15–17] duct-injected pancreas transplants and to the Pancreas Transplant Registry [2,5]. Isolated pancreatic islet transplantation has not been successful in humans thus far [18] and will not be discussed.

Pretransplant Pathologic Findings

A biopsy of the donor pancreas at transplantation should be performed, just as donor kidney, liver, and cardiac biopsies are often obtained, to assess not only the viability of the donor organ but to establish the absence of preexisting disease. The donor pancreas biopsy usually shows minor ischemic damage and saponification of the peripancreatic adipose tissue. A small number of T lymphocytes and macrophages as well as dendritic reticulum cells are found in the endocrine and exocrine pancreatic tissues [8]. There is weak expression of class I major histocompatibility antigen by the islets and acini and more prominent staining by endothelium and duct epithelium

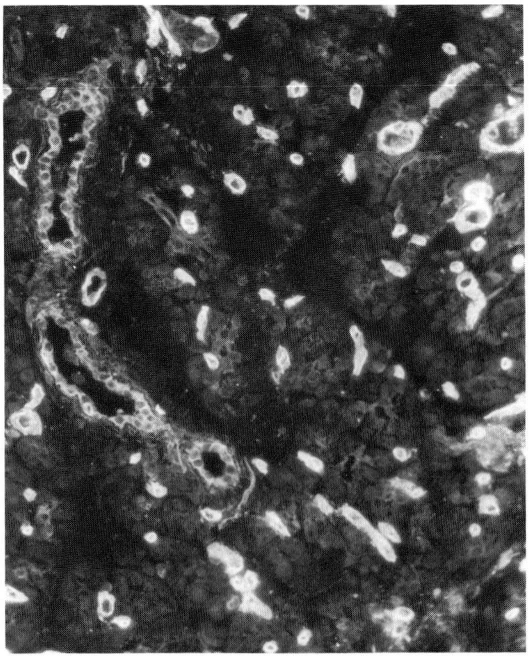

Figure 7.1
Normal pancreas. Class I antigen expression by the pancreatic acini is weak, while ducts, endothelium, and dendritic cells are strongly positive (immunofluorescence, class I antigen W6/32 ×144). (From Sibley RK, Sutherland DER. Pancreas transplantation. Am J Pathol 1987;128:151–70. With permission of the author and J.B. Lippincott.)

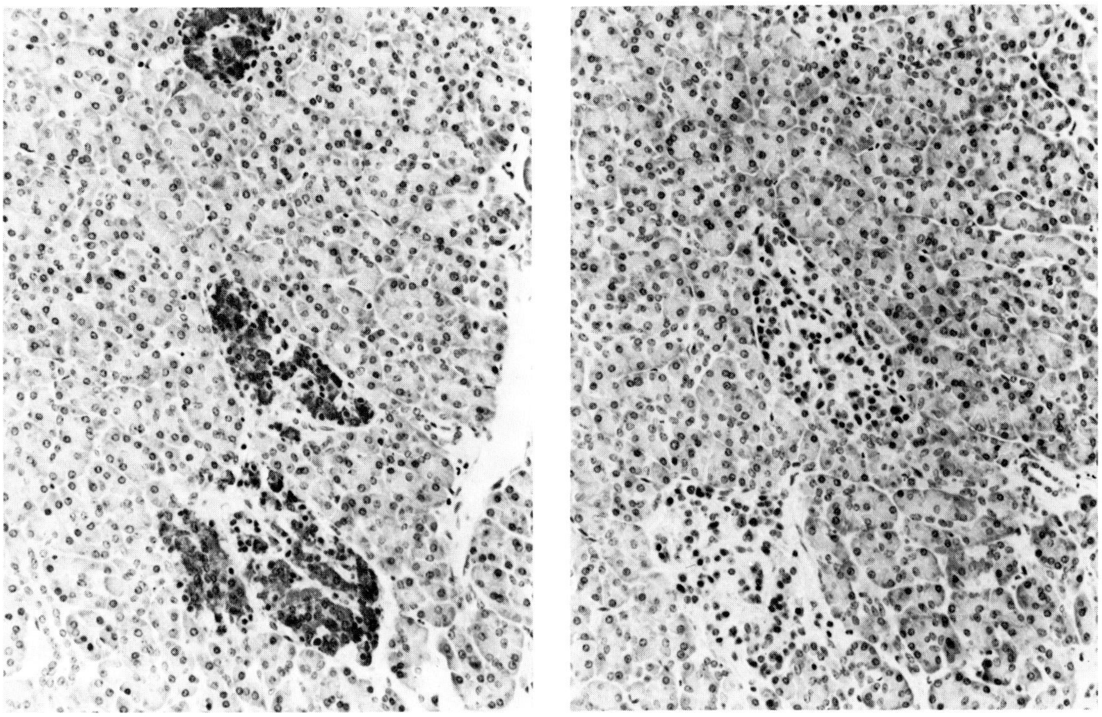

A *B*

Figure 7.2
Normal pancreas. A. The majority of endocrine cells in the normal islet are beta cells (immunoperoxidase, guinea pig antibovine insulin ×200). B. Alpha cells are distributed peripherally and along the intraislet vasculature (immunoperoxidase, rabbit antihuman glucagon ×200).

(Fig. 7.1). Class II antigen expression in the pancreas is normally limited to ductal epithelium and vascular endothelium, dendritic cells, lymphocytes, and macrophages [8,19,20].

Nearly all the native pancreases that were examined demonstrated a total lack of beta cells in the pancreatic islets [8], the cardinal feature of type I diabetes mellitus [21–23]. However, one patient in the Minnesota series was found to have type II diabetes [8].

To assess the status of the pancreatic islet properly, it is necessary to determine its structural integrity. On routine light microscopic examination the islets may appear normal, but with immunohistologic staining for pancreatic hormones they may display an abnormal number of alpha and beta cells. The normal islet of Langerhans in the beta-cell region consists of cells secreting insulin (65% to 75%) (Fig. 7.2A), glucagon (15% to 25%) (Fig. 7.2B), somatostatin (5% to 10%), and pancreatic polypeptide (1% to 3%), all arranged in a characteristic architectural distribution [24].

Post-Transplant Pathologic Findings

In pancreas transplantation, a large proportion of graft failures are "technical" [5], accounting for nearly 50% of 99 graft losses in the University of Minnesota series (Table 7.1). Acute and chronic rejection, recurrent disease, polymer duct injection–associated pancreatitis, viral-related graft hemor-

Table 7.1
Cause of 99 pancreatic graft losses (University of Minnesota)

	Functioning grafts	*Nonfunctioning grafts*
Technical		
Abscess	10	
Ascites	3	
Hemorrhage	2	
"Abscess"[a]	1	
"Pancreatitis[b]	9	
Thrombosis-infarction		23
Vesicocutaneous fistula	1	
Vascular anastomotic failure	1	
Viral		
Systemic cytomegalovirus	1	
Gastrointestinal/bladder hemorrhage	4	
Infarction — immunosuppression stopped		1
Polymer duct obstruction		
Silicone		4
Silicone/Infarction		1
Silicone/Rejection		9
Silicone/Rejection/Infarction		6
Prolamine		1
Other		
Type II diabetic[c]	1	
Death of patient	3	
Chronic pancreatitis/ Infarction		1
Recurrent disease		4
Recurrent disease/Rejection		4
Rejection/Thrombosis/ Infarction		6
Hyperacute rejection		1
Undetermined		1

[a]Mucinous cystadenoma found rather than abscess.
[b]Focal infarction rather than pancreatitis.
[c]High C-peptide level, but patient was insulin resistent.

rhage, patient death, and miscellaneous other causes account for the remaining graft losses.

Thrombosis-Infarction

One of the major "technical" factors accounting for pancreatic graft loss is arterial and venous thrombosis. Thrombosis with graft infarction occurred in 21% of failed grafts reported to the Pancreas Transplant Registry for 1983 to 1986 [5] and in nearly 25% of the Minnesota losses between 1978 and 1987. Arterial and venous thrombosis causes the sudden loss of graft function. It is a major early cause of graft loss, commonly occurring during the first day after transplantation. Kinking of the vessels and altered hemodynamics related to the implantation technique have been suggested as possible etiologies [8]. Other considerations include the release of pancreatic secretions, with damage of endothelium because of pretransplant ischemic damage, and manipulation of the graft during implantation. When arterial thrombosis is the cause of graft failure, the pancreas is gritty and yellow-white (Fig. 7.3A), whereas hemorrhagic infarction occurs with venous infarction (Fig. 7.3B).

Thrombosis with infarction may occur in the setting of acute pancreatitis [25,26]. One patient in the Minnesota series had clinical symptoms of acute

Figure 7.3
Thrombosis and infarction. Arterial thrombosis results in a shrunken white-yellow graft (A), while venous thrombosis results in a swollen, hemorrhagic organ (B).

A *B*

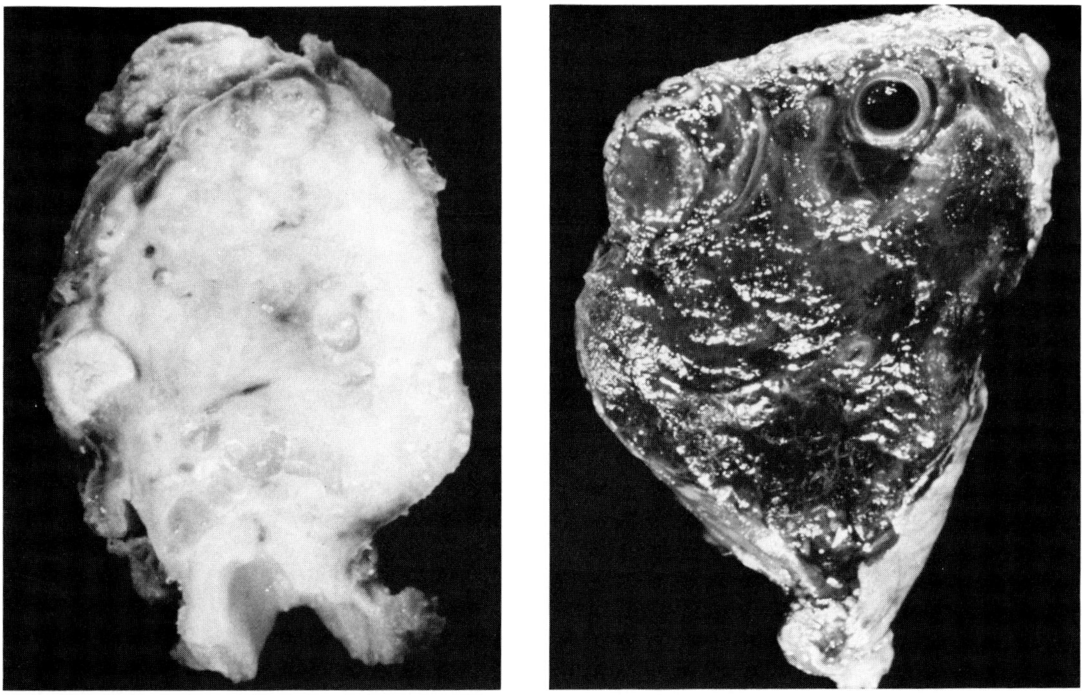

pancreatitis, but laparotomy demonstrated an infarcted graft and peripancreatic fat necrosis. It is conceivable that the thrombosis and infarction were preceded by acute pancreatitis, since fibrinoid necrosis and thrombosis of vessels occur as a complication of acute pancreatitis because of enzymatic digestion of vessel walls [25,26].

Focal-to-extensive graft necrosis commonly occurs in acute rejection. The pathogenesis may be the combination of endovasculitis related to rejection and rejection-induced pancreatitis with enzymatic damage to endothelial cells and pericytes.

Pancreatic grafts are not immune to chronic vascular rejection; symptoms manifest as slowly progressive hyperglycemia or acute graft failure. The latter event occurred in one patient from the Minnesota series 624 days after transplantation. This patient had no previous clinical evidence of graft malfunction. Although the sudden onset of severe hyperglycemia is dramatic, it is not as devastating as the sudden death of a cardiac transplantation patient who dies of an asymptomatic acute myocardial infarction secondary to severe chronic vascular rejection. One further cause of graft infarction is hyperacute rejection.

Pancreatitis

Acute Pancreatitis Nearly all patients have elevated serum amylase levels in the first few postoperative days; every graft that we have examined had saponification of peripancreatic adipose tissue, and examination of noninfarcted grafts in the first few days after transplantation revealed foci of acute pancreatitis. An elevated serum amylase does not necessarily indicate acute pancreatitis, since patients with acute rejection typically demonstrate transiently elevated serum amylase levels as well [6,7].

Three Minnesota patients with hyperamylasemia and hyperglycemia underwent pancreatic biopsy, which revealed acute pancreatitis in two patients and acute pancreatitis and acute rejection with focal infarction in the third patient. As is often the case in pancreas transplantation, there was no histologic explanation for the hyperglycemia in these three patients; the islets were entirely normal. The histologic features of acute pancreatitis in the transplant are inseparable from those occurring in the native pancreas (Fig. 7.4).

Chronic Pancreatitis Evidence of chronic pancreatitis is eventually found in all duct-obstructed grafts (see duct-injected grafts, below). Variable periductal and perilobular fibrosis, duct ectasia, acinar atrophy, and chronic inflammation without evidence of acute or chronic vascular rejection may also occur in enteric and bladder-drained grafts. The enteric or bladder-drained graft with obstruction initially has accentuated lobular architecture and a perilobular small lymphocytic, plasma cell, and macrophage infiltrate with edema and fibrosis. The larger ducts may show periductal concentric fibroplasia with edema and inflammation. The islets and vessels are usually normal. If the chronic pancreatitis is severe, extensive fibrosis and atrophy

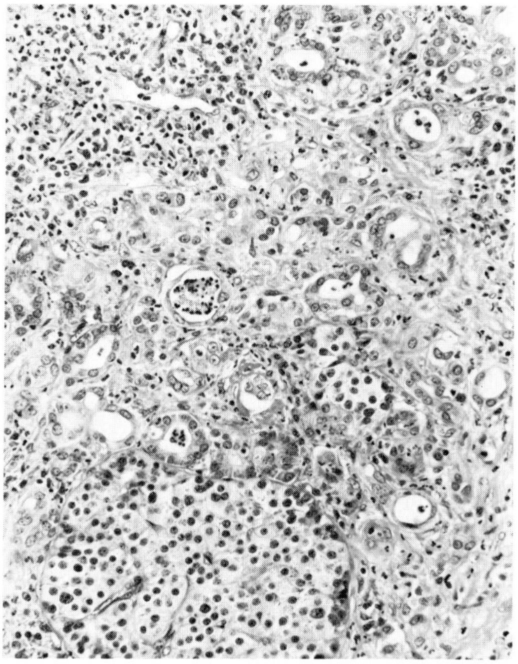

Figure 7.4
Acute pancreatitis is characterized by a predominantly acute polymorphonuclear leukocyte infiltrate and lesser numbers of plasma cells and lymphocytes (hematoxylin-eosin ×200).

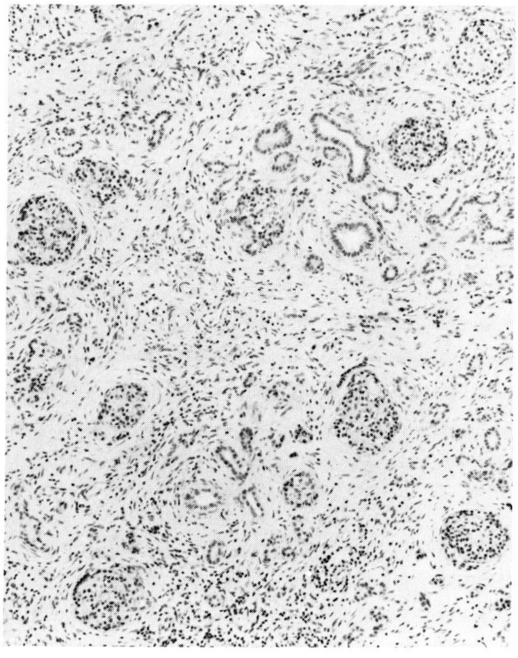

Figure 7.5
Chronic pancreatitis. This enteric-drained graft showed stenosis of the anastomotic site and extensive loss of the exocrine pancreas. Residual ducts, fibrosis, a modest inflammatory infiltrate, and coalesced islets are characteristic features (hematoxylin-eosin ×100).

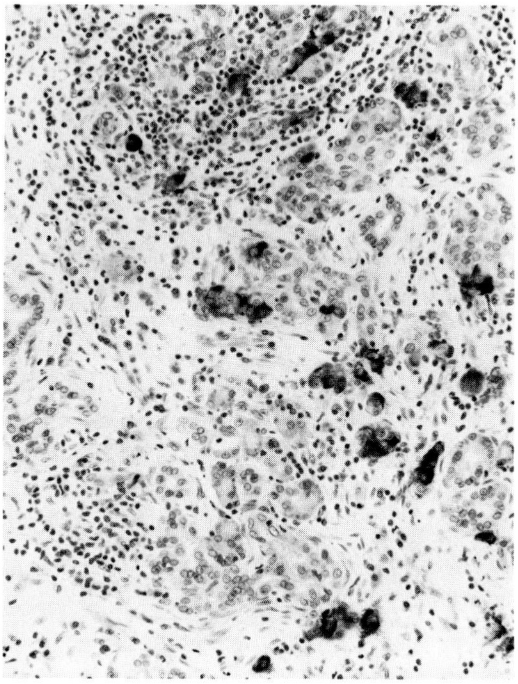

Figure 7.6
Chronic pancreatitis. Variable nesidioblastosis can be seen in grafts with both chronic rejection and chronic pancreatitis (immunoperoxidase, guinea pig antibovine insulin ×200).

of the exocrine pancreas are evident, and the islets coalesce (Fig. 7.5). The number of beta cells in the islets may be normal or decreased in number, a situation similar to that reported in the native pancreases of patients with severe, long-standing chronic pancreatitis [27]. In some cases the islets are fragmented and nesidioblastosis occurs (Fig. 7.6).

Endocrine Pancreas Only One open duct-drained graft, from which a biopsy was taken 4 years after transplantation because of mild hyperglycemia, remarkably demonstrated an endocrine pancreas only. The exocrine pancreas was completely atrophied, with minimal fibrosis and chronic inflammation (Fig. 7.7). Although there was mild loss of beta cells in some of the islets, the graft was still partially functioning 10 years after transplantation.

Rejection

Hyperacute Rejection Clinical and morphologic recognition of hyperacute rejection in the pancreas allograft is difficult because of the frequency of early graft loss due to arterial and venous thrombosis. A single patient in the Minnesota series had clinical and morphologic features compatible with hyperacute rejection. The patient developed graft failure in the first few hours after transplantation. The pretransplant crossmatch was negative, but the Panel Reactive Antibody was 80% when retested following removal of the graft, a feature not found with primary arterial and venous thrombosis. The

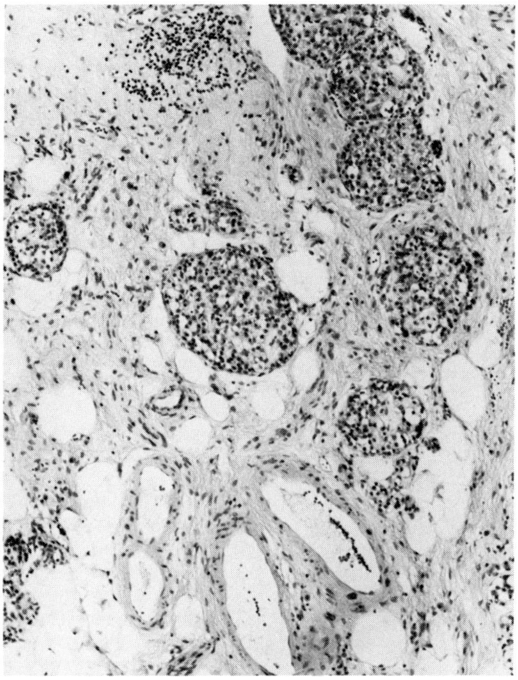

Figure 7.7
Endocrine only. This patient, with an open duct–drained graft, presented with mild postprandial hyperglycemia. Laparotomy revealed a nubbin of residual pancreas that demonstrated complete loss of the exocrine pancreas, minimal fibrosis, and chronic inflammation, normal blood vessels, and essentially normal but coalesced islets (hematoxylin-eosin × 100).

morphologic features were extensive fibrin thrombosis of small and medium-sized arteries, veins, and capillaries, with margination of polymorphonuclear leukocytes in the small vessels (Fig. 7.8A and B).

Acute Rejection Pancreatic graft function is monitored by measuring the plasma glucose and serum amylase levels. A presumptive diagnosis of acute rejection is made when there is a 25% increase above baseline fasting or postprandial glucose levels [28]. Hyperglycemia may, however, be drug induced, may occur because of recurrent disease, may be due to an infectious complication, or may occur in conjunction with polymer duct–obstructed chronic pancreatitis [8,28]. Acute irreversible hyperglycemia occurs with major vascular thrombosis and infarction of the graft.

Serum amylase levels are usually normal in the functioning pancreatic graft; thus a sudden increase of serum amylase followed by hyperglycemia suggests acute rejection [28,29]. Monitoring of urinary amylase has facilitated the diagnosis of early acute rejection in the bladder-drained graft [29,30,31]. Here, acute rejection is characterized by a sudden decrease of urinary amylase 1 to 2 days before hyperglycemia develops, and antirejection therapy has been quite successful in reversing the hyperglycemia of what is presumed to be early acute rejection in these grafts [30,31].

Acute rejection was thought to be the cause of graft loss in 37% of the failed procedures reported to the Pancreas Transplant Registry for 1983 to 1986 [5], but the diagnosis of acute rejection of the pancreatic graft is rarely made on the basis of biopsy because laparotomy is necessary to obtain the biopsy. In the Minnesota series, histologic evidence of acute rejection was

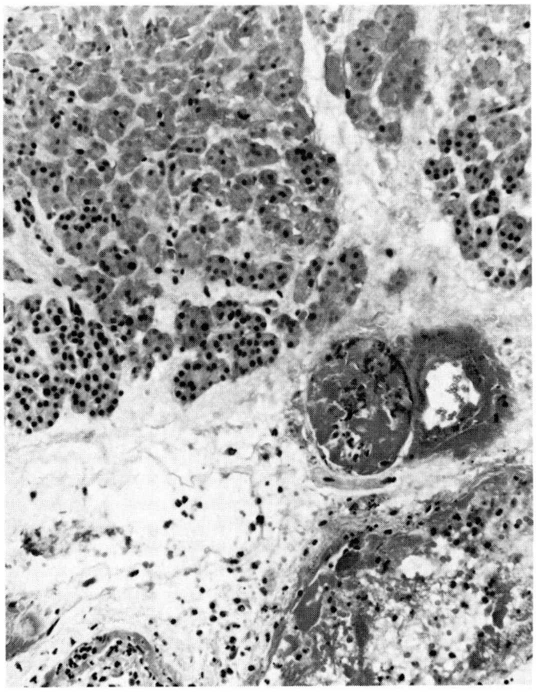
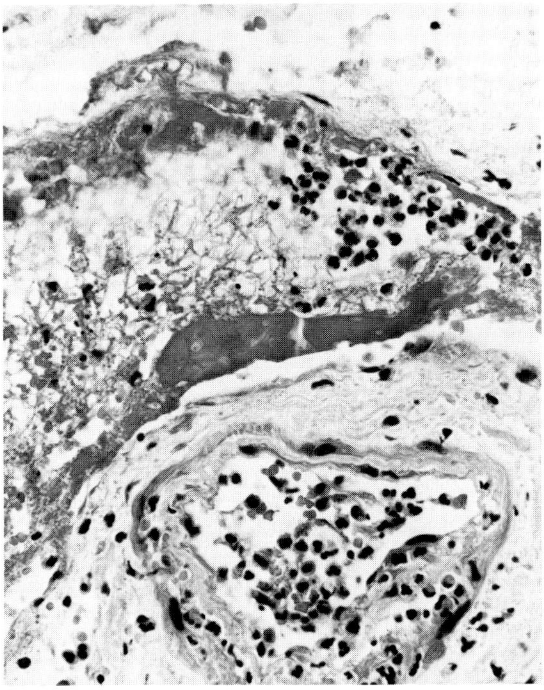

A *B*

Figure 7.8
Hyperacute rejection. This graft, removed 3 days after transplantation, never had adequate function. It is largely infarcted. The small vessels show thrombosis (A, hematoxylin-eosin ×200) and contain large numbers of polymorphonuclear leukocytes (B, hematoxylin-eosin ×400).

found in 36% of the grafts examined [8], and acute or chronic rejection was a contributing factor in 25% of graft failures [9].

Acute rejection is characterized by a pleomorphic infiltrate of polymorphonuclear and mononuclear cells that infiltrate the interstitial spaces, the epithelium of the exocrine pancreas (Fig. 7.9A and B), the walls of blood vessels (Fig. 7.10), and pancreatic nerves (Fig. 7.11). Similar features are reported in experimental models [32]. Although $CD8^+$ T lymphocytes predominate, $CD4^+$ and $CD38^+$ T lymphocytes, $CD68^+$ macrophages, and a few eosinophils, neutrophils, and plasma cells are also found. The lymphocytes consist of small cells with vesicular nuclei and prominent nucleoli (Fig. 7.12). The intensity of the cellular infiltrates in grafts with acute rejection is significantly increased when compared with donor and native biopsies and grafts with recurrent diabetes, duct-injected grafts without evidence of rejection, and grafts removed for technical reasons [8]. A few mononuclear cells may also be found in the islets. The "isletitis," beta-cell degranulation and destruction, if present, are best identified with immunohistochemical and electron microscopic studies because the infiltrates are usually sparse

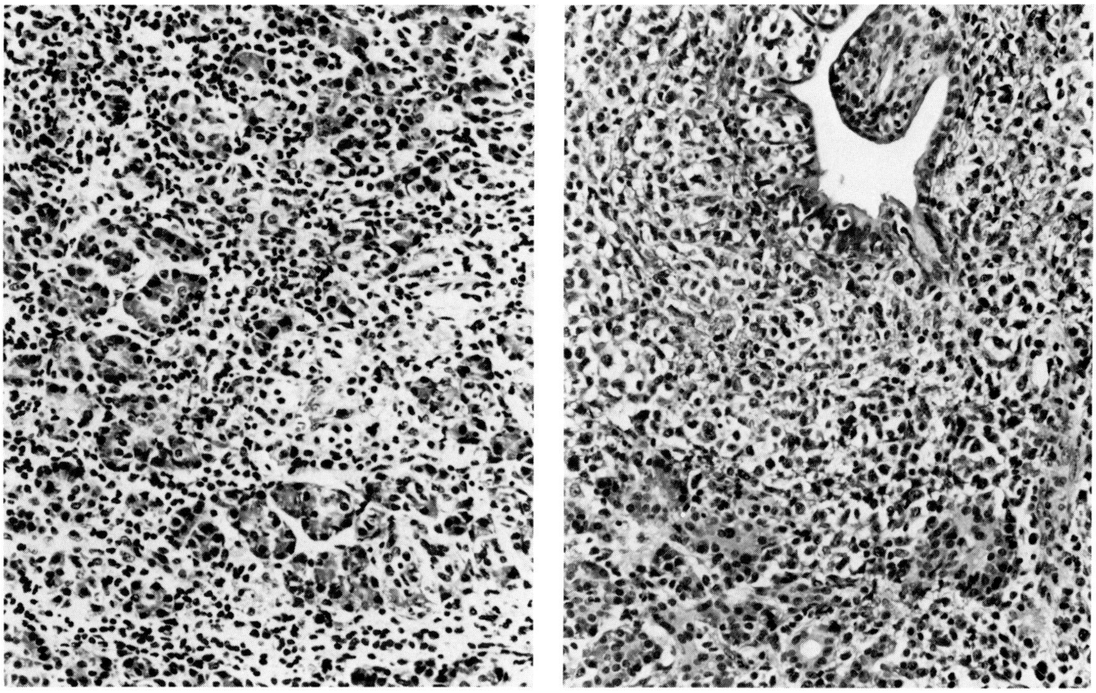

A *B*

Figure 7.9
Acute rejection. Patient presented with hyperglycemia, and biopsy demonstrated an intense diffuse mononuclear cell infiltrate within the exocrine pancreas. (A, hematoxylin-eosin ×200). The acinar and ductular epithelium was infiltrated by the mononuclear cells. (B, hematoxylin-eosin ×200).

and damage of beta cells difficult to identify. The exocrine pancreas typically shows varying degrees of zymogen granule loss, which is clinically manifested by decreased serum amylase production in patients with previously normal amylase levels.

The diagnosis of allograft rejection is supported if there is evidence of vascular involvement. As in other organ transplantation, mild and moderate acute vascular rejection are characterized by subendothelial infiltrates of transformed $CD8^+$ T lymphocytes and $CD68^+$ macrophages (see Fig. 7.10), and necrotizing vasculitis, fibrinoid necrosis, or thrombosis is characteristic of severe acute vascular rejection (Fig. 7.13).

The pathophysiology of fibrinoid necrosis and thrombosis of vessels that occurs in acute rejection may be either humoral or cellular mediated. Alternatively, it may be rejection-produced acinar damage, with release of zymogen products and digestion of vessel walls, which results in necrosis and thrombosis of the blood vessels. Whatever the etiology, these severe vascular lesions are associated with foci of graft necrosis that, if extensive, have unfavorable prognostic implications.

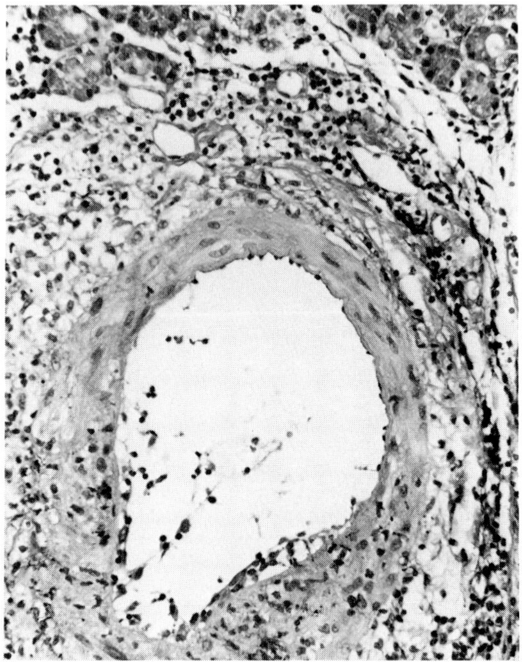

Figure 7.10
Acute vascular rejection. The finding of a mononuclear cell endovasculitis or necrotizing arteritis indicates acute rejection (hematoxylin-eosin ×200).

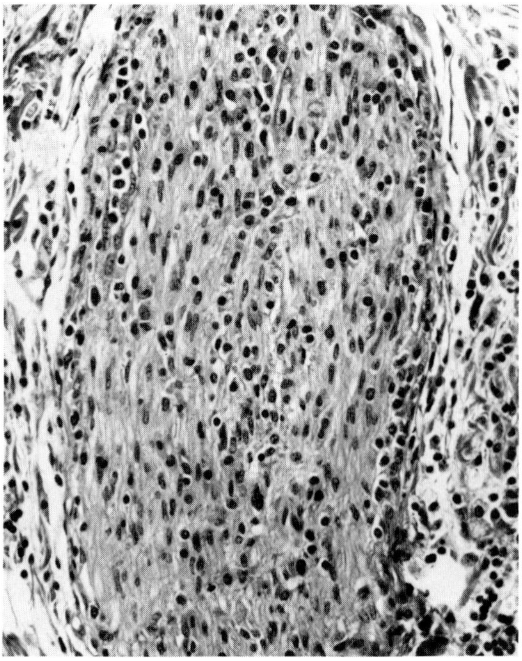

Figure 7.11
Acute rejection. The presence of a prominent mononuclear cell infiltrate of transformed lymphoid cells within graft nerves is helpful in identifying acute rejection in patients with severe chronic pancreatitis or chronic rejection (hematoxylin-eosin ×192).

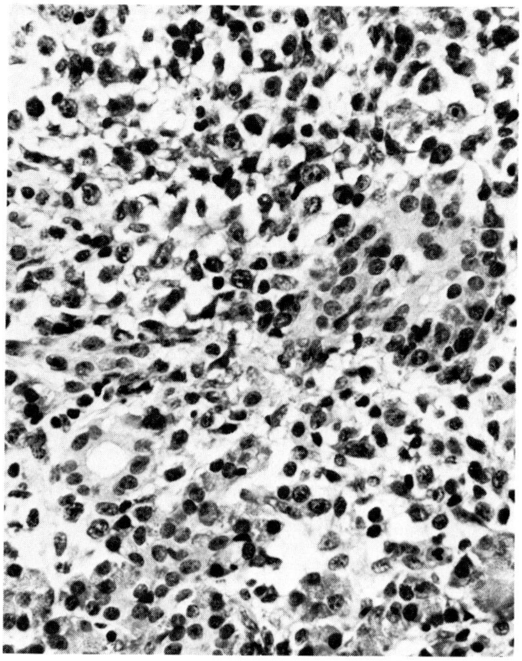

Figure 7.12
Acute rejection. The infiltrates in rejection consist predominantly of transformed lymphocytes (hematoxylin-eosin ×400).

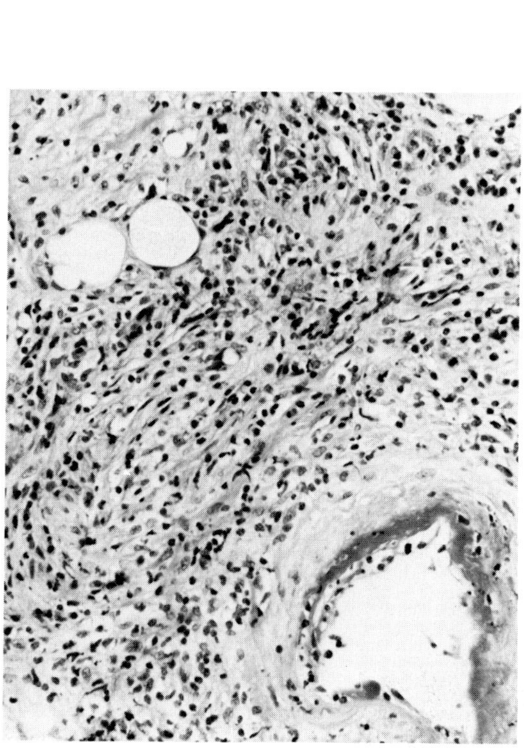

Figure 7.13
Acute vascular rejection. This silicone-injected graft demonstrates severe chronic pancreatitis. A prominent mixed inflammatory infiltrate and endovasculitis with fibrinoid necrosis suggests superimposed acute rejection (hematoxylin-eosin ×200). (From Sibley RK, Sutherland DER. In: Groth CG, ed. Pancreatic transplantation. London: Grune & Stratton, 1988;24.1 to 24.17.)

The histologic diagnosis of acute rejection is relatively clear-cut in the non-duct-obstructed graft. This is not the case in the enteric and bladder-drained graft with stricture of the duct or in duct-injected grafts where there is extravasation of the foreign material into the interstitial spaces and acute and chronic pancreatitis. An attempt should be made to separate the inflammatory changes of mild chronic pancreatitis from chronic superimposed acute rejection and severe chronic pancreatitis from chronic rejection. The distinction may not always be possible. Features that support the diagnosis of acute rejection, in addition to the changes of pancreatitis, include an intense transformed lymphocytic infiltrate within the exocrine pancreas as well as isletitis; lymphocytic endovasculitis indicates superimposed acute rejection (see Figs. 7.10 and 7.13).

It has been suggested that upregulation of class II or I major histocompatibility antigens in organ transplants precedes or is associated with the inflammatory infiltrate of acute rejection [33–36]. In the pancreatic allograft, upregulation of class I (Fig. 7.14A) and II (Fig. 7.14B) major histocompati-

Figure 7.14
In acute rejection there is hyperexpression of class I antigen on all pancreatic tissues (A, immunofluorescence, class I antigen W6/32 ×570). The exocrine pancreas and endothelial cells in acute rejection show prominent hyperexpression of class II antigens (B, immunofluorescence, HLA-DR ×570). (From Sibley RK, Sutherland DER. Pancreas transplantation. Am J Pathol 1987;128:151–70. With permission of the author and J.B. Lippincott.)

A *B*

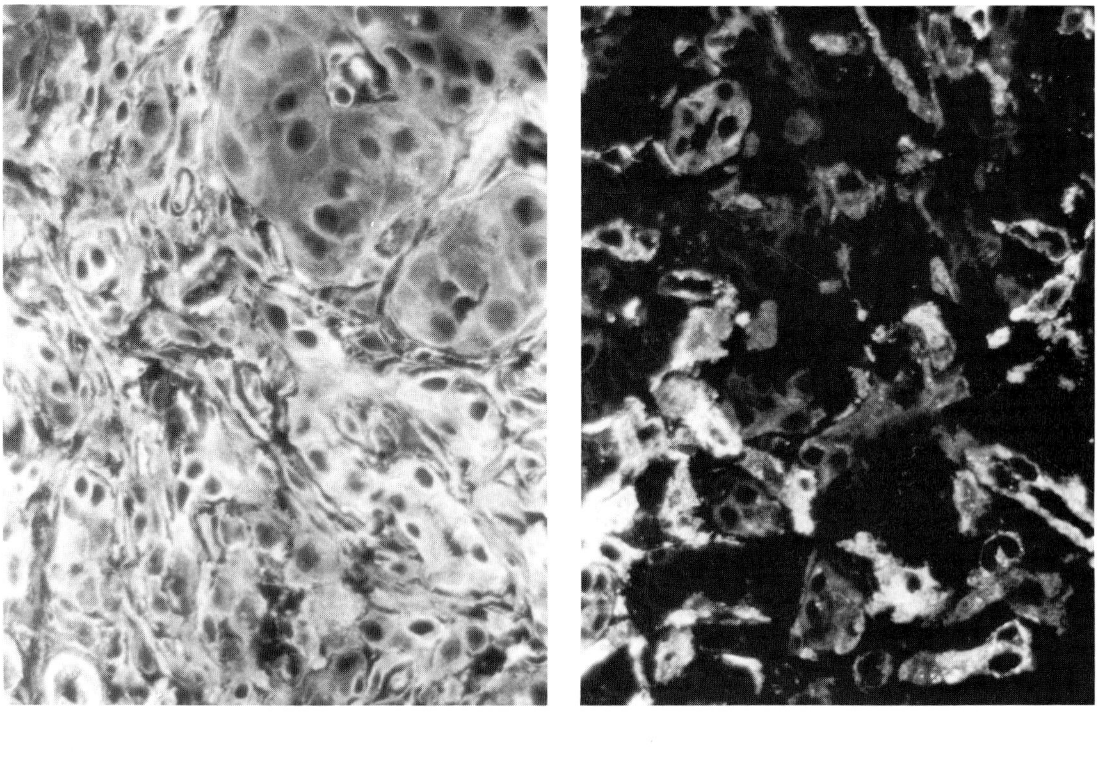

bility antigens occurred on the ducts, acini, and endothelial cells in grafts with acute rejection. Cases with acute rejection and isletitis had mild to moderate upregulation of class I antigens in the islets, but none of the endocrine cells expressed detectable class II antigens [8]. The upregulation of major histocompatibility antigens in pancreatic grafts, however, does not indicate acute rejection, since similar features occurred in polymer-injected grafts without evidence of acute rejection and in HLA-identical-twin donated grafts, where rejection does not occur [8]. Moreover, Bovo et al. [37] reported upregulation of major histocompatibility molecules in nontransplanted pancreases with acute pancreatitis.

Chronic Rejection To implicate chronic rejection in addition to polymer-induced chronic pancreatitis in the etiology of graft failure, it is necessary to have previous evidence of acute rejection or histologic evidence of chronic vascular rejection. Chronic vascular rejection in the transplanted pancreas is identical to that found in cardiac, renal, and hepatic grafts with chronic vascular rejection and is characterized by variable narrowing of arterial lumens by a concentric fibroproliferative endarteritis (Fig. 7.15). In some grafts it is difficult to separate chronic vascular rejection from organized thrombus, but recanalized vessels, rarely found in rejection-associated thrombosis, or low-grade lymphocytic endovasculitis are helpful in the differential diagnosis. The islets in the graft with chronic rejection may be difficult to identify. Alloimmune destruction or infarction is probably responsible for their disappearance.

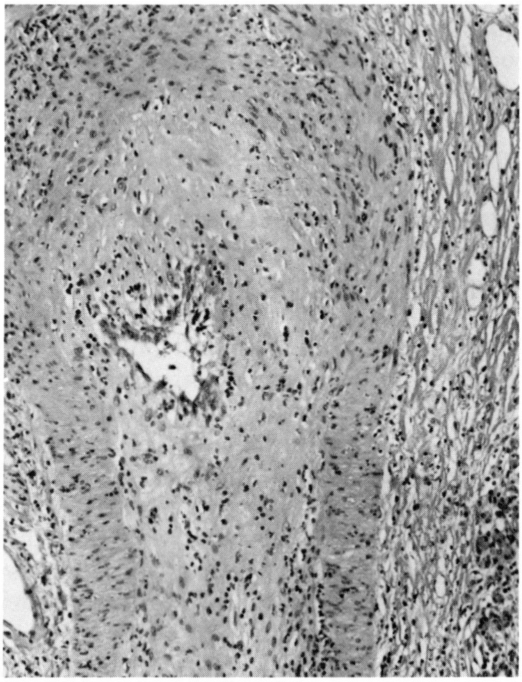

Figure 7.15
Chronic vascular rejection is characterized by a prominent obliterative fibrous endarteritis (hematoxylin-eosin ×192).

Figure 7.16
Cytomegalovirus infection of the graft anastomotic site may result in intractable hemorrhage secondary to ulceration of the mucosa (immunoperoxidase, human anti-CMV ×200).

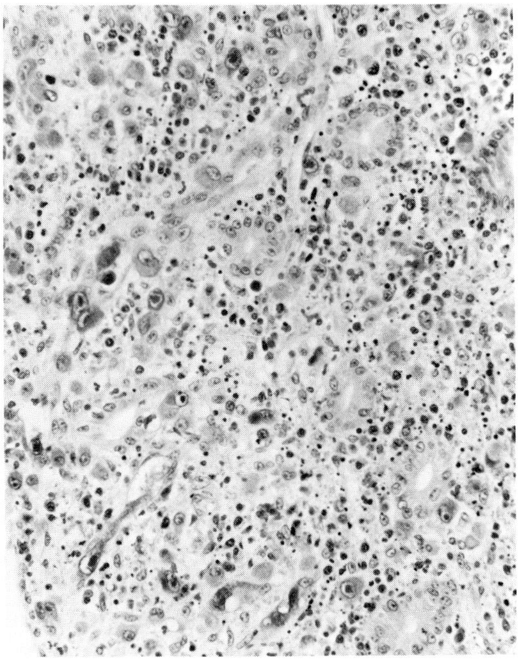

Figure 7.17
CMV disease. The significance of the cytomegaloviral inclusions in this silicone-injected graft with histologic evidence of acute rejection is uncertain. Both islet and, more typically, acinar inclusions can be found in patients without systemic evidence of viral infection (immunoperoxidase, human anti-CMV ×200).

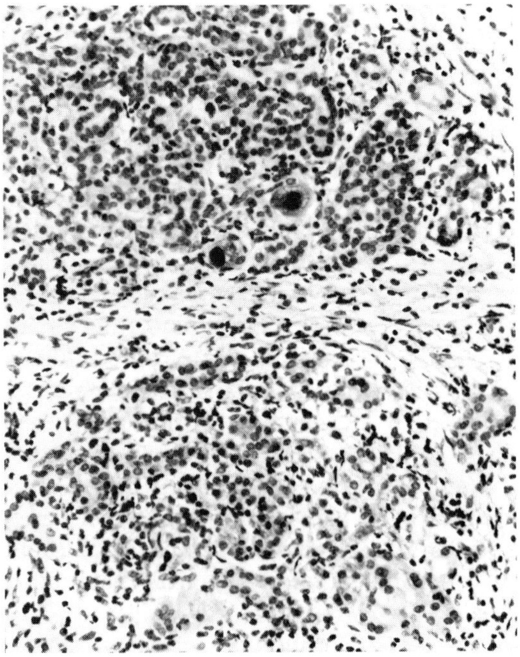

In ten patients the CMV inclusions were found in grafts with histologic evidence of acute rejection or in grafts with silicone-associated pancreatitis (Fig. 7.17). Whether the intensity or the phenotype of the inflammatory infiltrates in these grafts was altered by the viral infection is unknown.

Duct Injection–Associated Pancreatitis

One of the major complications of pancreas transplantation is anastomotic leak. Numerous techniques have been developed to prevent this complication [3, 4], including the injection of liquid synthetic polymers into the pancreatic duct. These substances harden immediately after injection to form a solid cast within the major duct and its branches [46–48]. This destroys the exocrine pancreas and eliminates the exocrine function without adversely affecting endocrine function in short-term analyses [11,46]. An absorbable biologic glue, prolamine, has also successfully been used to obliterate the pancreatic ducts of dogs and patients with chronic pancreatitis [49] or a transplanted pancreas [15–17]. Of the synthetic compounds introduced into persons who have undergone pancreas transplantation, two of the synthetic polymers, silicone and neoprene, and the biodegradable prolamine, have been extensively used. Injection of a large amount of the synthetic material into the pancreatic duct is usually associated with transiently elevated serum amylase levels, whereas lesser amounts are often associated with low-grade chronic hyperamylasemia. The number of infectious complications and the number of anastomotic leaks have been lower than in the non-duct-obstructed grafts [7], and graft function at 1 year compares with other duct management techniques [5]. The long-term effects of the chronic pancreatitis on graft function are presently unknown.

The results of polymer duct injection at the University of Minnesota are quite poor. Only 3 of 41 duct-injected grafts (36 silicone, 4 prolamine, 1 neoprene) are still functioning 5.5 to 8 years after transplantation; only 7 grafts functioned longer than 1 year.

Dubernard and colleagues [12,13] had better results with a neoprene duct-injection technique. One third of their neoprene-injected grafts were functioning at 2 years and 20% were functioning at 4 years after transplantation [13]. However, many of the patients had an abnormal OGTT, raising concern for the long-term function of these grafts.

Management of the pancreatic secretions in the Munich series is based on prolamine duct obliteration [15–17]. In this series, pancreas-kidney transplantations have been much more successful than pancreas transplantation alone. The actuarial 5-year graft survival in the combined group was 50%. Nearly 40% of the patients with functioning grafts, however, had abnormal OGTTs, and the 5- and 10-year survival rates are presently unavailable.

Causes of graft failure in duct-injected grafts include patient death (31%), rejection (43%), thrombosis with infarction (18%), and infection (8%) [12, 16,50]. The possibility that the chronic pancreatitis associated with polymer duct injection might play a role in the development of the abnormal OGTT or eventual graft failure is considered but not listed as a cause of graft failure. In the Minnesota series, however, pancreatic biopsies were often performed to determine the cause of post-transplant hyperglycemia or graft failure in the duct-injected grafts. Transplantectomies were also examined to evaluate the cause of graft loss. The causes of graft loss were chronic pancreatitis alone or associated with infarction (19%); chronic pancreatitis and rejection, often with infarction (55%); thrombosis and infarction (7%); patient death, infection, and recurrent disease (4% each); and unknown (7%).

Pathologic Features of Injection-Associated Pancreatitis In neoprene- and silicone-injected grafts, the synthetic material obliterates the ductal system and extravasates into the interstitial spaces [8,11]. Initially an acute inflammatory infiltrate of varying severity, edema, fat necrosis, and foci of necrotizing pancreatitis are found (Fig. 7.18). Eventually a mononuclear cell infiltrate predominates, and perilobular edema and progressive fibrosis develop (Fig. 7.19A and B). The extravasated polymer elicits a foreign body giant cell reaction (Fig. 7.20). Finally the graft consists of inflamed cicatrix, foreign material with giant cell reaction, and coalesced islets (Fig. 7.21). In some cases there is extensive allograft infarction; acute, organizing, or chronic small vessel thrombosis may be found. The etiology of the thrombotic process may be related to enzymatic digestion of vessel walls secondary to pancreatitis.

Prolamine not only causes necrosis of the ductal epithelial cells but permeates and rapidly destroys the exocrine tissue as well [8,49,51]. There is a

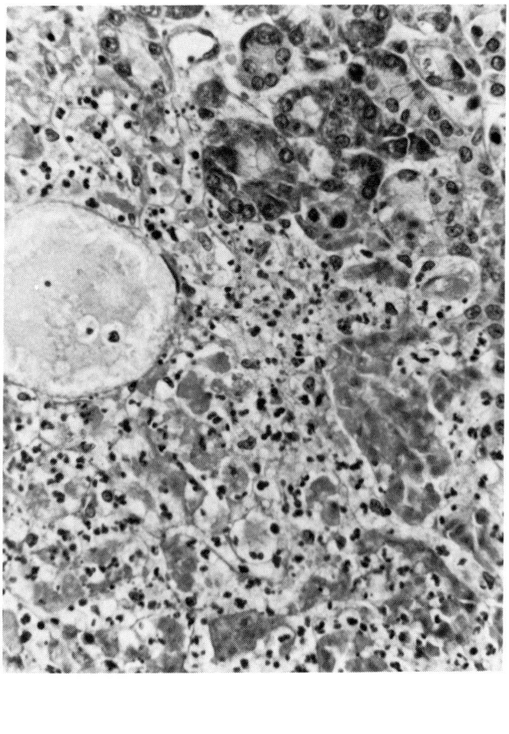

Figure 7.18
Acute pancreatitis, with minimal clinical features, occurs early in polymer duct–injected grafts (hematoxylin-eosin ×400).

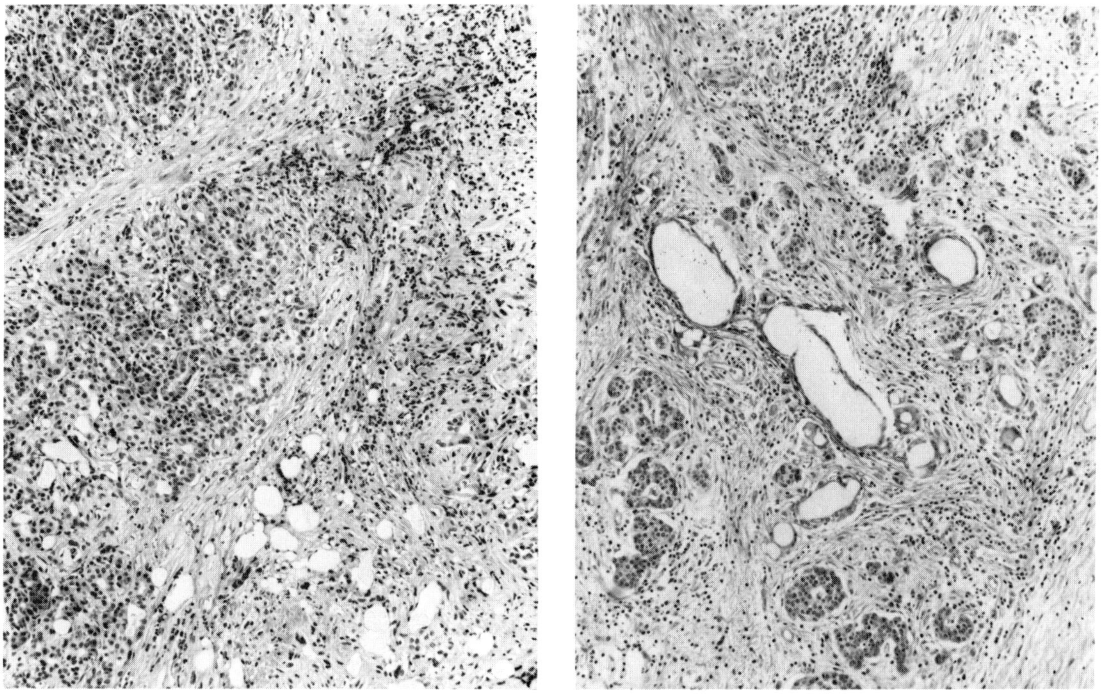

A *B*

Figure 7.19
This patient with a silicone duct–injected graft presented with mild hyperglycemia. Extravasated foreign material, perilobular fibrosis, inflammation, and focal necrosis are evident (A, hematoxylin-eosin ×100). This neoprene duct–injected graft shows residual islets, foreign body giant cell reaction, mononuclear cell infiltrate, and prominent fibrosis (B, hematoxylin-eosin × 100). (From Sibley RK, In: Dubernard JM, Sutherland DER, eds. International handbook of pancreas transplantation. Kluwer Academic Publishers, 1989;203–23.)

moderate mixed inflammatory cell infiltrate and collections of foreign body giant cells, although the foreign material is not visible because it is biodegradable (Fig. 7.22A). Later biopsies or transplantectomies reveal islets set within a moderately dense and modestly inflamed cicatrix. A few residual ductules and collections of giant cells may also be evident (Fig. 7.22B).

In the duct-injected transplanted pancreas, a biopsy performed because of hyperglycemia or a transplantectomy performed because of technical factors typically reveals chronic pancreatitis of varying severity. There may be evidence of superimposed acute or chronic rejection. Features suggesting the former include an intense, predominantly lymphoid infiltrate within the residual exocrine pancreas, or an endovasculitis (Fig. 7.23), while concentric fibrointimal endarteritis is compatible with chronic vascular rejection. In the severely atrophic and infarcted gland it is often difficult to discern whether rejection or polymer-associated chronic pancreatitis, or both, are responsible for the destructive process [8,52–54] (Fig. 7.24).

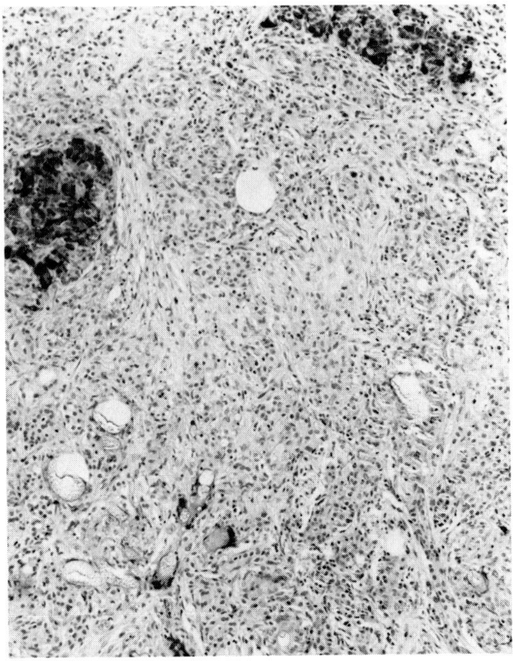

Figure 7.20
This failed silicone duct–injected graft contained islets with numerous beta cells, a prominent inflammatory infiltrate, and foreign body giant cell reaction. (Immunoperoxidase, guinea pig antibovine insulin ×100). (From Sibley RK, In: Dubernard JM, Sutherland DER, eds. International handbook of pancreas transplantation. Kluwer Academic Publishers, 1989;203–23)

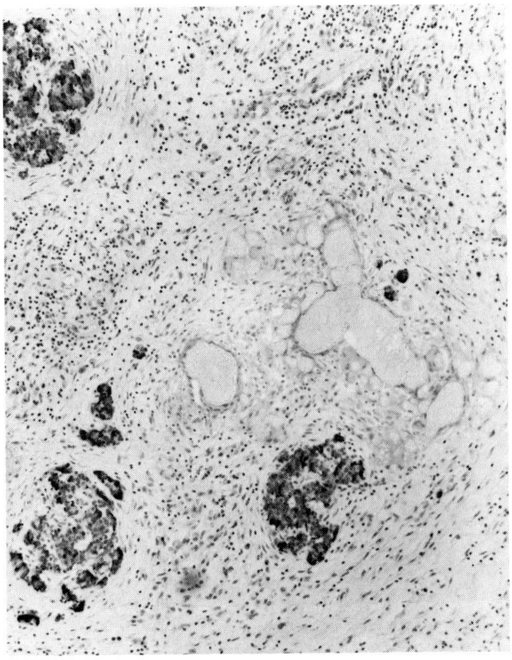

Figure 7.21
This failed neoprene duct–injected graft showed extensive destruction of the exocrine pancreas, the extravasated neoprene, and islets containing abundant beta cells (immunoperoxidase, guinea pig antibovine insulin ×100). (From Sibley RK, In: Dubernard JM, Sutherland DER, eds. International handbook of pancreas transplantation. Kluwer Academic Publishers, 1989;203–23)

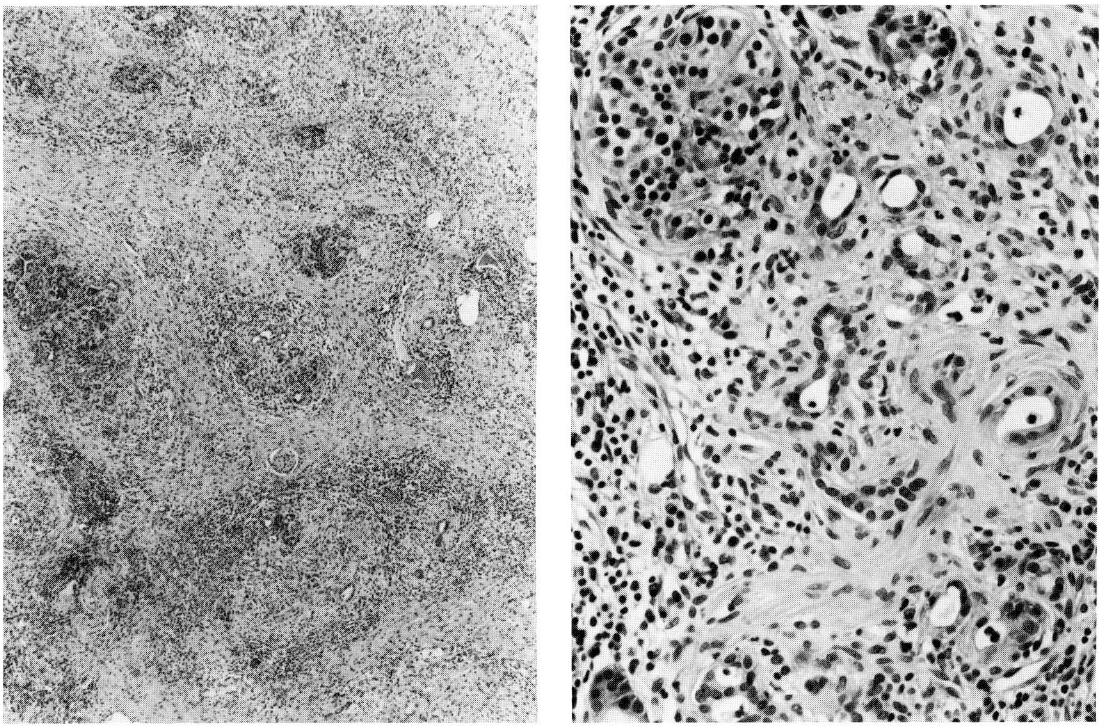

A *B*

Figure 7.22
This prolamine duct–injected graft shows atrophy of the exocrine pancreas, residual pancreatic ductules, a moderate mononuclear cell infiltrate, and normal islets (A, hematoxylin-eosin ×40. B, hematoxylin-eosin ×200). (From Sibley RK, In: Dubernard JM, Sutherland DER, eds. International handbook of pancreas transplantation. Kluwer Academic Publishers, 1989;203–23.)

Examination of the islets in patients with hyperglycemia usually reveals normal islets or mildly degranulated beta cells. The islets in grafts that are no longer functioning can appear entirely normal (see Figs. 7.20 and 7.21; Fig. 7.25), certainly a disconcerting feature when there is no evidence of graft function, or no islets, which corresponds with the lack of function (Fig. 7.24). The latter grafts usually show evidence of superimposed acute or chronic rejection and extensive infarction. Other grafts show prominent fragmentation of the islets and nesidioblastosis (see Fig. 7.6).

Major histocompatibility antigen expression by the islets and exocrine pancreas in two silicone-injected grafts without histologic features of rejection was similar to the findings in grafts showing evidence of acute rejection. The number of inflammatory cells in grafts with acute rejection, however, was five times that found in the nonrejecting silicone duct–injected graft [8].

Pathophysiology of Hyperglycemia in Chronic Pancreatitis and Polymer-Related Chronic Pancreatitis The pathophysiology of the hyperglycemia and the lack of function in grafts with essentially normal-appearing islets is uncertain, but several hypotheses have been proposed. IL-1, in this situation produced by inflammatory cells in response to the synthetic polymers or duct obstruction from other causes, may modulate insulin secretion [38] or directly damage beta cells [39,55]. In the graft with severe fibrosis, the microcirculation of the islets may be adversely affected, blunting the normal response of beta cells to a glucose load. Severe chronic pancreatitis associated with an abnormal OGTT, and even exogenous insulin dependence, is a well-recognized phenomenon in the native pancreas [56,57].

Recurrent Diabetes Mellitus

The occurrence of recurrent disease in the renal graft is well recognized [58,59]. Recurrence of the disease, which originally led to end-stage liver failure, has also been reported [60]. Thus it is not surprising that a similar event occurs in the transplanted pancreas [8,61,62]. Unlike the multiple disorders associated with end-stage renal, cardiac, and hepatic disease, all type I diabetic patients have selective destruction of the beta cell of the islet of Langerhans [21–23,63]. Mild chronic pancreatitis is another feature of the type I diabetic pancreas [22].

The pathogenetic mechanism(s) of beta-cell destruction have not been entirely elucidated. Nearly all type I diabetic patients are HLA-DR3 or DR 4 genotypic [64]. This may predispose these individuals to beta-cell damage by some exogenous environmental factor [65] or endogenous inflammatory process that promotes beta-cell damage and destruction by cellular- and humoral-mediated mechanisms [66]. That cellular-mediated immunity plays a role in beta-cell destruction is suggested by the finding of "insulitis" [21–23, 63] in recent-onset type I diabetic patients. The insulitis consisted of T and B lymphocytes in a single type I diabetic studied at autopsy [67]. The role of humoral-mediated immunity in beta-cell destruction is supported by the finding of granular deposits of immune globulin and C9 in the islets [67], and islet cell cytoplasmic and surface antibodies are found in a high proportion of early type I diabetic patients [68,69]. The finding of HLA-DR$^+$ beta cells, the hyperexpression of class I antigen on islet cells, and the presence of gamma interferon in beta cells in early type I diabetic patients lend credence to the immune theory of beta-cell destruction [67,70,71]. More recently, Nerup and colleagues [72] have proposed that the release of IL-1 by cells either infiltrating (lymphocytes, macrophages), or native to (dendritic cells, endothelial cells) the pancreas may play an early role in beta-cell damage. Gamma interferon may also play an early role in the development of beta-cell destruction, since the in vitro exposure of rat endocrine cells to gamma interferon induces Ia molecules on the endocrine cells [73]. The upregulation or induction of class I and II antigens on a cell is thought to increase the number of CD4 and CD8 receptors, allowing specific lymphocytes and cytotoxic antibodies to recognize the cell [35,67,70,71,74].

The immunologic and histologic features of beta-cell destruction that occur in the BB/W rat are remarkably similar to those seen in humans [75,76]. There is extensive literature concerning the diabetic BB/W rat, but we shall comment only on two recent reports. The experiment of Weringer and Like [77] suggests that beta-cell destruction may not be MHC restricted; contrariwise, Woehrle et al. [78] found that cultured and noncultured MHC-identical islets from Wistar-Firth rats were destroyed in the BB/W rat, although survival of MHC-nonidentical Lewis rat islets in these same animals was in some cases permanent. These findings may have important implications in human pancreas transplantation.

Whatever the mechanisms of selective beta-cell destruction, the process has been reenacted in four HLA-identical twin recipients and five HLA-identical sibling pancreas transplant recipients [8,61]. The clinical features were (1) progressive hyperglycemia unresponsive to antirejection therapy, when instituted, requiring exogenous insulin treatment; (2) the return of serum and urine C-peptide levels to pretransplant baseline levels; or (3) the necessity of intermittent use of insulin in patients with C-peptide levels reduced from post-transplant levels but above pretransplant levels.

All the patients had type I diabetes of 12 to 27 years' duration (Table 7.2). Each patient had normalization of glucose metabolism in the post-transplant period. Three HLA-identical and one HLA-identical sibling developed hyperglycemia 4 to 8 weeks after transplantation and resumed insulin treatment

Table 7.2
Clinical data on 9 HLA-compatible pancreatic transplant recipients in whom diabetes mellitus recurred postoperatively

Sex	*Duration of diabetes (yr)*	*Donor*	*Immunosuppression*	*Duration of normoglycemia (mo)*	*Resumed insulin (mo)*
F	22	Id twin	None	1	2.5
F	26	HLA-Id sis	CsA	2	6
F	17	Id twin	None	1.25	9
F	27	Id twin	None	2	26
F	21	Id twin	AZA	32	PF–51
F	12	HLA-Id sis	CsA	7	58
M	22	HLA-Id bro	CsA + Pred	9	15
M	13	HLA-Id bro	CsA + Pred	23	29
M	18	HLA-Id bro	CsA + Pred	21	SL–21

Id twin, identical twin; HLA-Id sis/bro, HLA-identical sister/brother; CsA, cyclosporine A; AZA, azathioprine; Pred, prednisone; SL, sudden loss; PF, partial function.

2.5 to 26 (mean 11) months after transplantation. The efficacy of antilymphocyte globulin, azathioprine, prednisone, and cyclosporine, which were given to these four patients in varying combinations, dosages, and duration, is uncertain. Two were insulin dependent 6 weeks and 4 months after the initial symptoms, but the other two patients appeared to have at least a partial response to the immunotherapy. Both eventually became insulin dependent 7 and 24 months after hyperglycemia first appeared.

Four other HLA-identical siblings developed hyperglycemia 7 to 23 (mean 15) months after transplantation, necessitating insulin therapy at 21 to 58 (mean 41) months after transplantation. One HLA-identical twin was treated with low-dose azathioprine from the time of transplantation and had normal function until 32 months later, when hyperglycemia was noted. She presently has partial function, 54 months after transplantation.

It is of course necessary to rule out the possibility of diabetes mellitus in the donor pancreas. Each donor was normoglycemic after transplantation and has remained so. Furthermore, biopsy of five of the donated segmental isografts and allografts showed normal endocrine and exocrine pancreas, while the native biopsies of three patients showed features typical of type I diabetes mellitus.

Sixteen biopsies and one transplantectomy were examined at various times after transplantation. Five biopsies were obtained soon after hyperglycemia first appeared. Other biopsies were performed to evaluate the effect of treatment or to establish the end-stage nature of the recurrent disease. One biopsy was performed prospectively to evaluate the islets, although the patient showed no clinical evidence of endocrine disease [8,61].

The major feature in the biopsies obtained at initial hyperglycemia was a prominent collection of mononuclear cells within and around the islets (Fig. 7.26). An average of 85 mononuclear cells per islet was found, which resulted in architectural disarray, prominent degranulation, and destruction of beta cells (Fig. 7.27). Electron microscopic study demonstrated both lymphocytes and macrophages within the islets, and phagocytized beta cells were easily identified (Fig. 7.28). The majority of the inflammatory cells within the islets were $CD8^+$ lymphocytes (Fig. 7.29), with lesser numbers of $CD4^+$ lymphocytes and OKM1 reactive macrophages. None of the endocrine cells stained with antisera against immune globulins, complement, or HLA-DR antigen, but all of the endocrine cells showed strong class I antigen expression (Fig. 7.30). Intraislet endothelial cells demonstrated marked increase in HLA-DR antigen expression. Biopsies performed when there was poor or no residual function demonstrated further loss of beta cells from the islets. Immunohistochemical staining revealed either (1) complete lack of beta cells in the islets (Fig. 7.31A and B) with return of class I antigen hyperexpression by the endocrine cells and HLA-DR antigen hyperexpression by endothelial cells to normal or (2) islets with residual beta cells, mononuclear cell infiltrates, and increased class I and class II antigen expression.

Unlike the three preceding HLA-identical twins, a fourth HLA-identical twin received azathioprine from the time of transplantation. This drug did not, by itself, prevent recurrence, although the patient remained asymptomatic for 32 months, when hyperglycemia first appeared. This patient under-

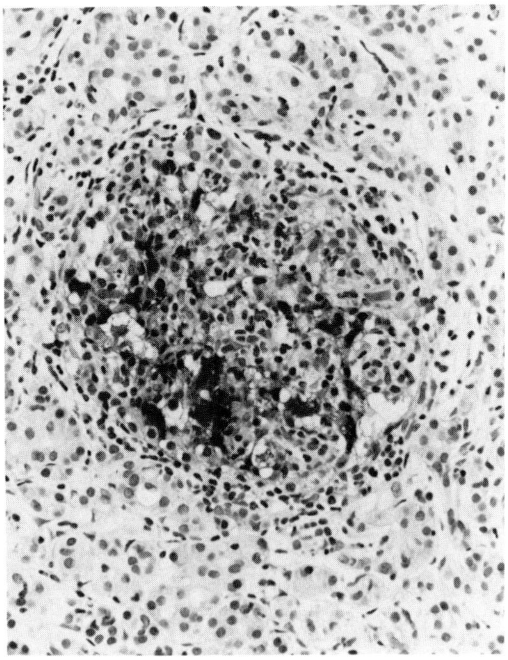

Figure 7.27
Early recurrent diabetes demonstrates degranulation or destruction of beta cells with prominent architectural disarray (immunoperoxidase, guinea pig antibovine ×200).

went a prospective biopsy two months after transplantation, and although endocrine function was normal, a mild isletitis was evident and there was hyperexpression of HLA-DR antigen by intraislet endothelial cells. The number of beta cells in the islets appeared to be normal. In the second biopsy, the islets appeared normal on light microscopy, but nearly 90% lacked beta cells. Even though there was no residual inflammatory infiltrate in the islets, those containing residual beta cells showed a prominent increase in class I antigen expression.

Transplant biopsies or pancreatectomies in the other four HLA-identical sibling recipients demonstrated acute and chronic rejection as well as recurrent disease. A mild chronic pancreatitis [22] is often found in the type I diabetic pancreas, but these grafts showed not only prominent acinar inflammation but acute vascular or chronic vascular rejection as well. It is possible that the isletitis present in these grafts was also a rejection phenomenon; however, as previously noted, the islets in patients with acute rejection are normal, show degranulation of beta cells, or display infarction of the islets, while in chronic rejection the islets typically reveal the loss of all endocrine cells, not the selective loss of beta cells as seen in these four patients and in the native pancreatic islet of the type I diabetic patient.

Peripancreatic Lymph Nodes

The peripancreatic lymph nodes may be entirely normal but, more often, are remarkably abnormal. A focal to diffuse necrotizing lymphadenitis with foci

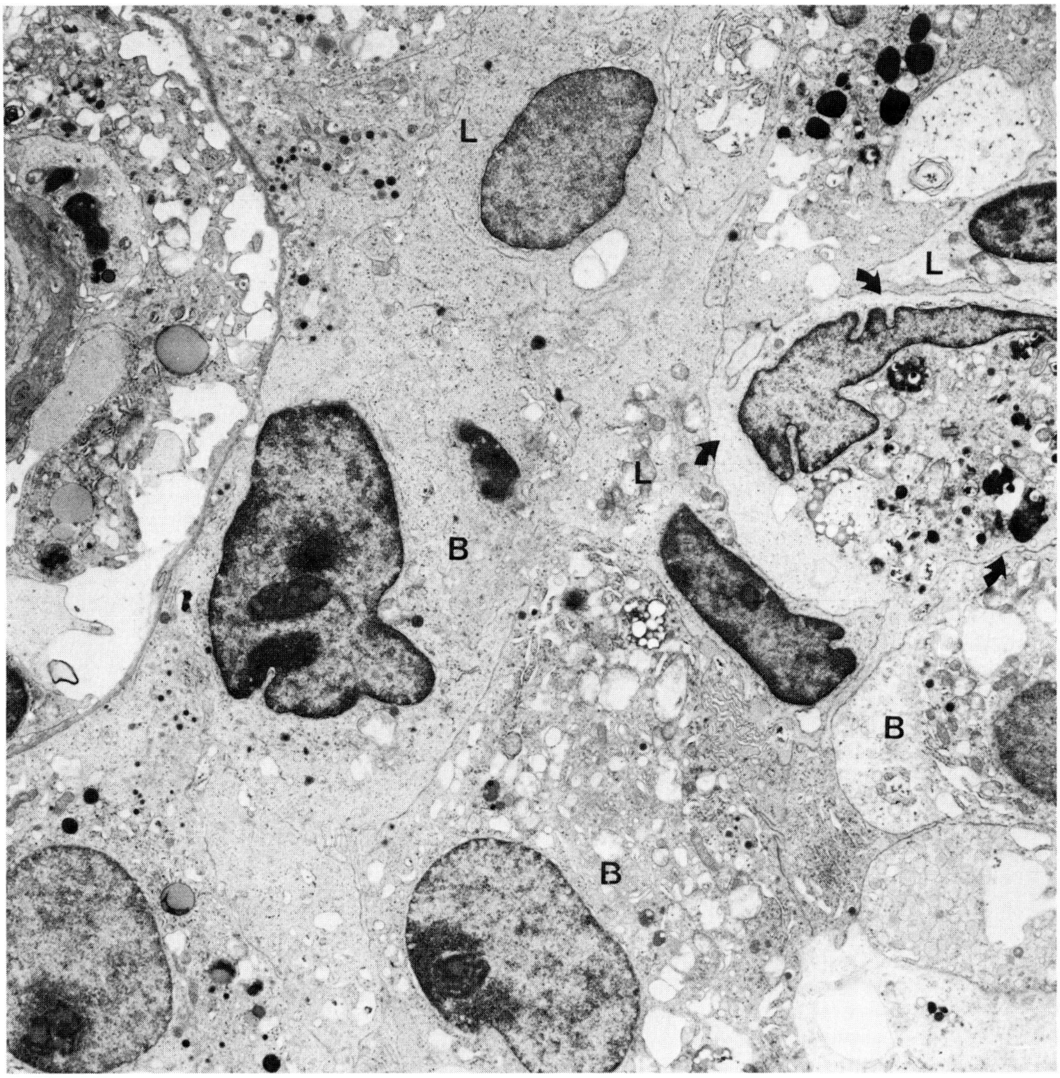

Figure 7.28
Lymphocytes, L, degranulated beta cells, B, and phagocytized beta cells (arrows) are evident in early recurrent disease (×5260). (From Sibley RK et al. Lab Invest 1985;53:132–44. © by U.S. & Canadian Academy of Pathology, Inc. With permission of the author and Williams & Wilkens.)

of fibrinoid necrosis and fibrin thrombosis of vascular spaces occurs in many cases (Fig. 7.32). The sinuses may contain large numbers of macrophages containing cellular debris (see Fig. 7.32). These changes probably are secondary to enzymatic digestion of the nodes but theoretically could represent host versus graft disease. Some lymph nodes show diffuse effacement of nodal architecture, with a proliferation of plasmacytoid lymphocytes and immunoblasts, and occur in patients with evidence of viral infection [79].

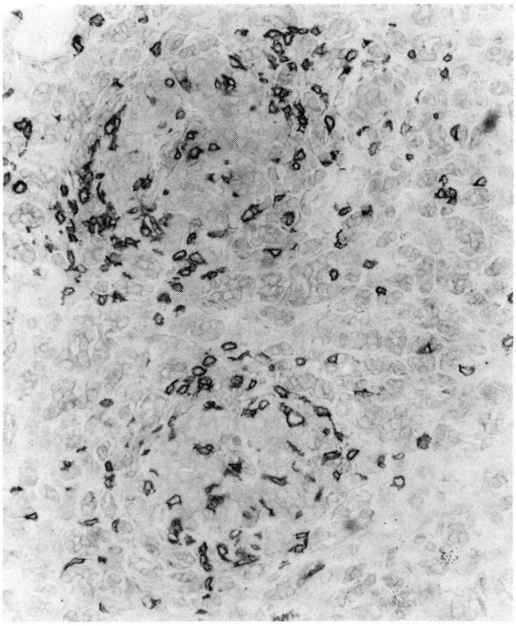

Figure 7.29
The mononuclear cells in early recurrent disease consist predominantly of CD8$^+$ T lymphocytes (immunoperoxidase, OKT8 ×200). (From Sibley RK et al. Lab Invest 1985;53:132–44. © by U.S. & Canadian Academy of Pathology, Inc. With permission of the author and Williams & Wilkens.)

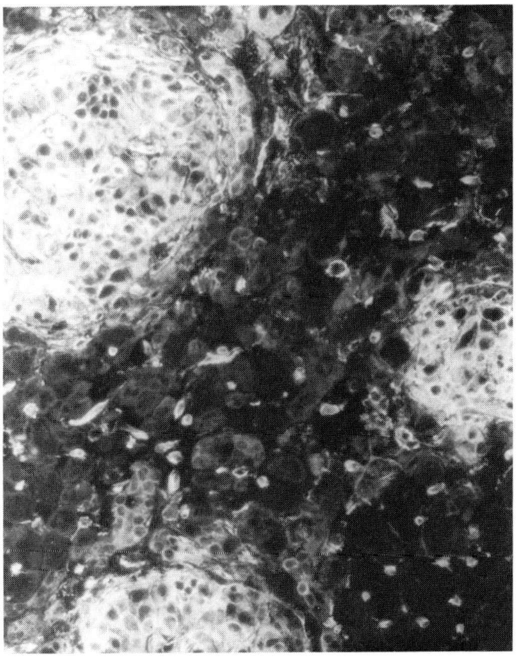

Figure 7.30
The islets in early recurrent diabetes mellitus demonstrate strong expression with class I antigen (immunofluorescence, class I antigen W6/32 ×85). (From Sibley RK, Sutherland DER. Pancreas transplantation. Am J Path 1987;128:151–70. With permission of the author and J.B. Lippincott.)

2. Sutherland DER, Kendall D. Clinical pancreas and islet transplant registry report. Transplant Proc 1985;17:307–11.
3. Sutherland DER. Pancreas and islet transplantation. I. Experimental studies. Diabetologia 1981a;20:161–85.
4. Sutherland DER. Pancreas and islet transplantation. II. Clinical trials. Diabetologia 1981b;20:435–50.
5. Sutherland DER, Moudry KC. Pancreas transplant registry: history and analysis of cases 1966 to October 1986. Pancreas 1987;2:473–88.
6. Sutherland DER, Goetz FC, Najarian JS. Pancreas transplantation at the University of Minnesota: donor and recipient selection, operative and postoperative management, and outcome. Transplant Proc 1987;19:63–74.
7. Sutherland DER, Goetz FC, Najarian JS. One hundred pancreas transplants at a single institution. Ann Surg 1984;200:414–40.
8. Sibley RK, Sutherland DER. Pancreas transplantation: an immunohistologic and histopathologic examination of 100 grafts. Am J Pathol 1987;128:151–70.
9. Sibley RK. Pathology of pancreas graft. In: Dubernard JM, Sutherland DER, eds. International handbook of pancreas transplantation. Dordrecht: Kluwer Academic Publishers, 1989;203–23.
10. Secchi A, Pontirole AE, Traeger J, et al. A method for early detection of graft failure in pancreas transplantation. Transplantation 1983;35:344–8.
11. Blanc-Brunat N, Dubernard JM, Toraine JL, et al. Pathology of the pancreas after intraductal neoprene injection in dogs and diabetic patients treated by pancreatic transplantation. Diabetologia 1983;25:97–107.
12. Dubernard JM, Traeger J, Piatti PM, et al. Report of 54 human segmental pancreas allografts prepared by duct obstruction with neoprene. Transplant Proc 1985;17:312–4.
13. Dubernard JM, LaRocca E, Gelet A, et al. Simultaneous pancreas and kidney transplantation: long-term results and comparison of two surgical techniques. Transplant Proc 1987;19:2285–7.
14. Cantarovich D, Traeger J, LaRocca E, et al. Evolution of metabolic and endocrine function in ten neoprene-injected segmental pancreas allografts at three to 54 months after transplantation, versus preliminary results in nine whole pancreas allografts with enteric division. Transplant Proc 1987;19:2310–3.
15. Land W, Gebhardt CH, Gall FP, et al. Pancreatic duct obstruction with prolamine solution. Transplant Proc 1980;12:72–5.
16. Land W, Landgraf R, Illner W-D, et al. Improved results in combined segmental pancreatic and renal transplantation in diabetic patients under cyclosporine therapy. Transplant Proc 1985;17:317–24.
17. Land W, Landgraf R, Illner W-D, et al. Clinical pancreatic transplantation using the prolamine duct occlusion technique—the Munich experience. Transplant Proc 1987;19:75–83.
18. Gray DWR, Morris PJ. Developments in isolated pancreatic islet transplantation. Transplantation 1987;43:321–31.
19. Natali PG, De Martino C, Quaranta V, et al. Expression of Ia-like antigens in normal human nonlymphoid tissues. Transplantation 1981;31:75–8.
20. Daar AS, Fuggle SV, Fabre JW, et al. The detailed distribution of MHC class II antigens in normal human organs. Transplantation 1984;38:293–8.
21. Gepts W, Lecompte PM. The pancreatic islets in diabetes. Am J Med 1981;70:105–15.
22. Foulis AK, Stewart JA. The pancreas in recent-onset type I (insulin-dependent) diabetes mellitus; insulin content of islets, insulitis and associated changes in the exocrine acinar tissue. Diabetologia 1984;26:456–61.

23. Foulis AK, Liddle CN, Farquharson MA, et al. The histopathology of the pancreas in type I (insulin-dependent) diabetes mellitus: a 25-year review of deaths in patients under 20 years of age in the United Kingdom. Diabetologia 1986;29:267–74.
24. Kloppel G, Lenzen S. Anatomy and physiology of the endocrine pancreas. In: Kloppel G, Heitz PU, eds. Pancreatic pathology. Edinburgh: Churchill Livingstone, 1984;133–53.
25. Phat VN, Guerrieri MT, Alexandre JH, Camilleri JP. Early histological changes in acute necrotizing hemorrhagic pancreatitis. Pathol Res Pract 1984;178:273–9.
26. Gyr K, Heitz PU, Beglinger C. Pancreatitis. In: Kloppel G, Heitz PU, eds. Pancreatic pathology. Edinburgh: Churchill Livingstone, 1984;44–72.
27. Kloppel G, Bommer G, Commandeur G, Heitz PU. The endocrine pancreas in chronic pancreatitis. Virchows Arch A Pathol Anat Histol 1978;377:157–74.
28. Sutherland DER, Casanova D, Sibley RK. Role of pancreas graft biopsies in the diagnosis and treatment of rejection after pancreas transplantation. Transplant Proc 1987c;19:2329–31.
29. Prieto M, Sutherland DER, Fernandez-Cruz L, et al. Rejection in pancreas transplantation. Transplant Proc 1987;19:2348–9.
30. Prieto M, Sutherland DER, Fernandez-Cruz L, et al. Experimental and clinical experience with urine amylase monitoring for early diagnosis of rejection in pancreas transplantation. Transplantation 1987;43:73–9.
31. Dafoe DC, Campbell DA Jr., Rocher L, et al. Diagnosis of rejection in simultaneous renal/pancreas (urinary bladder drained) transplantation. Transplant Proc 1987;19:2345–7.
32. Steiniger B, Klempnauer J. Distinct histologic patterns of acute, prolonged, and chronic rejection in vascularized rat pancreas allografts. Am J Pathol 1986;124:253–62.
33. Koene RAP, de Waal RMW, Bogman JJT. Variable expression of major histocompatibility antigens: role in transplantation immunology. Kidney Int 1986;30:1–8.
34. Pober JS, Collins T, Gimbrone MA, et al. Inducible expression of class II major histocompatibility complex antigens and the immunogenicity of vascular endothelium. Transplantation 1986;41:141–6.
35. Steiniger B, Klempnauer J, Wonigeit K. Altered distribution of class I and class II MHC antigens during acute pancreas allograft rejection in the rat. Transplantation 1985;40:234–9.
36. Fabre JW, Milton AD, Spencer S, et al. Regulation of alloantigen expression in different tissues. Transplant Proc 1987;19:45–9.
37. Bovo P, Mirakian R, Merigo F, et al. HLA molecule expression on chronic pancreatitis specimens: is there a role for autoimmunity? A preliminary study. Pancreas 1987;2:350–6.
38. Comens PG, Wolf BA, Unanue ER, et al. Interleukin 1 is potent modulator of insulin secretion from isolated rat islets of Langerhans. Diabetes 1987;36:963–70.
39. Spinas GA, Hansen BS, Linde S, et al. Interleukin 1 dose-dependently affects the biosynthesis of (pro)insulin in isolated rat islets of Langerhans. Diabetologia 1987;30:474–80.
40. Mandrup-Poulsen T, Egeberg J, Nerum J, et al. Ultrastructural studies of time-course and cellular specificity of interleukin-1 mediated islet cytotoxicity. Acta Pathol Microbiol Immunol Scand C 1987;95:55–63.
41. Pukel C, Baquerizo H, Rabinovitch A. Destruction of rat islet cell monolayers

by cytokines: synergistic interactions of interferon-gamma, tumor necrosis factor, lymphotoxin, and interleukin 1. Diabetes 1988;37:133–6.
42. Oppenheim JJ, Kovacs EJ, Matsushima K, Durum SK. There is more than one interleukin-1. Immunol Today 1986;7:45–56.
43. Schienvold FL, Alejandro R, Mintz DH. Identification of Ia-bearing cells in rat, dog, pig, and human islets of Langerhans. Transplantation 1986;41:364–72.
44. Laprini A, Valente U, Celada F, et al. Morphology, cytochemical features, and membraned phenotype of HLA-DR interstitial cells in the human pancreas. Pancreas 1987;2:127–35.
45. Foucar E, Mukai K, Foucar K, et al. Colon ulceration in lethal cytomegalovirus infection. Am J Clin Pathol 1981;76:789–801.
46. Dubernard JM, Traeger J, Neyra P, et al. A new method of preparation of segmental pancreatic grafts for transplantation: trials in dogs and in man. Surgery 1978;84:633–9.
47. Baumgartner D, Sutherland DER, Heil J, et al. Long-term canine segmental pancreas transplants with the duct left open, neoprene-injected duct, and pancreatico-ureterostomy: a comparative study. Transplant Proc 1981;13:812–4.
48. Gooszen HG, Bosman FT, van Schilfgaarde R. An analysis of long-term histologic changes leading to decreased endocrine function after duct obliteration of the canine pancreas. Transplant Proc 1984;16:776–7.
49. Gebhardt CH, Stolte M. Pankreasgang-okklusion durch Injektion einer Schnellhartenden Aminosaurenlosung. Langenbecks Arch Chir 1978;346:149–66.
50. Munda R, First MR, Weiss MA, Alexander JW. Pancreas transplantation—University of Cincinnati. Transplant Proc 1987;19:17–23.
51. Gokel JM. Simultaneous pancreas and kidney transplantation in man—graft morphology. Hormone Metab Res 1983;13:76–7.
52. Dubernard JM, Traeger J, Touraine JL, et al. Rejection of human pancreatic allografts. Transplant Proc 1980;12:103–6.
53. Munda R, Alexander JW, First MR, et al. Synchronous transplantation of a kidney and duct-obliterated segmental pancreas: report of a case. Transplant Proc 1980;12:98–102.
54. Lindsey NJ, Nolan MS, Slater DN, et al. Rat pancreas allotransplantation; a short-term comparison of rejection patterns with different methods of exocrine drainage. Pathology 1983;139:259–74.
55. Mandrup-Poulsen T, Bendtzen K, Nerup J, et al. Affinity-purified human interleukin I is cytotoxic to isolated islets of Langerhans. Diabetologia 1986;29:63–7.
56. Bank S, Marks IN, Vinik AI. Clinical and hormonal aspects of pancreatic diabetes. Am J Gastroenterol 1975;64:13–22.
57. Vinik AI, Jackson WPU. Endocrine secretions in chronic pancreatitis. In: Podolsky S, Viswanathan M, eds. Secondary diabetes: the spectrum of the diabetic syndromes. New York: Raven, 1980;165–89.
58. Cameron JS. Glomerulonephritis in renal transplants. Transplantation 1982;34:237–45.
59. Sibley RK, Payne P. Morphologic findings in the renal allograft biopsy. Semin Nephrol 1985;5:294–306.
60. Neuberger J, Portmann B, MacDougall RD, et al. Recurrence of primary biliary cirrhosis after liver transplantation. N Engl J Med 1982;306:1–4.
61. Sibley RK, Sutherland DER, Goetz F, Michael AF. Recurrent diabetes mellitus in the pancreas iso- and allograft. Lab Invest 1985;53:132–44.
62. Sibley RK, Sutherland DER. Recurrence of diabetes mellitus in the pancreas graft. In: Groth CG, ed. Pancreatic transplantation. London: Grune & Stratton, 1988;24.1 to 24.17.

63. Gepts W. Pathological anatomy of the pancreas in juvenile diabetes mellitus. Diabetes 1965;1:619–33.
64. Wolf W, Spencer KM, Cudworth AG. The genetic susceptibility to type 1 (insulin-dependent) diabetes: analysis of the HLA-DR association. Diabetologia 1983;24:224–30.
65. Yoon J-W, Austin M, Onodera T, Notkins AL. Virus-induced diabetes mellitus. N Engl J Med 1979;300:1173–9.
66. Nerup J, Lernmark A. Autoimmunity in insulin-dependent diabetes mellitus. Am J Med 1981;70:135–41.
67. Bottazzo GF, Dean BM, McNally JM, et al. In situ characterization of autoimmune phenomena and expression of HLA molecules in the pancreas in diabetic insulitis. N Engl J Med 1985;313:353–60.
68. Bottazzo GF, Dean BM, Gorsuch AN, et al. Complement-fixing islet-cell antibodies in type 1 diabetes: possible monitors of active beta cell damage. Lancet 1980;1:668–72.
69. Irvine WJ, McCallum CJ, Gray RS, et al. Pancreatic islet-cell antibodies in diabetes mellitus correlated with the duration and type of diabetes, coexistent autoimmune disease, and HLA type. Diabetes 1977;26:138–47.
70. Foulis AK, Farquharson MA, Hardman R. Aberrant expression of class II major histocompatibility complex molecules by B cells and hyperexpression of class I major histocompatibility complex molecules by insulin containing islets in type 1 (insulin-dependent) diabetes mellitus. Diabetologia 1987;30:333–43.
71. Foulis AK, Farquharson MA, Meager A. Immunoreactive gamma-interferon in insulin-secreting beta cells in type 1 diabetes mellitus. Lancet 1987;2:1423–7.
72. Nerup J, Mandrup-Poulsen T, Molvig J. The HLA-IDDM association: implications for etiology and pathogenesis of IDDM. Diabetes Metab Rev 1987;3:779–802.
73. Markmann JF, Hickey WF, Kimura H, et al. Gamma interferon induces novel expression of Ia antigens by rat pancreatic islet endocrine cells. Pancreas 1987;2:258–61.
74. Pober JS, Ginhone MA Jr, Collins T, et al. Interactions of T lymphocytes with human vascular endothelial cells: role of endothelial cell surface antigens. Immunobiology 1984;168:483–94.
75. Kakhooda AF, Like AA, Chappel CI, et al. The spontaneously diabetic Wistar rat: metabolic and morphologic studies. Diabetes 1977;26:100–12.
76. Marliss EB, Nakhooda AF, Poussier P, Sima AAF. The diabetic syndrome of the 'BB' Wistar rat: possible relevance to type 1 (insulin-dependent) diabetes in man. Diabetologia 1982;22:225–32.
77. Weringer EJ, Like AA. Immune attack on pancreatic islet transplants in the spontaneously diabetic biobreeding Worcester (BB/W) rat is not MHC restricted. J Immunol 1985;134:2383–6.
78. Woehrle M, Markmann JF, Silvers WK, et al. Transplantation of cultured pancreatic islets to BB rats. Surgery 1986;100:334–40.
79. Frizzera G, Hanto DW, Gajl-Peczalska KJ, et al. Polymorphic diffuse B-cell hyperplasias and lymphomas in renal transplant recipients. Cancer Res 1981; 41:4262–79.

8

Intestinal Transplantation

JAMES L. MADARA

Multiple obstacles to small intestinal transplantation in humans exist that largely have not been overcome (and often not even systematically studied). Thus it is not surprising that only a handful of attempts at transplanting human small intestine have been made [1]. Furthermore, it is not surprising that these few attempts have not met with great success.

The first such attempts failed almost immediately after surgery presumably due, in large part, to technical problems [2,3]. However, even after small intestinal transplantation had been performed that was technically successful from a surgical point of view [4–6], multiple complications ensued. Such transplants tended to become infiltrated with mononuclear cells [4] or were frankly necrotic [5] within 1 to 2 weeks, suggesting that acute rejection had taken place. One interesting exception was a transplantation in which the donor was an HLA-identical sibling and in which the patient was treated for rejection with immunosuppressive therapy [6]. This patient did reason-

I wish to acknowledge Dr. Robert Kirkman of the Department of Surgery, Brigham and Women's Hospital. Dr. Kirkman collaborated in the experiments in which I was involved; they are outlined in this chapter. I also thank Ms. Virginia Hamel for her skills in preparing this manuscript. This work was supported in part by NIH grant DK 35932.

ably well and was able to ingest food for 2 months. Since the donor intestinal segment was in continuity with the host intestine and practically the entire host small intestine had been resected, it is clear that the donor loop came in contact with meal-related lumenal substances during this time, and it is likely (but unproved) that the donor loop provided some absorptive function. The general medical condition of this patient subsequently deteriorated, and she died approximately 2.5 months after undergoing transplantation.

Potential Problems with Transplantation of the Small Intestine

In general, the sequential morphologic and functional alterations accompanying presumptive rejection in the above cases were not precisely defined. However, it is clear that multiple potential obstacles in addition to rejection may complicate attempts to successfully transplant the small intestine.

The first and most obvious potential problem is graft-vs-host disease (GVHD). The small intestine contains numerous clusters of mucosal and submucosal lymphoid cells [7] that can recognize and process foreign proteins and mount immune responses against these targets [8]. Such cells may enter into the general circulation [8]. Aggregates of lymphoid cells are most obvious in the distal ileum and appear as the macroscopic Peyer's patches. However, similar but smaller aggregates occur along the length of the small intestine [7], and thus one is not able to exclude these cells from the donor loop by selectively avoiding macroscopic Peyer's patches. Evidence suggests that the severity of clinical GVHD can be reduced by decreasing the amount of lymphoid tissue transplanted, i.e., transplanting shorter lengths of intestine [13]. In addition, data suggest that the lymphoid tissue in the mesenteric lymph nodes may be equally or even more important than lymphoid tissue in the intestinal wall in the development of GVHD [14]. In the rat GVHD does complicate small intestinal transplantation and, in fact, may be lethal [9].

An additional problem area potentially confounding successful small intestinal transplantation is enteric motility. For example, it has been shown that simply by autotransplantation, abnormalities in small intestinal motility occur [10]. If disorders of enteric motility occur in transplanted loops, complications ranging from diarrhea induced by dysmotility to bacterial overgrowth could be encountered.

Another example of a factor that perhaps should be better understood before attempts at transplantation in humans is the effect of lymphatic transection. Absorbed dietary lipid is largely packaged as chylomicrons, which are taken up through lacteals [7]. Blockade of this system by masses, such as tumors, may result in abnormal fat absorption. Thus unless transected lymphatic channels in allografts recanalize—and this may occur [11]—it is possible that defects in fat absorption might follow transplantation. Likely, other confounding factors hindering transplantation of the small intestine will be highlighted as we better understand the physiologic consequences of this procedure. For example, only recently has it been appreciated that denervation, which occurs with transplantation, may impair water absorption [11].

Is the need of small intestinal transplantation great enough to justify the expense necessary to study and resolve the obstacles outlined above? I really do not know. Dr. Robert Kirkman of the Brigham and Women's Hospital Department of Surgery recently pointed out to me that data on home total parenteral nutrition suggest that about 200 new patients require such support each year in the United States. Given that such therapy costs tens of thousands of dollars a year per patient, there might be an economic gain if small intestinal transplantation could be performed without costly associated morbidity. As important, significant morbidity is associated with total parenteral nutrition.

Structure and Function of Small Intestinal Epithelium Following Transplantation

Graft-vs-Host Disease

The pathology GVHD involving the intestine due to bone marrow transplantation in humans is well recognized and described in Chapter 9. It remains to be shown whether GVHD accompanying small bowel transplantation has comparable sequelae in the host intestine (and in other organs). Virtually nothing is known with certainty regarding small bowel transplant–stimulated GVHD in humans. In animal models it is clear that the syndrome of GVHD occurs after small intestinal transplantation [9]. However, most experimental studies judge GVHD on the basis of clinical features (e.g., hair and weight loss, death). Similarly, little is known concerning the histologic appearance of GVHD lesions following intestinal transplantation. Thus it is impossible to state whether GVHD associated with this procedure will be identical to GVHD following bone marrow transplantation.

Rejection

Histologic Appearance The experience with the histologic appearance of rejection of small intestinal allograft in humans is obviously limited. Sketchy reports suggest that, not surprisingly, mononuclear cell infiltration of the wall and mucosal necrosis occur [5] in the presence of patent large arteries. In dog models villus atrophy, thickening of the muscular wall, and sloughing of the mucosa have been described [15]. In my opinion, histologic descriptions of rejection-associated lesions are limited and generally not documented with photomicrographs. For this reason I will rely heavily on our own experience with this lesion as derived from experiments performed in rats [16]. It remains to be seen whether the lesions that develop in this model faithfully recapitulate those which develop in humans after transplantation. In these experiments we transplanted small intestinal segments from Lewis X Brown Norway F_1 hybrids into adult male Lewis rats. The allografts were not in continuity with the host intestine but were opened to stoma on the abdominal wall. We then sequentially obtained host and graft jejuna for histologic and functional studies.

As seen at low magnification by light microscopy, mucosa of allografts is

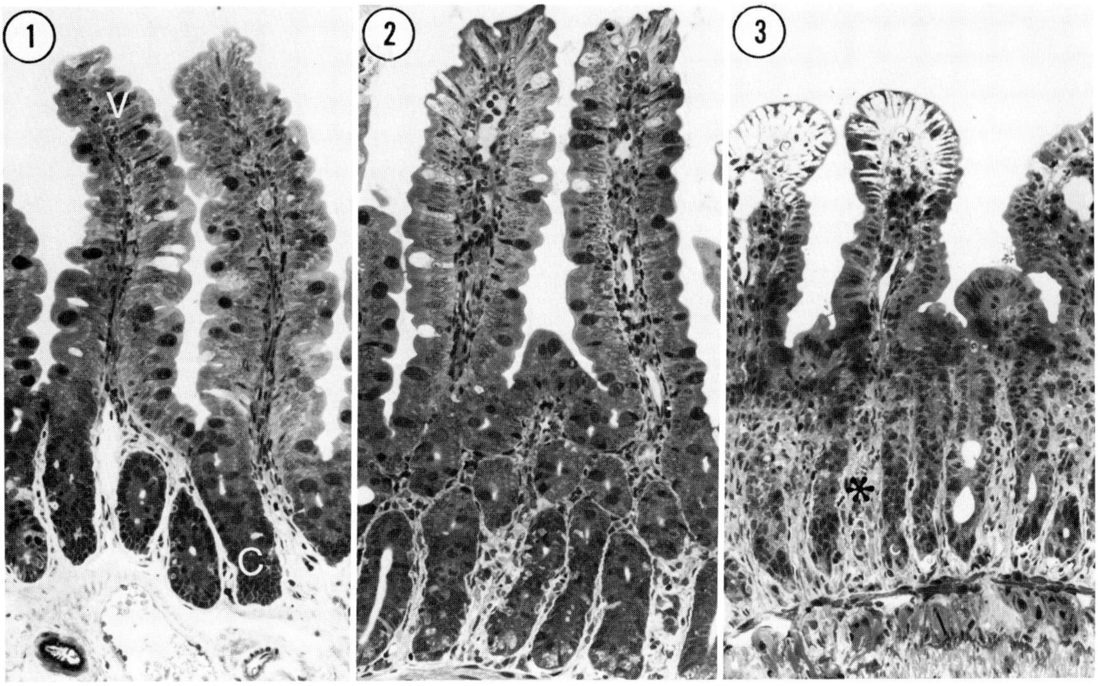

A *B* *C*

Figure 8.1
Light photomicrographs of 1 μm resin-embedded sections of jejunal mucosa at various intervals after transplantation. A. Control jejunal mucosa showing short crypts, C, *and tall villi,* V, *lined by columnar villus absorptive cells. B. Jejunal mucosa 3 days after transplantation. The morphologic appearance of the mucosa is similar to that of the control mucosa. Although some animal-to-animal variation in mucosal depth was noted, morphometric analysis revealed that mucosal surface amplification was not significantly different from controls. C. Jejunal mucosa 6 days after transplantation. Villi are shortened, and crypts appear to be minimally elongated. In addition, the paracellular spaces at the villus tips are dilated and the lamina propria adjacent to the crypt has increased numbers of mononuclear cells.*

structurally normal 3 days after transplantation (Fig. 8.1A and B). However, by day 6 structural abnormalities consisting of diminished villus height and mild elongation of crypts occurs (Fig. 8.1C). By 9 days the jejunal mucosa of allografts (but not of the host) is markedly affected (Fig. 8.1D and E): in areas that are least affected, villi and crypts are short, but in most areas villi-crypt architecture is ablated and a simple cuboidal epithelium of vacuolated cells lines this organ. In such areas infiltration by mononuclear cells is intense and fine mucosal and submucosal blood vessels display cellular walls and compromised lumens (Fig. 8.1D). Also, vesiculation and atrophy of the smooth muscle cells of the muscularis propria may be seen by day 9. Such changes are largely prevented with cyclosporine therapy (Fig. 8.1F). Figure 8.2 depicts the degree of structurally defined epithelial injury that can occur between days 3 and 9. Although absorptive cells at day 3 retain their usual columnar appearance and exhibit lush brush borders, by day 9 epithelial

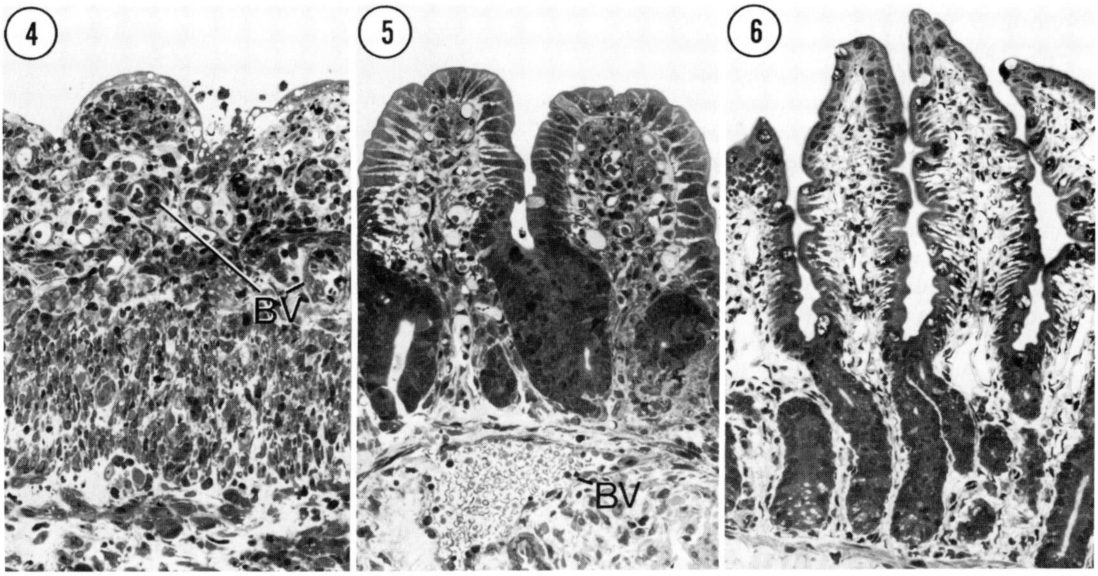

D E F

Figure 8.1 *(continued)*
D and E. Jejunal mucosa 4 days after transplantation. The degree of mucosal "atrophy," as indicated by crypt and villus shortening, was always striking. However, the degree of cytologic abnormality was occasionally only mild (5). Note that the more commonly seen severely affected areas with the cuboidal villus epithelial cells (4) display fine blood vessels, BV, *with compromised lumens, but the least affected areas (5) have fine blood vessels that appear relatively unremarkable. F. Jejunal mucosa 9 days after transplantation from an animal treated with cyclosporine. The mucosal structure in cyclosporine-treated animals was remarkably preserved, although morphometric analysis did reveal a substantial overall decrease in mucosal surface amplification (toluidine blue stain ×20). (From Madara JL, Kirkman RL. J Clin Invest 1985;75:502–12. Reproduced by copyright permission of the American Society for Clinical Investigation.)*

morphology is often low cuboidal, brush borders generally are not detectable by light microscopy, and cellular vacuolization is prominent. Of interest, acute rejection of human small intestinal allografts follows a similar temporal course [2,3,5] to that we describe in the rat.

Further analysis of the structural evolution of this lesion at higher magnification as seen by light and electron microscopy shows that subtle abnormalities consisting of rare foci of crypt epithelial cell destruction associated with mononuclear cell infiltration of the lamina propria can be detected at day 3. Such alterations are more prominent by day 6 (Fig. 8.3) even though cells lining the villi are cytologically normal at this time. Of interest, microvascular alterations occurred with a time course paralleling the crypt lesion. As shown in Figure 8.4, rarely by day 3, and prominently by day 6, endothelial cells of the microvasculature assumed swollen "activated" morphology and are often closely associated with large mononuclear cells. Often the lumens of such vessels are completely occluded. Such observations suggest

testinal GVHD following bone marrow transplantation is similarly directed toward the crypt epithelial lining [20,21].

Pathophysiologic Findings The above outline of the morphology of jejunal allograft rejection can also be placed into a functional perspective (for an overview of the principles of jejunal epithelial structure-function relationships, outlined below, see Madara and Trier [7]). The crypt epithelium is the only site at which jejunal epithelial cells move through the cell cycle; thus this is the "proliferative compartment" of this epithelium. Furthermore, after division, crypt cells migrate to the villus base, rapidly differentiate into villus absorptive cells (and other villus adult cell types), and finally migrate up the villus and are eventually sloughed into the lumen from the villus tip. The life span of the villus absorptive cell is approximately 3 to 5 days. Thus it is not surprising that injury to the proliferative crypt compartment would be followed by villus shortening. Alternatively, villus shortening and villus cell injury that occur late in the course of rejection could primarily result from ischemic injury induced by the microvascular lesion.

Cell proliferation is not the only function of the crypt epithelium. This is also the site of fluid and electrolyte secretion (see Madara and Trier [7]). Secretion by the crypt is an electrogenic mechanism due to the presence of chloride channels on the apical membranes of undifferentiated crypt cells. Thus one can detect an electrical signal on stimulation of chloride secretion with agents such as the phosphodiesterase inhibitor theophylline. As shown in Figure 8.5A, theophylline-induced chloride secretion in allografts is reduced as assessed by measurement of either transepithelial potential difference response or transepithelial short circuit current (I_{sc}). Furthermore, the temporal sequence of reduction in the ability to secrete (Fig. 8.5A) parallels nicely the evolution of the above described crypt injury. Comparable effects on chloride secretion were not seen in either host intestine or isografts [16]. Thus such functional alterations are clearly due to rejection.

Although the structure and function of crypt epithelium was affected early in the course of rejection, significant alterations in the structure of villus absorptive cells were not recognized until day 9. This structural feature also paralleled the evolution of alterations in function that specifically relate to the villus compartment. For example, absorptive cells on the villi absorb glucose through a sodium glucose co-transport mechanism. Since the net result is transepithelial absorption of a cation without an accompanying anion, electrical signals are again generated. As shown in Figure 8.5B, the electrical potential difference and I_{sc} occurring as a result of stimulated absorption of glucose is not significantly diminished in jejunal allografts until day 9. Again, such alterations do not occur in host jejuna or in isografts [16] and thus must be attributed to the rejection process. Finally, these alterations in epithelial transport are largely ablated with cyclosporine therapy, which, as noted above, also prevents the structural manifestations of rejection [16]. Unfortunately, cyclosporine is less effective in pigs than in rats [23] at ameliorating the structural effects of rejection. Thus the potential efficacy of this agent in suppressing small intestinal transplant rejection in humans is uncertain.

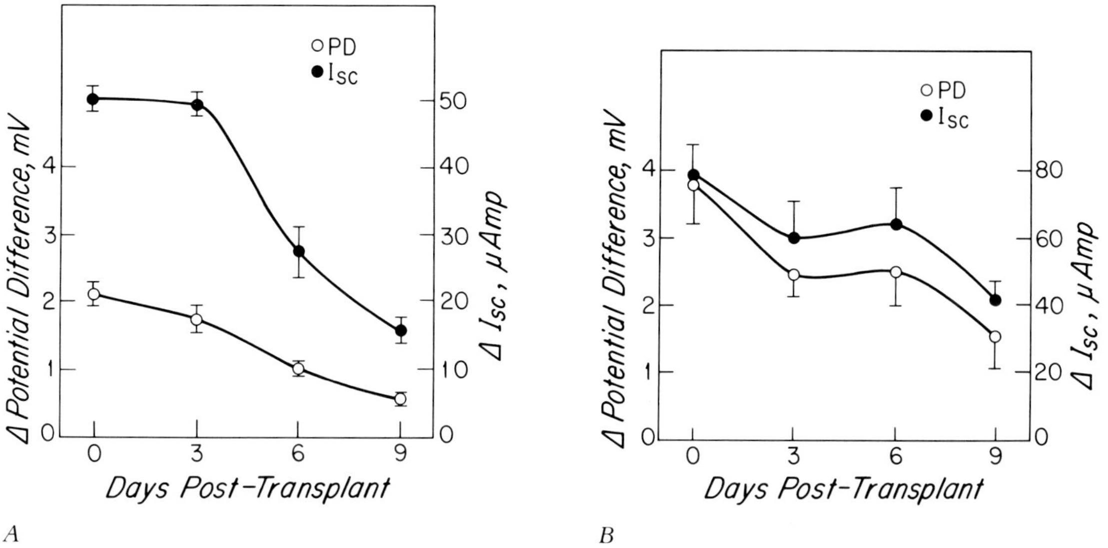

Figure 8.5
A. Effect of transplantation on stimulated chloride secretion of graft jejuna as assessed by measurement of electrical responses to 5 mM serosal theophylline. Marked impairment of active chloride secretion was present by the sixth postoperative day in graft jejunum. B. Effect of transplantation on stimulated sodium-coupled glucose transport of graft jejuna as assessed by measurement of electrical responses to 20 mM mucosal glucose. Impaired absorptive responses could be detected by measurements of I_{sc} *at 9 days or of* PD *by 3 days.* (PD, *transepithelial potential difference;* I_{sc}, *transepithelial short circuit current.) (From Madara JL, Kirkman RL. J Clin Invest 1985;75:502–12. Reproduced by copyright permission of the American Society for Clinical Investigation.)*

Summary and Conclusions

The available data concerning small intestinal transplantation both in humans and in experimental models are very limited compared with knowledge in other organs, such as the heart, lung, and kidney. In my view, one of the least developed aspects of the limited literature on small intestinal transplantation is the area of the pathology of rejection. The available data from the rat model suggest that with acute first-set rejection of jejunal allografts, the major initial targets are the endothelium of the microvasculature and the crypt epithelial cells. Later in rejection villus absorptive cells are affected, presumably indirectly. Functional sequelae, including diminished active secretory and absorptive functions, parallel these structural alterations, as does diminution in epithelial barrier function [16]. In some species, but not necessarily in all, structural and functional sequelae of rejection can be significantly ameliorated by cyclosporine therapy.

Of importance to pathologists is the microvascular and crypt injury that occurs early in the rejection process. These features, combined with the presence of unaffected columnar villus absorptive cells, are not characteristic of other diseases that affect the small intestine and that would enter into the clinical differential diagnosis for a patient who underwent intestinal transplantation. These features are also readily recognized in 1 μm sections prepared from mucosal biopsies and thus presumably could be used clinically in following patients with intestinal allografts. However, as can be distilled from this brief review, our knowledge in the area of small intestinal transplantation is presently cursory at best; much basic work remains to be done before such a procedure could be deemed a useful clinical tool.

References

1. Ruiz JO, Lillehei RC. Intestinal transplantation. Surg Clin North Am 1972;52:1075–91.
2. Lillehei RC, Idezuki Y, Feemster JA, et al. Transplantation of stomach, intestine, and pancreas: experimental and clinical observations. Surgery 1967;62:721–41.
3. Okumura M, Fujimura I, Ferrarri AA, et al. Transplante del intestino delgrado; apresentacao de um caso. Rev Hosp Clin Fac Med Sao Paolo 1969;24:39–54.
4. Olivier G, Rettori R, Olivier CH, et al. Homotransplantation orthotopique de l'intestine grêle et des côlons droight et transverse chez l'homme. J Chir 1969;98:323–30.
5. Alican F, Hardy JD, Mukadder C, et al. Intestinal transplantation: laboratory experience and report of a clinical case. Am J Surg 1971;121:150–9.
6. Fortner JG, Sichuk G, Litwin SD, Beattie EJ. Immunological responses to an intestinal allograft with HLA identical donor-recipient. Transplantation 1972;14:531–5.
7. Madara JL, Trier JS. Functional morphology of the mucosa of the small intestine. In: Johnson LR, ed. Physiology of the gastrointestinal tract, ed 2. New York: Raven, 1987;1209–51.
8. Kagnoff MF. Immunology of the digestive system. In: Johnson LR, ed. Physiology of the gastrointestinal tract, ed 2. New York: Raven, 1987;1699–1728.
9. Monchik GJ, Russell PS. Transplantation of small bowel in the rat: technical and immunological considerations. Surgery 1971;70:693–702.
10. Sarr MG, Kelley KA. Myoelectric activity of the autotransplanted canine jejunileum. Gastroenterology 1981;81:303–10.
11. Reznick RK, Craddock GH, Langer B, et al. Structure and function of small bowel allografts in the dog: immunosuppression with cyclosporine A. Can J Surg 1982;25:51–5.
12. Watson AJM, Lear PA, Ellot EJ, et al. Impaired water absorption in rat small bowel transplants is due to graft denervation. Gastroenterology 1987;92:1687.
13. Deltz E, Muller Hermelink HK, Ulrichs KK, et al. Development of GVH reaction in various target organs after small intestine transplantation. Transplant Proc 1981;13:1215–6.
14. Theide A, Deltz E, Schack T, Ulrichs K. Successful manipulation of GVHD-reaction in semi-allogeneic intestinal transplantation in rat by treatment of the donor recipient. (Abstr.) Presented at the Seventh International Congress in Microsurgery, Lyon, France: 1982.
15. Ruiz JO, Uchida H, Schultz LS, Lillehei RC. Problems in absorption and im-

munosuppression after intestinal allotransplantation. Am J Surg 1972;123:297–307.

16. Madara JL, Kirkman RL. Structural and functional evolution of jejunal allograft rejection in rats and the ameliorating effects of cyclosporine therapy. J Clin Invest 1985;75:502–12.
17. Forbes RDC, Guttman RD, Gomersall M, Hibberd J. A controlled serial ultrastructural tracer study of first-set cardiac allograft rejection in the rat. Am J Pathol 1983;111:184–6.
18. Dvorak M, Mihm M, Dvorak A, et al. Rejection of first-set skin allografts in man: the microvasculature is a critical target of the immune response. J Exp Med 1979;150:322–32.
19. Anderson ND, Wyllie RG, Shaker IJ. Pathogenesis of vascular injury in rejecting rat renal allografts. Johns Hopkins Med J 1977;144:135–47.
20. Sale GE, Shulman HM, McDonald GB, Thomas ED. Gastrointestinal GVH disease in man: a clinicopathologic study of the rectal mucosa. Am J Surg Pathol 1979;3:291–9.
21. Epstein RJ, McDonald GB, Sale GE, et al. The diagnostic accuracy of rectal biopsy in acute GVH disease: a prospective study of thirteen patients. Gastroenterology 1980;78:764–71.
22. Pritchard TJ, Madara JL, Tapper O, et al. Failure of cyclosporine to prevent small bowel allograft rejection in pigs. J Surg Res 1985;38:553–8.

9

Bone Marrow and Thymic Transplantation

GEORGE E. SALE

Marrow transplantation has achieved spectacular success over the last 20 years [1–3]. Because it is the most complicated transplant biologically yet the simplest surgically, it occupies a unique position among transplants. As in heart transplantation, high drama accompanies the total ablation of a vital organ and its attempted replacement. Before the marrow transplant, two systems are really ablated—hematopoietic and lymphoid. The complexity of postoperative care is so different in degree that it sets marrow transplantation clinically apart from the other types. It can also be argued that marrow transplantation has approached the broadest range of diseases and has provided more immunologic information in experimental and clinical studies than have the other forms.

Marrow transplantation generates different problems than does transplantation of most solid organs for two important reasons. The first is that the procedure is so simple that no "surgeon" is required. The resulting take or rejection of a graft cannot be diagnosed grossly and is understandable only in relatively abstract immunologic terms. The second is that rejection in this

This work was supported in part by grants CA 15704 and CA 18029 from the National Cancer Institute and HL 36444 from the National Heart and Lung Institute, NIH.

setting is less important (because less frequent) than its bizarre diametric opposite, graft-vs-host disease (GVHD), perhaps the strangest iatrogenic disease to come along in the twentieth century. This is, in stark language, the rejection of the patient by potent immunodestructive capabilities contained within or initiated by the T lymphocytes of the engrafted donor cells themselves. When the immunodeficiency caused by GVHD is superimposed on the lymphoid ablation caused by radiation and chemotherapy, the most severely immunosuppressed of humans results.

Thymic transplantation is included in this chapter for the obvious reason that it, too, can produce GVHD and has a similar aim: to replace cells of the immunohematopoietic system that are absent because of naturally occurring disease or therapeutic manipulations such as irradiation used in treating malignant disease.

Transplantation and Toxicity

Indications for Marrow Transplantation

Theoretically, marrow transplantation could be done for any disease in which marrow or immune cell replacement is needed, such as severe combined immune deficiency or after heavy irradiation and chemotherapy for treatment of tumors thought to have a steep enough dose/response curve to warrant the risk. In practice, transplantation has generally been carried out for aplastic anemia and acute leukemias, particularly myeloblastic. In addition, transplantation has been used to approach some inborn errors of metabolism that have a high mortality, such as major thalassemia and malignant osteopetrosis.

Severe combined immune deficiency and aplastic anemia were the first diseases in which major clinical successes were reported. After enough transplantation had been performed in end-stage leukemia patients, it became evident that a small number were being "cured" (evidenced by flat survival probability curves) and that good clinical condition was important to improve the prognosis. Then a major advance resulted from transplanting adult acute myelogenous leukemia patients while they were still in first remission. This yielded a stunning 60% long-term survival rate that became a major stimulus for performing the procedure in many new centers worldwide. Meanwhile, major advances had been made against rejection in aplastic anemia (the group at greatest risk for rejection) when studies by Storb et al. [4] revealed presensitization due to prior blood transfusions to be associated with a 30% risk of rejection. Early transplantation before transfusions in this severely aplastic group cut the rejection rate to 5%. Subsequently, transplantation in patients with chronic myelogenous leukemia while still in the chronic phase has become more common, since these patients have a short median survival with any prior conventional regimen. This has been another major success.

More recent studies have focused on allogeneic transplantation for patients with resistant forms of lymphoma and Hodgkin's disease. Efforts to deplete the donor bone marrow of mature T lymphocytes to prevent GVHD have generally been successful in that aim but have been associated with very disappointing increases in both the rejection and relapse rates in a large number of centers, prompting a major reassessment of this approach. Meanwhile, great interest in "purging" tumor cells from bone marrow, primarily by using monoclonal antibodies to antigenic determinants on tumor cell surfaces, has been of widespread interest, especially associated with use of autologous cryopreserved bone marrow.

Technique and HLA Matching

The theoretically ideal donor of bone marrow is an identical twin, whose marrow cells should be neither rejected nor capable of mounting a graft-vs-host reaction. Identical twin transplantations are indeed among the most successful but are obviously rare. The next best donor is a sibling matched at the major histocompatibility loci (chromosome 6 and the A, B, and D loci). A patient with siblings has a good chance of finding a match (>25% per sibling) and in more than half the cases can avoid significant GVHD or rejection.

Most patients have neither a twin nor a matched sibling donor. For these patients, the possibility of an unrelated matched donor has recently been opened up by an international cooperative blood banking effort to provide such donors [5]. More than a hundred such transplantations will have been reported by the publication of this book. Results have been very promising. Even without a matched donor, a person has the additional two options of a partially mismatched transplant with one or two determinants unmatched (a higher risk procedure still under investigation) or autologous transplant with marrow stored while in remission and treated to attempt the removal of residual tumor cells without damaging stem cells.

The marrow transplant procedure itself is simple. Donor marrow is obtained with multiple needle aspirations from iliac crests and occasionally femoral or other sites, usually under general anesthesia. The marrow is anticoagulated and strained through fine mesh, then infused intravenously into the recipient, who has just been treated with irradiation or chemotherapy to ablate host rejection responses as well as tumor in some cases. Extensive supportive care is given until engraftment produces good peripheral white blood cell counts, usually at 3 weeks. The major difficulties causing disease in these patients relate to the toxicity of irradiation and chemotherapy, alloimmune diseases (rejection, GVHD), and temporary but severe immune deficiency associated with infection. Some of the bone marrow samples undergo manipulation before reinfusion, such as removal of T cells with monoclonal antibodies plus complement, or tumor cell killing with antibodies or chemotherapeutic agents.

Bone Marrow Before and After Transplantation

Before transplantation, rapid and thorough reevaluation of the bone marrow is important. Awareness of relapse status must be accurate and current. The primary diagnosis must be confirmed. In aplastic and dysmyeloplastic states, as well as chronic myelogenous leukemia, chromosome analysis must be repeated. Such diseases as hairy-cell leukemia and atypical myelodysplasia in apparent aplastic anemia must be ruled out.

After transplantation, marrow examinations at days 7, 14, 21, and 28 are routine. On day 7, severe fat necrosis of the marrow is common, with residual macrophages, mast cells, and fibroblasts. In some cases, early engraftment may be evident in the form of hematopoietic precursors or colonies in sections or smears. Some colonies of myeloid, erythroid, and megakaryocytic lineage are usually seen by day 14. Absolute peripheral granulocyte counts greater than $500/mm^2$ are usually seen before week 3. If blasts are persistent at day 7 or 14, even if they are not seen on day 21 and 28, chances of relapse are much increased. Platelet counts are usually the latest to recover but are usually adequate by day 30 [6].

True rejection occurs in 5% to 30% of aplastic patients and (until the advent of marrow T-cell depletion) in less than 4% of leukemia patients [7]. "True" rejection requires evidence of engraftment on bone marrow morphology followed by its loss. In most such cases, rejection is evident by day 60 but may occur later. Primary failure to engraft is defined by absent evidence of a graft at any time after infusion and is thought by some to be mediated by natural killer (NK) cells. The morphology of rejection is nonspecific marrow damage with marked loss of cellularity, usually in three lines simultaneously, although occasionally heralded by pure red cell or granulocytic aplasia. Mortality is high, and second transplantation attempts are not usually successful after rejection.

Toxicity of Radiation and Chemotherapy

The doses of irradiation and chemotherapy given marrow transplant recipients for leukemia are set at deliberately superlethal ranges that require rescue for marrow aplasia. Consequently, although the marrow toxicity is redressed by the new marrow, toxicity to gut, liver, lung, skin, and other organs can present severe problems. Immediate toxicity to the gastrointestinal tract includes a brief pancreatitis and an acute "mucositis" involving most mucosal surfaces. The histologic expression of the latter is atypia of mucosal epithelia followed by regeneration due to the agents' acute cytotoxic effects. Mouth, conjunctiva, throat, esophagus, and intestines suffer similar lesions. Our data on sequential recovery of the mucosa observed on rectal biopsy suggest that, as with skin and bone marrow, it takes about 3 weeks for these organs to recover from the insults inflicted by the preconditioning regimens. Occasional cases will be very severe, for example, pseudomembranous colitis occurring by day 0 associated with bacterial or fungal superinfection. Similarly, severe, often protracted cystitis may be attributed to mucosal damage caused by cyclophosphamide. Cardiotoxicity is an occasional problem associated usually with previous daunomycin administration. When the ejection fraction is low, nitrogen mustard may be substituted for cyclophosphamide in the preconditioning regimen for such reasons.

Perhaps the most puzzling problem in the area of toxicity is the fact that about 11% of patients in both the allogeneic and syngeneic recipient population develop an idiopathic, probably noninfectious interstitial pneumonitis. Epidemiologic indications are that this entity is most tightly linked to radiation as a risk factor. The patients show a nonspecific interstitial pneumonia with diffuse alveolar damage. Fractionation of the radiation dosages to approximately 200 rad (two Gray) fractions delivered in five to seven daily doses has decreased the relative toxicity of this irradiation to the lung.

Hepatic toxicity, in the form of veno-occlusive disease, has emerged as an extremely common and important dose-limiting toxicity for these radiochemotherapeutic regimens. In 1976, this entity had not been separated clearly from the centrolobular congestion associated with terminal cardiac failure, nor had its clinical manifestations, such as bilirubin elevation, been distinguished from those of severe GVHD. It was therefore not surprising that careful histologic studies by Berk et al. [8] led to the suggestion that centrilobular venous damage of this sort was a manifestation of GVHD. Further study established that veno-occlusive disease was associated with the dose and type of chemoradiotherapy, but did not segregate with manifestations of GVHD, as defined clinically and histologically in the major extrahepatic target organs (skin and gut) [9]. Further clinical and histologic studies have clearly defined the diagnostic features and some of the pathophysiologic mechanisms of veno-occlusive disease [10–12].

Veno-occlusive disease usually occurs before day 15 to 20 after transplantation; ascites, a tender enlarged liver, weight gain, and elevated total bilirubin tip off the clinician to the disease. Hepatorenal syndrome requiring dialysis is frequent. Aggressive fluid management often reverses the course, but mortality is relatively high at 33%. If the patient develops liver GVHD in addition, the prognosis worsens.

Histologically, veno-occlusive disease consists of damage to the central vein of the lobule, characterized by endothelial damage and loss, subendothelial edema and hemorrhage, and subsequent accumulation of some coagulation factors. The initial lesion is a functional obstruction of the postsinusoidal endothelial pores entering the small venules. This is seen as due to acute edema and hemorrhage and is not thrombotic in the classic sense. The eventual fibrosis of the venular wall or extravenular tissue and centrolobular region that develops is subtle and requires a trichrome stain to appreciate. The lesion is easily missed in all its stages. Shulman and colleagues have demonstrated factor VIII and fibrinogen in the lesions by immunohistochemistry [12]. Early veno-occlusive disease is hard to distinguish from congestive changes. Late veno-occlusive disease may be confused with nonspecific centrolobular collagenization.

Graft-vs-Host Disease

The unique complication of marrow transplantation (or transplantation of any living allogeneic lymphoid cells) is GVHD. There is a bewildering array of literature on the graft-vs-host reaction as it is operationally defined in many different in vitro and in vivo systems. For the purposes of this chapter it can be defined as a syndrome of skin, liver, and gut disease with immunodeficiency caused by allogeneic T lymphocytes given during a transplantation containing allogeneic lymphocytes (e.g., a blood, marrow, spleen, liver, or gut transplant).

As implied in Chapter 1, the pathology of GVHD should in theory shed light on the rejection of individual organ transplantation. To a degree this is true. Comparing skin and liver transplants to GVHD of these organs has been fruitful in identifying cellular targets in endothelium and epithelium. Now it appears that the lung may teach us similar, although hard-learned, lessons as we compare the bronchiolar lesions of heart-lung transplant recipients (Chapter 6) with the bronchiolar lesions statistically associated with chronic GVHD [14,15].

To paraphrase a classic lecture by R.E. Billingham [16], the fundamental requirements for a true graft-vs-host reaction are (1) a donor with one or more genetically determined differences from the host, (2) the introduction of living immunocompetent cells (e.g., lymphocytes or stem cells from the donor into the host), (3) survival of the donor cells in the host at least long enough to undergo an immunologic reaction, and (4) end-point assessable evidence of an immunologic reaction by the donor cells against host tissues (e.g., target cell damage). A shorthand but perhaps inaccurate way of describing GVHD is to suggest that it is the diametric opposite of rejection in which the graft rejects the host. Graft-vs-host "disease" as opposed to "reaction" refers to the syndrome of clinical features caused by the attack of immunocompetent donor lymphoid cells against certain target organs in the host. In humans, GVHD has been separated into an early acute form occurring in the first 3 months after transplantation and a later chronic form. Although this is partially arbitrary, distinct immunologic and histologic differences between the two syndromes may indicate differing pathogenesis.

Diagnosis and Management

The most common time of onset for acute GVHD is in the third to fourth week after transplantation, when engraftment is becoming established. However, the range of onset can be between 1 week and as long as 60 to 80 days. The cases that occur during the first 4 weeks pose the greatest diagnostic difficulty because of the toxicity reactions from chemotherapy and radiation that can mimic the signs and symptoms of GVHD in the skin, liver, and gut as well as the fact that these patients undergo infections during this period that may mimic one or another clinical feature of GVHD [17,18]. Fortunately, in most patients, GVHD can be sorted out from these other elements by combining clinical judgment, histologic findings, and repeated observation. The pathologist's role is usually to indicate whether the histologic findings are compatible with the diagnosis of GVHD, but he or she may not always be able to render a pathognomonic statement, since even the highly characteristic histologic features are not 100% specific (Table 9.1).

Typical clinical features of acute GVHD are skin rash, diarrhea, and jaundice with fever. The initial target organ and severity of involvement vary. In

Table 9.1
*Unifying diagnostic features of graft-versus-host disease following bone marrow transplantation**

	Skin	*Liver*	*Intestine*	*Squamous mucosa of lip or mouth*	*Ducts of salivary or lacrimal gland*	*Conjunctiva and tarsal plate*
Consistent lesion	Basal vacuolar degeneration	Hepatocyte degeneration; eosinophilic necrosis	Crypt abscess	Basal vacuolar degeneration with mononuclear infiltrates	Abnormal periductal mononuclear infiltrates	Mononuclear cell infiltration
"Diagnostic" lesion	Eosinophilic bodies (after day 20)	Atypical degeneration of small bile ducts	Individual crypt cell necrosis and mononuclear cell infiltration ("exploding crypt") (see Sale et al., ref. 18)	Eosinophilic bodies (as in skin)	Ductal epithelial cell necrosis, often with dilatation and attenuation or obliteration	Basal cell necrosis in epithelium of conjunctiva or tarsal plate

*Unifying diagnostic lesions of graft-vs-host disease are individual cell death (apoptosis) based on a "threshold" concept of diagnosis in which the "diagnostic" lesion is the minimum degree of change needed for diagnosis. The "consistent" lesion is suspicious but insufficient for a diagnosis.
Source: Adapted from Sale GE, Shulman HM. The pathology of bone marrow transplantation. New York: Masson Publishing USA, 1984.

the initial reports, 70% of the patients who were transplanted by matched allografts developed GVHD. Frequency fluctuated thereafter, and the overall incidence is approximately 55% without T-cell depletion of bone marrow in HLA-matched recipients. Clinical severity of GVHD is graded as designated in Table 9.2. In general, grades II through IV have prognostic significance, whereas grades 0 and I are nondiagnostic. Severe acute GVHD may result in fatal infection by denudation of the gut mucosa or by general immunodeficiency, producing greater susceptibility to threatening infections such as pneumonia or disseminated fungus. Early liver disease with ascites (day 0 to 15) is usually veno-occlusive disease rather than GVHD, although initially this was misdiagnosed. This is treated differently than GVHD, making the distinction important. Treatment of patients with acute GVHD has varied over the years but usually employs steroids, cyclosporine, methotrexate in low doses, and antibodies to T cells in the form of antithymocyte globulins and monoclonal antibodies to known specific epitopes.

Chronic GVHD, a late sequel, also involves multiple systems and seems to be a superimposition of some features of autoimmunity on the preexisting alloimmune state [19–21]. Recent data from Parkman and colleagues suggest that in addition to alloimmune reactivity, some host cells may react against host fibroblasts [22]. The onset of chronic GVHD may be progressive from a prior state of acute GVHD, or it may follow a quiescent period of clinical inactivity of acute GVHD. Alternatively, it may occur de novo without preceding evidence of acute GVHD. In the absence of specific therapy, clinical signs of chronic GVHD were reported to develop between day 70 and 250 and occasionally as late as day 500. The most frequent time for this disease to develop is between days 120 and 150. Earlier recognition has occurred

Table 9.2
Overall clinical grading of severity of GVHD

Grade	*Degree of organ involvement*
I	+ to + + skin rash; no gut involvement; no liver involvement; no decrease in clinical performance
II	+ to + + + skin rash; + gut involvement or + liver involvement (or both); mild decrease in clinical performance
III	+ + to + + + skin rash; + + to + + + gut involvement or + + to + + + + liver involvement (or both); marked decrease in clinical performance
IV	similar to grade III with + + to + + + + organ involvement and extreme decrease in clinical performance

Source: Adapted from Thomas ED, Storb R, Clift RA, et al. Bone marrow transplantation. N Engl J Med 1975;292:832–43, 895–902.

recently as a result of studies obtained at days 80 to 100 routinely in follow-up of patients in an outpatient clinic.

In some patients the onset of chronic GVHD is associated with sun exposure, febrile illnesses, or viral infections. The initial sites involved may correspond to sun exposure, trauma, venous stasis, viral exanthemas, or prior local irradiation. Although a minority of patients have limited GVHD that does not progress, most cases are eventually disseminated. Typical manifestations of chronic GVHD include scleroderma, chronic liver disease, sicca syndrome, and esophagitis, with less frequent syndromes including myositis, serositis, arthritis, and vaginal stenosis. Circulating autoantibodies were reported in approximately two thirds of untreated patients with chronic GVHD, including antinuclear antibody, rheumatoid factor, antimitochondrial antibody, and direct Coombs' reactivity. Treated patients have far fewer autoantibody manifestations. Eosinophilia occurs in 75% of chronic GVHD patients. Approximately 20% will fulfill the criteria of the American Rheumatological Association for the diagnosis of systemic lupus erythematosus despite the fact that the overall similarity to scleroderma is the most striking. The limited form of chronic GVHD has skin lesions that resemble localized scleroderma. The more frequent extensive disease shows generalized inflammatory involvement of skin beginning with lichenoid lesions and followed by sclerodermatous lesions, sicca syndrome, and eventual development of scleroderma in some patients.

There is a high morbidity and mortality particularly associated with immune deficiency. Morbidity is due to cosmetic deformities from skin contractures, ulcerations, xero-ophthalmia, and weight loss; mortality is due to frequent infections, predominantly with gram-positive organisms. Weight loss and failure to thrive are frequent, probably due to multiple factors including poor caloric intake secondary to xerostomia and the dysphagia of esophagitis and occasionally from malabsorption. Therapeutic trials have so far concluded that prednisone alone is superior to the combination of prednisone and azathioprine for the care of these patients and that cyclosporine has a distinct role in some other patients.

Pathophysiology

The pathogenesis of GVHD is a complex topic that here can be only outlined. Allogeneic donor bone marrow contains a mixture of hematopoietic cells and lymphocytes of both mature B and T phenotype as well as less mature lymphoid cells. A number of animal and other studies have clearly indicated that the T lymphocytes within the bone marrow graft are the responsible initiating cells for the graft-vs-host reaction and that of particular importance (at least for acute GVHD) are the mature T cells that have achieved a phenotype of the T8:T4 level. Animal studies indicate that either the T4- or the T8-positive cell groups can subserve a graft-vs-host reaction [23,24]. If mature T cells are removed from bone marrow of rats and mice before marrow transplantation, graft-vs-host reaction is largely prevented. Similar results, although less uniform, have occurred in human beings.

The method by which these T cells produce the graft-vs-host reaction is unknown. The "lymphoid suicide" reaction is thought to be one of the first events that is a pitched battle between donor and host T lymphocytes, predominantly killers, producing a massive suicide or mutual fratricide of lymphocytes. This is thought to be an in vivo reflection of the mixed lymphocyte reaction, which has been used to determine the DR locus incompatibilities. These are oversimplifications for several reasons, but it is clear that profound lymphoid depletion occurs even in F1 hybrid situations in which radiation is not necessary to produce engraftment. Thus, in both the radiation chimera and the F1 hybrid, the destruction of immune system cells is profound in the lymph nodes, spleen, and thymus of the hosts; profound immune deficiency follows.

Some authors have suggested that there is a specific attack not only by donor lymphocytes against host lymphocytes but by donor lymphocytes against host epithelial cells of the thymus, skin, liver, gut, and other targets. Seemayer and colleagues [25] have postulated that a specific damaging effect by donor T-cell killer lymphocytes or NK cells may cause severe damage to thymic epithelium, producing severe immunodeficiency for long periods. Similarly, other authors have suggested that these killer lymphocytes kill epithelial cells in the skin, liver, and gut directly and have published photographs of satellite cell dyskeratosis of the skin and crypt cell necrosis in the gut as evidence, albeit indirect. Some have argued that the GVHD or wasting syndrome is entirely secondary to immunodeficiency and that the lesions of skin, liver, and gut are simply secondary to infection. This view is no longer widely held; most investigators agree that there is a component not only of lymphoid but also of epithelial destruction that may be directly cytotoxic. Evidence in humans is to date almost entirely circumstantial, but animal studies have shown direct cytotoxic effects in a number of systems. Relevant studies by Steinmuller and colleagues showed direct cytotoxic activity of T cells in mice against a minor histocompatibility antigen expressed in epidermal cells [26,27].

In tandem with recent studies on autoimmunity in humans and animals, it has become evident that there are not only circulating autoantibodies that may be normal or physiologic expressions of the immune system but also circulating autocytotoxic T cells and NK cells that may represent a physiologic mechanism. In this regard, the confusing issue of "pseudo GVHD," in which graft-vs-host–like syndromes were reported and evaluated in autologous and syngeneic graft recipients, may be more easily explained as an aberrant autoimmune phenomenon associated with an imbalance of the regulatory mechanisms of normal T-cell physiology. Thus, although it is a misnomer to term such reactions GVHD, they can now be more easily understood in light of modern immunology's concept of autocytotoxic cells in normal physiology.

A particularly interesting line of thought suggests that mechanisms are different in acute versus chronic GVHD. The issue is whether chronic GVHD is simply the sequel of prolonged activity of the same mechanisms (largely cytotoxicity directed at host alloantigen) as obtain in acute GVHD or whether it operates by a second mechanism that is largely autoimmune rather than alloimmune and involves altered regulation of collagen synthesis by fibroblasts, resulting in the fibrosis seen in the sclerodermatous skin and salivary, lacrimal, and hepatic connective tissue.

Recent studies in a mouse minor histoincompatible GVHD model provide evidence that lymphoid cells cloned from the spleens of animals with chronic GVHD are able to increase the amounts of collagen synthesized per fibroblast in affected mice and that these lymphocytes may be directed against autologous (host) D (Ia) locus determinants on the fibroblast surface [21]. The most recent data suggest that IL-3 or IL-4 may be very important effector molecules in this process. Tending to confirm a role of altered immunoregulatory cell circuits alone in GVHD-like phenomena (unrelated to alloimmune differences between donor and host) is the syngeneic "pseudo GVHD" syndrome, which can be induced by cyclosporine in mice and rats [28]. Thus, some evidence is now available to implicate autoimmunity (superimposed on alloimmunity) as an important process in chronic GVHD. That chronic GVHD spares the gut in both humans and mice remains unexplained.

Clinical and Pathologic Findings

The histologic findings in GVHD following bone marrow transplantation are summarized in Table 9.2. The histology of skin GVHD is that of a lichenoid skin reaction with a relatively sparse lymphoid infiltrate, exocytosis of mononuclear cells into the epidermis, and "satellite cell dyskeratosis" (in which lymphoid cells surround epidermal cells, many of which undergo keratinization and destruction or what has been described by Weeden and Searle as apoptosis, and die). The reaction is often associated with basal cell vacuolization and spongiosis and with a surprisingly sparse perivascular dermal infiltrate. Hair follicles and surface epidermis are often attacked simultaneously. Follicular necks and the cells at the bases of the epidermal rete ridges are usually attacked first, which has given rise to our hypothesis that stem cells or their early progeny may be targets in this reaction [29].

Distinguishing the skin lesions of GVHD during the first 3 weeks after transplantation from less specific infectious, immunologic, or toxic reactions to radiation and chemotherapy is a guessing game within a nightmare. So far the only approach that seems to be logical is serial skin biopsies and careful clinicopathologic correlation. Occasionally, sweat ducts are involved early in the process, but usually this is found in patients with chronic GVHD. Cytologic atypia is considered the basic hallmark of radiation and chemotherapy reactions and usually wanes after 3 to 4 weeks after the transplant (Fig. 9.1). A minor form of post-transplant dermatitis with eczematous histologic features has been described by Sloane and colleagues, who consider it unrelated to GVHD [30]. Chronic GVHD usually presents with a more acanthotic lichenoid picture similar to lichen planus. With varying degrees of rapidity these patients develop papillary dermal sclerosis and then may develop deep sclerodermatous collagenization of the dermis associated with inflammatory lesions of the sweat glands and ducts and a panniculitis of the

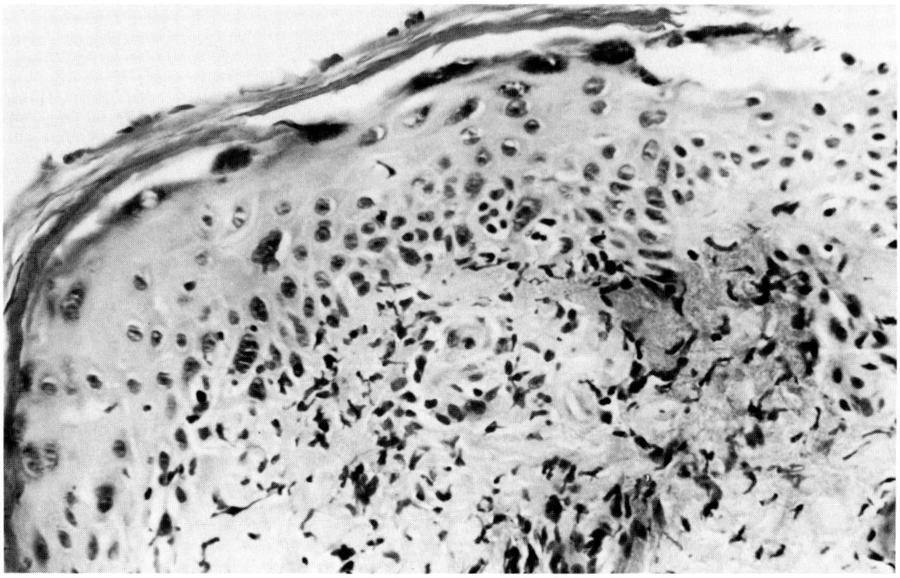

Figure 9.1
Medium-power photograph of skin biopsy obtained day 19 after identical twin graft in patient preconditioned with cyclophosphamide and 1000 rad of total body irradiation for leukemia. There is an inflammatory infiltrate of lymphocytes at the dermal-epidermal junction. Two foci in the center show individual epidermal cell necrosis with adjacent lymphocytes compatible with satellitosis and lymphocytes around dying individual epithelial cells. Note the moderate cytologic atypia manifested by variation in nuclear size and shape (hematoxylin-eosin ×700). This illustrates the difficulty associated with diagnosing GVHD in the first 3 weeks after transplantation. Such cases have been interpreted by other authors as evidence of a pseudo-GVHD reaction in twins.

subcutaneous fat with the production of new bands of fibrous tissue between fat lobules (Figs. 9.2 to 9.7). This eventuates in dense deep scleroderma and a hidebound skin. Pigmentation abnormalities and severe atrophy of the epidermis accompany these changes. Often the atrophy is so severe that the skin is ulcerated.

The gut lesions of GVHD usually appear within a few days of skin lesions and evidence of liver function test abnormalities. Anorexia, nausea, and secretory diarrhea are cardinal signs. Volume of diarrhea may range from 1 to 4 liters per day. The initial lesion histologically is individual cell necrosis in the crypts of ileal, rectal, jejunal, or duodenal tissue. Typically, the distal small bowel is involved maximally, but involvement of the gastrointestinal tract in acute GVHD is much more generalized than has been usually appreciated. Multiple individual cell death within crypts produces the appearance of the "exploding crypt" followed by crypt abscess formation and (in severe cases) total loss of the epithelium of the gastrointestinal tract with ensuing disseminated gram-negative septicemia and often uncontrollable endotoxic death (Figs. 9.8 to 9.10). Gastrointestinal bleeding is also a serious hazard at this time. The cause of death in acute GVHD is usually from this severe

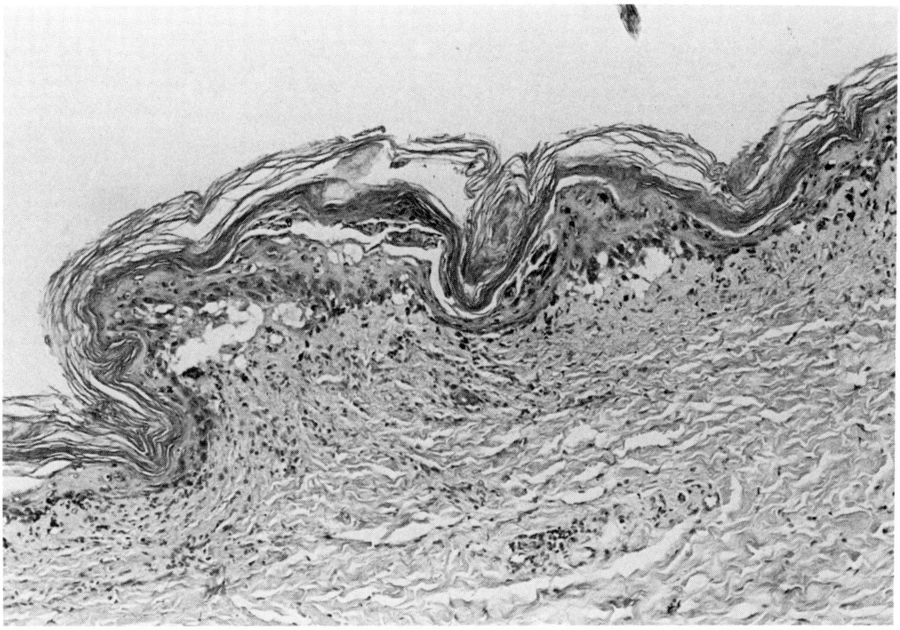

Figure 9.2
Severe acute GVHD of the skin with gross features resembling those of toxic epidermal necrolysis 18 days after mismatched allogeneic transplant. Despite the paucity of infiltrating mononuclear cells, there is necrosis of most of the stratum spinosum of the epidermis, and the basal layers show separation from dermis. Simultaneously there was frank ulceration in other areas of the skin as well as less severe lesions of grade II GVHD in the skin with simultaneous liver and gastrointestinal tract involvement (UPN 640). (From Sale GE, Shulman HM. The pathology of bone marrow transplantation. New York: Masson Publishing USA, 1984.)

gut involvement and only occasionally due to predominantly severe skin involvement with an appearance of second-degree burns.

Protracted gut GVHD can resemble Crohn's disease on x-ray film and gross appearance but histologically has no resemblance. Superinfection with cytomegalovirus (CMV) fungi and bacteria is frequent. Esophagitis during the period of maximal risk for acute GVHD is often due to reflux or to *Candida* or CMV infection but can be due to acute GVHD. If the patient recovers, the usual only remaining target organ for chronic GVHD within the gut is the esophagus, which may show some chronic changes in the distal third but particularly web formation in the proximal third, an event whose site predilection remains unexplained. The lesions that develop in this region arise from severe chronic inflammation and fibrosis.

Liver lesions in GVHD are more clearly understood due to clarification of two areas of controversy in this field. Small bile duct lesions with mononuclear cell infiltration and individual cell destruction had been observed in GVHD since the earliest histologic studies. Van Bekkum and De Vries in 1967 reported such lesions in both nonhuman primates and human recipi-

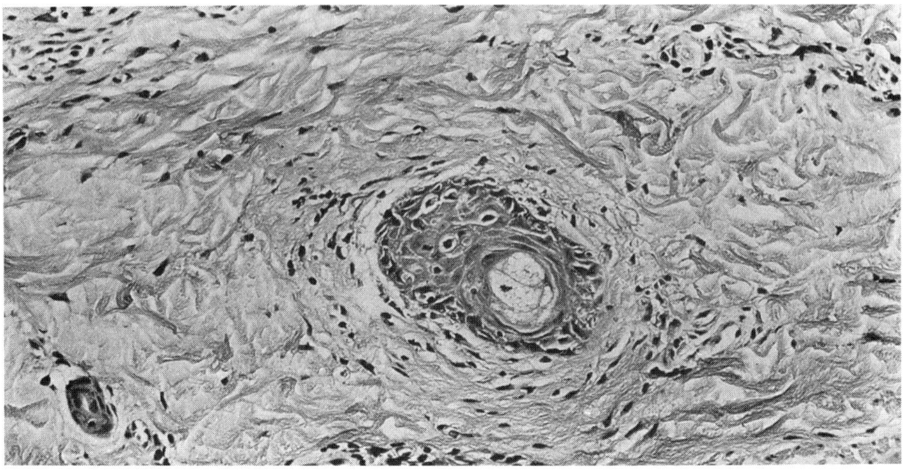

Figure 9.3
GVHD involving hair follicle in leukemia patient 80 days after allograft showing typical infiltrating lesions of the hair follicle and some perivascular involvement of adjacent dermis. Sweat duct in the lower left corner also shows initial involvement (hematoxylin-eosin × 250).

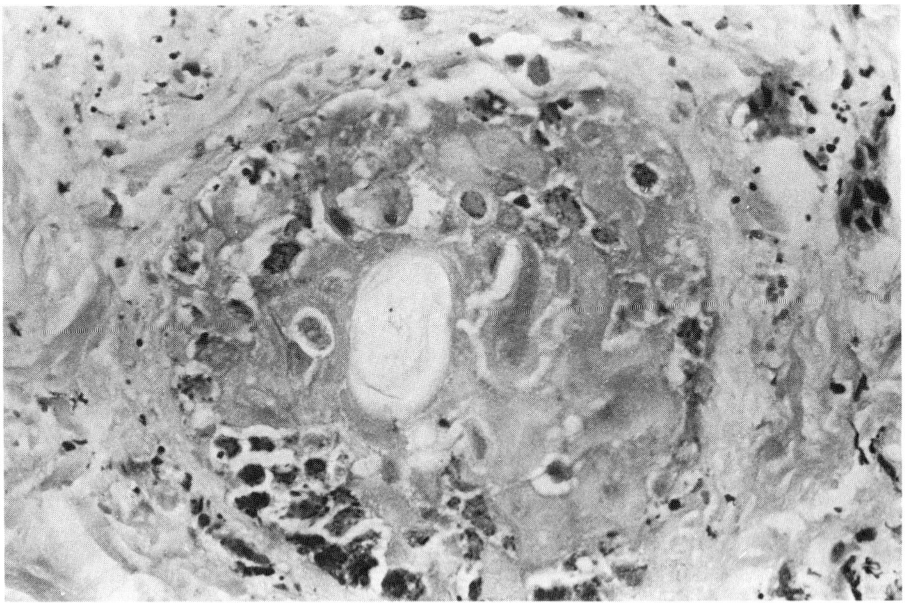

Figure 9.4
One of the differential diagnoses of skin GVHD is early viral involvement, particularly with herpes zoster. This hair follicle shows relatively advanced invasion by herpes zoster in a patient who initially presented with maculopapular lesions that progressed to vesicles. Note marginated chromatin in many of the involved cells of this hair follicle. At this stage, the differential diagnosis between this and GVHD is simple, but before this it can be quite difficult. This emphasizes the need for careful clinical and pathologic correlation (hematoxylin-eosin × 700).

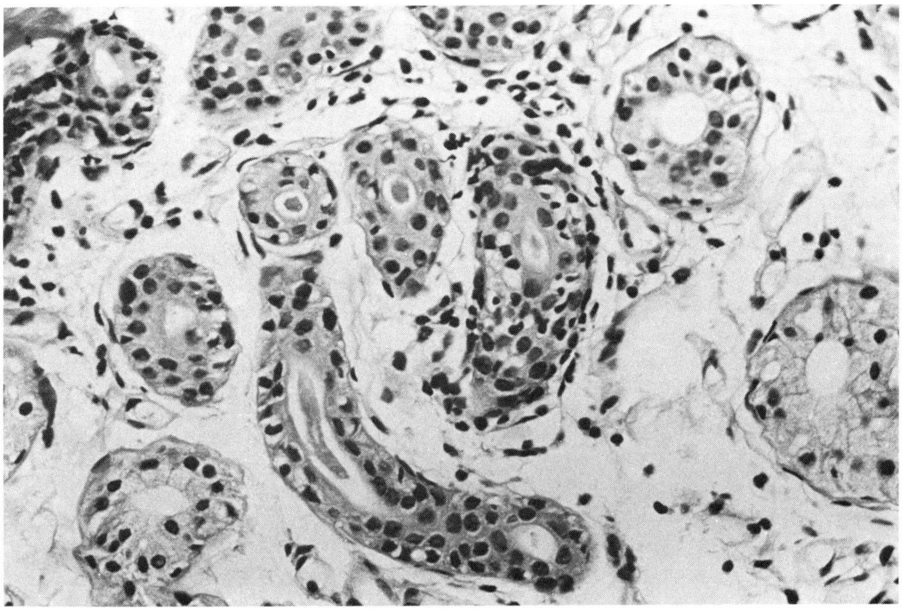

Figure 9.5
Medium-power photograph of early chronic GVHD showing characteristic infiltrating lesions and destruction of epithelial cells in several sweat ducts in this eccrine coil approximately day 85 after allograft for leukemia (hematoxylin-eosin × 450).

ents. Lerner and colleagues in 1974 proposed that the small bile duct lesions be used as diagnostic and grading criteria. Woodruff and Slavin suggest that these lesions were not specific and were more likely viral in origin. A coded study of canine marrow transplant recipients reported that small bile duct lesions occur with high frequency in mismatched allograft combinations and are absent in autografts and radiation controls [31]. Subsequent separate studies by Berman, Berneau, Sloane, and Shulman have strongly supported the disease specificity of small bile duct lesions for GVHD [32–36]. Furthermore, Fennell [37] and Snover [38] have subsequently clearly demonstrated that chronic liver allograft rejection also shows small bile duct lesions indistinguishable from those of GVHD. Progressive GVHD of the liver produces a picture of bizarre periportal ductules containing inspissated bile. Recent data have shown that small bile ducts in rats and humans express class II antigen when immunologically stimulated in GVHD, as do the enterocytes and epidermal cells. The fact that the small bile ductule shares this type of individual cell necrosis and the facultative production and expression of class II antigen is a unifying pathogenetic feature of the lesions of GVHD (Figs. 9.11 to 9.17).

The second major controversy that has been clarified in the last few years arose from the eventual ability to distinguish clearly between GVHD and veno-occlusive disease, already discussed. It will suffice to add the footnote

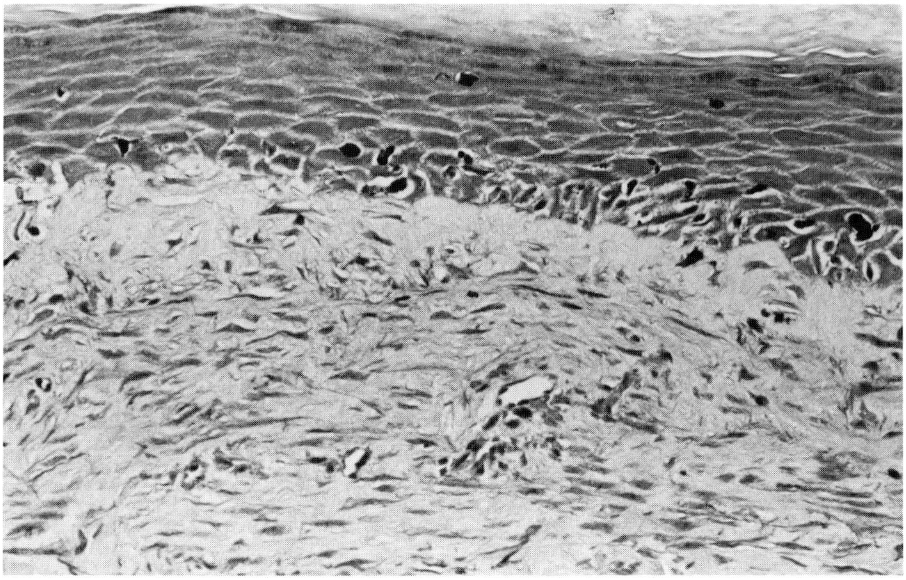

A

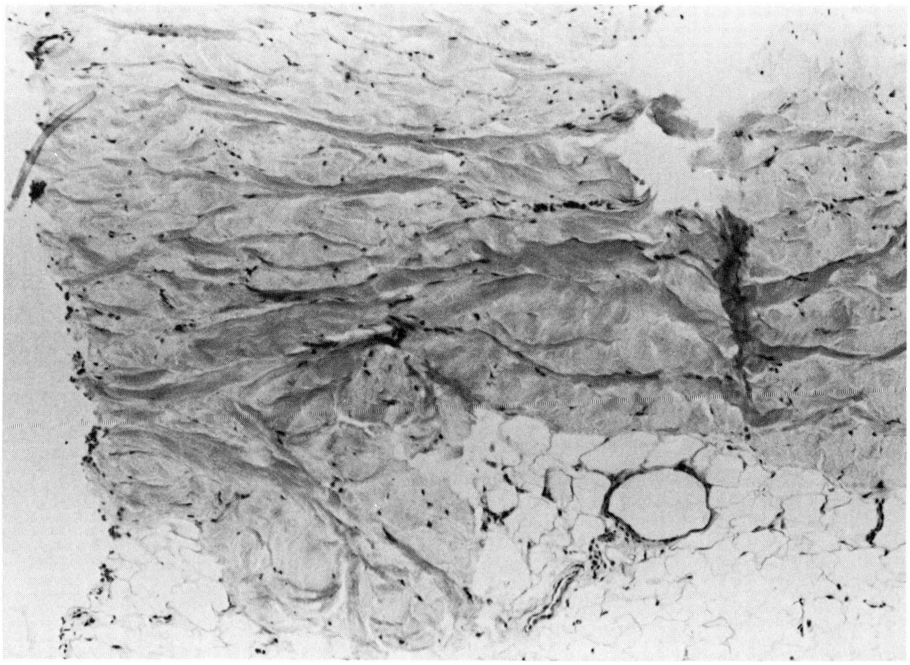

B

Figure 9.6
Skin biopsy at day 247, four months after the de novo onset of generalized chronic GVHD and 40 days after institution of immunosuppressive therapy. A. Evidence of ongoing GVHD includes infiltration by lymphocytes and injured basal cells. The rete ridges have been destroyed, producing a flat border. Papillary dermal sclerosis is evident (hematoxylin-eosin × 350). B. Dense reticular dermal alterations with elongated and straightened collagen bundles illustrate the substitutive collagenosis (hematoxylin-eosin × 500). (From Sale GE, Shulman HM. The pathology of bone marrow transplantation. New York: Masson Publishing USA, 1984.)

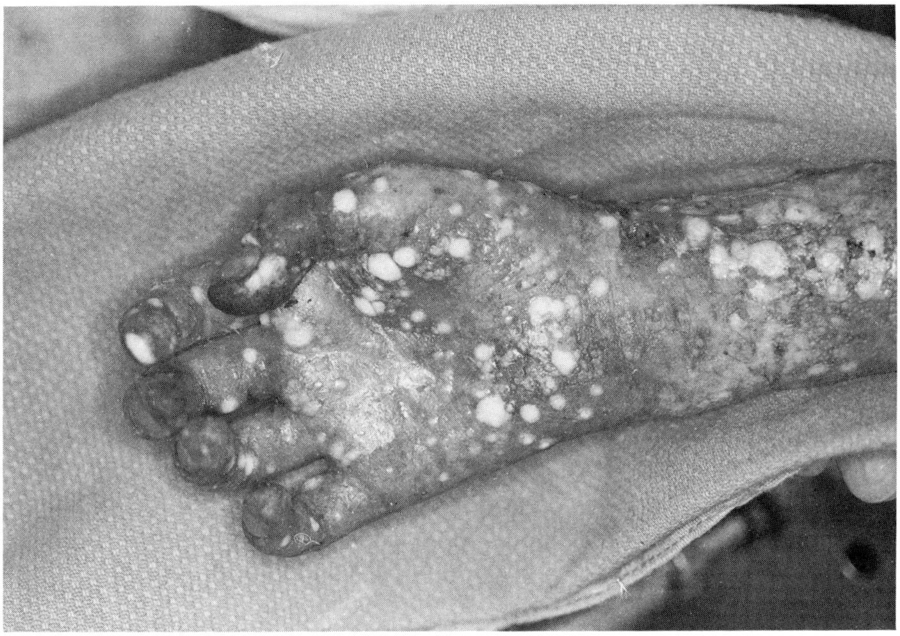

Figure 9.7
Gross photograph at autopsy of severe case of aggravated skin GVHD in patient who developed GVHD during a first transplantation for aplastic anemia, rejected his graft, and then developed a severe GVH reaction of the skin after a second graft from the same donor and died day 56 after the second graft. In this rare case, the features of acute and chronic GVHD are superimposed, with severe lichenoid lesions as well as diffuse ulceration of the skin, which was the primary cause of death in this individual. Luckily, severity of this degree is rare.

that endothelialitis, that is, the infiltration and destruction of endothelial cells by lymphocytes, has been described by Snover in both liver graft rejection and GVHD. The lesion is relatively infrequent in treated patients but may provide some overlap between the lesions of GVHD and veno-occlusive disease. The lesions described by Snover are predominantly in the portal vein, but it is interesting to note that dogs with GVHD often have lesions of the central veins [39] and that allografted patients have a higher incidence of veno-occlusive disease than do syngeneically or autologously grafted patients. This implies some allogeneic risk factor affecting the central venous region indirectly.*

Sicca Syndrome

The sicca syndrome associated with chronic GVHD is an interesting chapter in the understanding of this disease. Both oral and ocular morbidity are se-

*Dulley et al., personal communication.

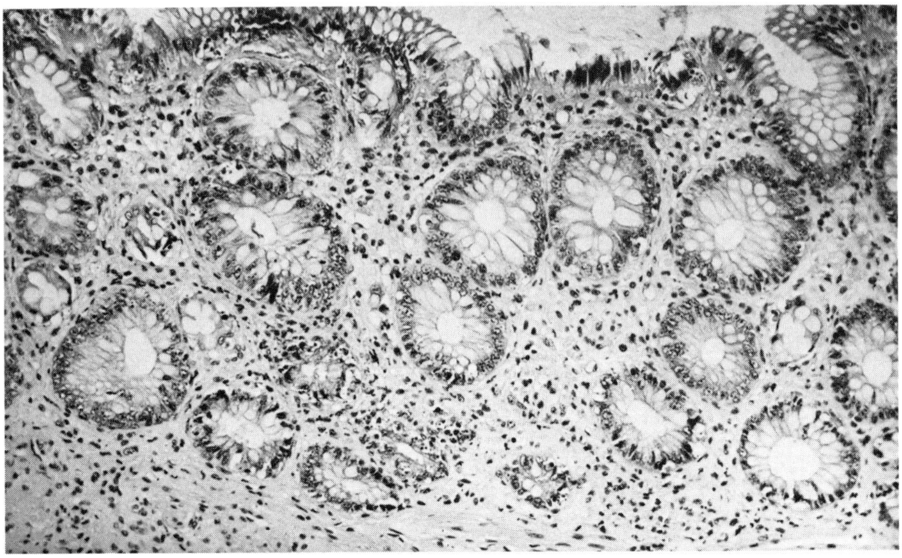

A

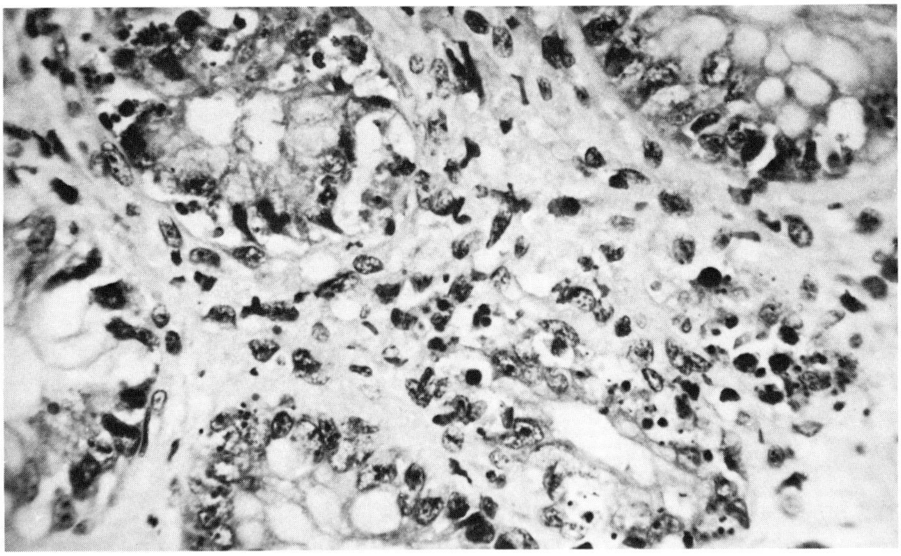

B

Figure 9.8
A. Low-power view of rectal biopsy 40 days after allograft showing infiltration and destruction of crypts, particularly at lower left with lymphocytes and apoptosis. (From Sale GE, Shulman HM, McDonald GB, et al. Am J Surg Pathol 1979;3:291–9.) B. High-power view of the same field showing one of the involved crypts that has the characteristic appearance of the exploding crypt of GVHD. Note the marked cellular degeneration evident in both the crypt at the upper left and at the lower right as well as the edges of the crypt in the lower left and upper right. This lesion is believed more specific than the crypt abscess (Figure 9.9) for GVHD of the gut. Similar changes are seen in stomach, duodenum, ileum, and jejunum.

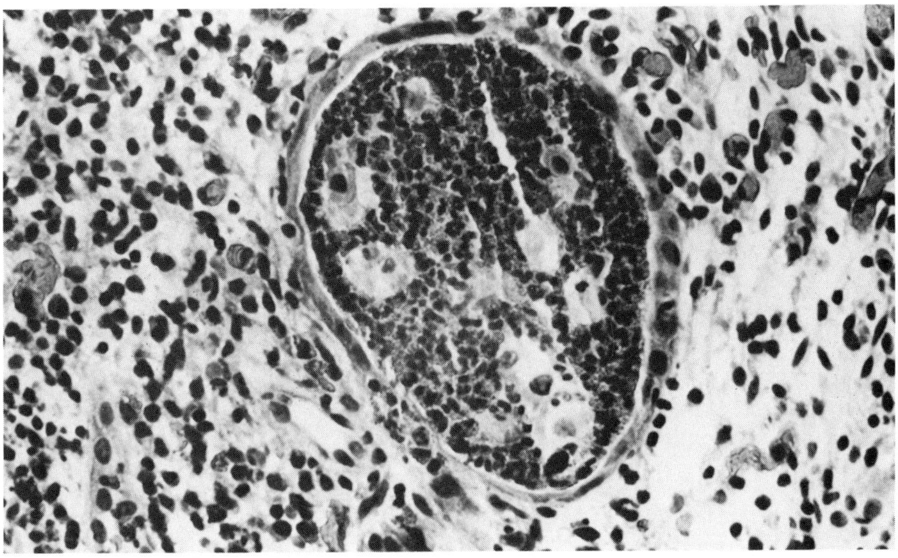

Figure 9.9
Day 42 after allograft. This patient with peripheral eosinophilia showed a bizarre eosinophilic crypt abscess as an interesting variant of the usual polymorphonuclear leukocytic crypt abscess seen in acute GVHD (medium-power view, hematoxylin-eosin). (From Sale GE, Shulman HM, McDonald GB, et al. Am J Surg Pathol 1979;3:291–9.)

rious problems. Keratoconjunctivitis sicca associated with loss of lacrimal gland function invites blinding herpes infections either by loss of IgA production and antibody protection or by loss of antigen-presenting cells of the Langerhans cell family in the limbus and cornea. The oral and ophthalmic lesions of both acute and chronic GVHD include epithelial necrosis of the squamous epithelium lining the mouth, the intercalated ducts of the salivary and lacrimal glands, and the conjunctival mucosa and other adnexal structures of the tarsal plate (Figs. 9.18 to 9.20). Oral and conjunctival epithelium is affected in both acute and chronic GVHD as shown by careful studies of autopsy material. Primary involvement of the limbus but not the cornea has been demonstrated by Beschorner and colleagues in rats and by us in humans. Chorioditis strongly associates with GVHD according to Jabs and colleagues. Izutsu et al. [40,41] have shown that sodium handling by the salivary glands is markedly abnormal in these patients, which strengthens the general hypothesis that the injury focuses on intercalated ducts. They also demonstrated that salivary IgA is markedly reduced.

Lung After Bone Marrow Transplantation

Controversy has centered around the problem of sorting out the various bronchopulmonary lesions associated with marrow transplantation. The

Figure 9.10 (right)
Low-power view of grade III GVHD of the gut showing loss of crypts and marked attenuation of surface epithelium with dilatation of vessels in the lamina propria. This is the stage just preceding total denudation of the gut that is the life-threatening feature of acute GVHD. (From Sale GE, Shulman HM, McDonald GB, et al. Am J Surg Pathol 1979;3:291–9.)

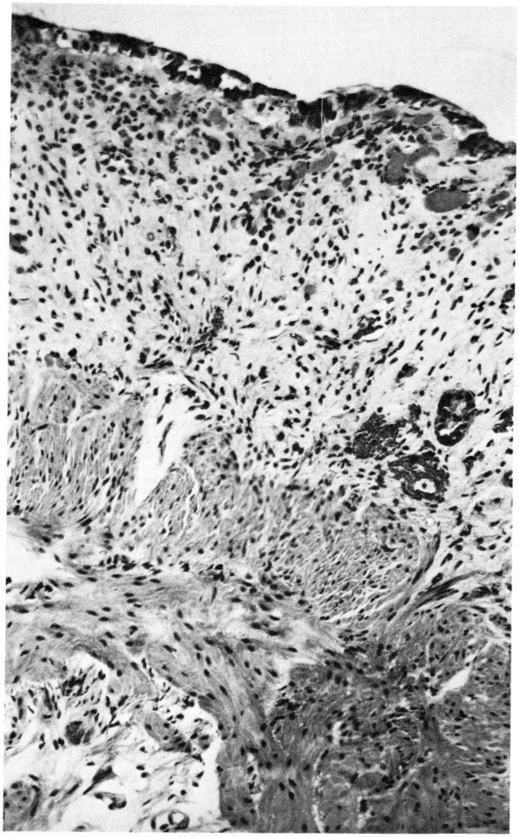

Figure 9.11 (below)
Day 57 after second bone marrow allograft, veno-occlusive disease showing damage to the venous endothelium with considerable embolization of hepatocytes inside the subendothelial zone of this sublobular vein. (From Sale GE, Shulman HM. The pathology of bone marrow transplantation. New York: Masson Publishing USA, 1984.)

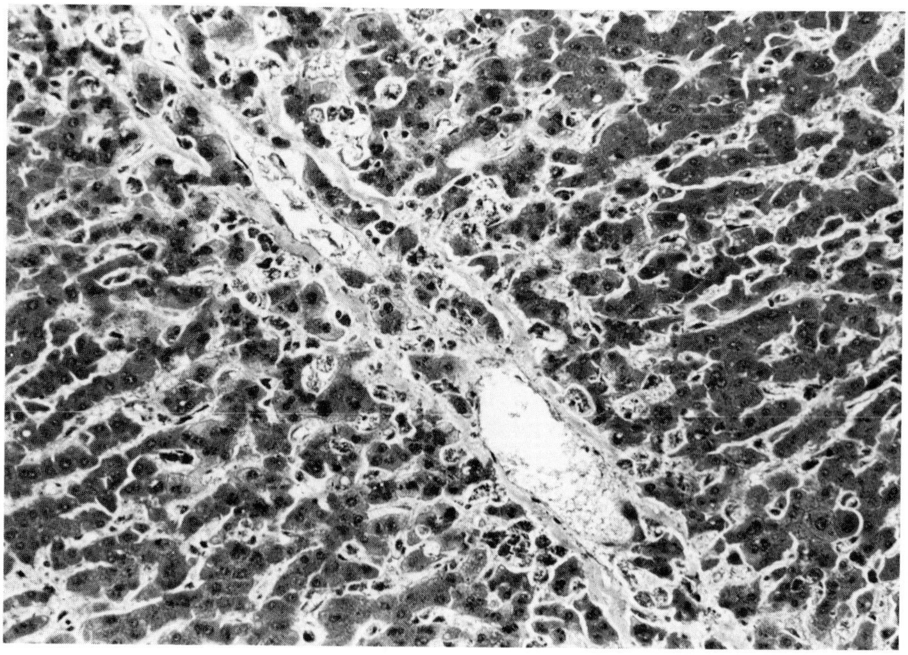

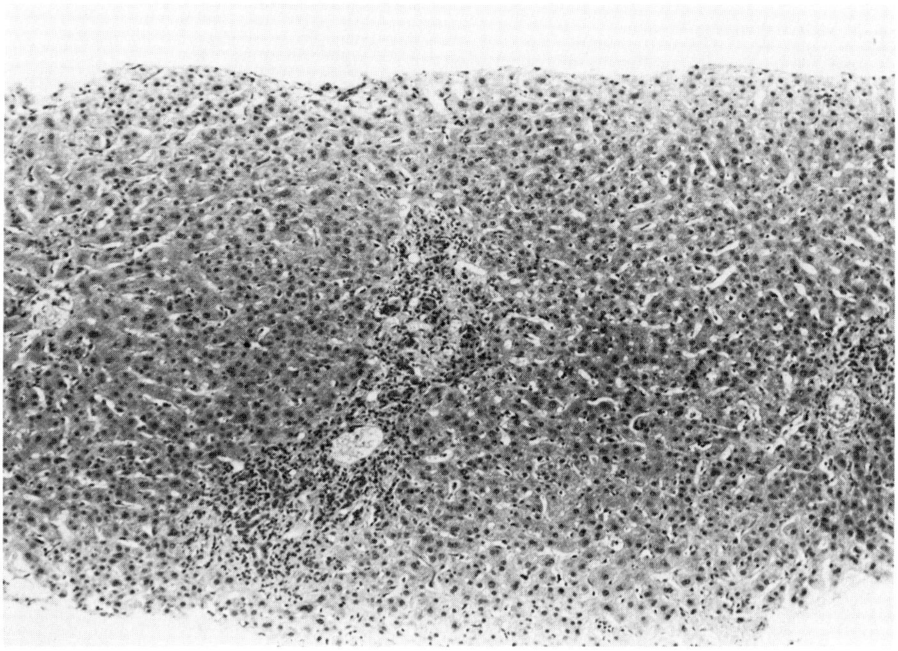

Figure 9.12
Low-power view of needle biopsy of liver showing pattern of triaditis and lobular hepatitis of GVHD on day 72 after transplantation. (From Sale GE, Shulman HM. The pathology of bone marrow transplantation. New York: Masson Publishing USA, 1984.)

three major risk factors in the etiology of bronchopulmonary lesions are chemoradiotherapy, GVHD, and infection. There seems to be general agreement that the bronchial mucous glands are a target of the sicca syndrome in GVHD. Interstitial pneumonitis, a frequent problem in these patients, has no established direct causative connection with GVHD. However, in 1978 a lesion known as lymphocytic bronchitis was identified by Beschorner and colleagues and associated with bronchospasm, bronchopneumonia, and ciliary paralysis in patients with GVHD [42]. A lesion indistinguishable from lymphocytic bronchitis has been found in a similar percentage of autologous and syngeneic graft recipients as well as patients without transplants with viral pneumonia and simple endotracheal intubation [15]. This casts serious doubt on the specificity of the *large* airway lesion for GVHD. However, a number of studies have shown that patients with chronic GVHD can develop severe obstructive pulmonary function test abnormalities that have been (in some cases) associated with the *small* airway histologic lesion of bronchiolitis obliterans [14]. As emphasized by Drs. Yousem and Tazelaar in Chapter 6, the circumstantial evidence therefore strongly points to a specific immunologic lesion of GVHD and of lung rejection that centers on small bronchioles. It remains difficult to rule out secondary infection in these lesions.

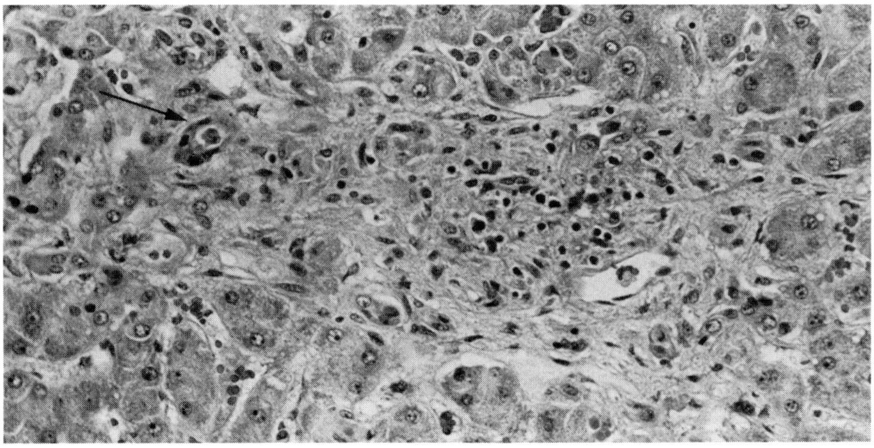

Figure 9.13
Medium-power liver biopsy 1 week after onset of hyperacute GVHD in a patient who received a mismatched allogeneic graft (biopsy day 18). The portal triad shows degenerative, partly necrotic small bile duct containing luminal debris (arrow). There is a slight mononuclear infiltrate and periportal acidophilic bodies. (From Sale GE, Shulman HM. The pathology of bone marrow transplantation. New York: Masson Publishing USA, 1984.)

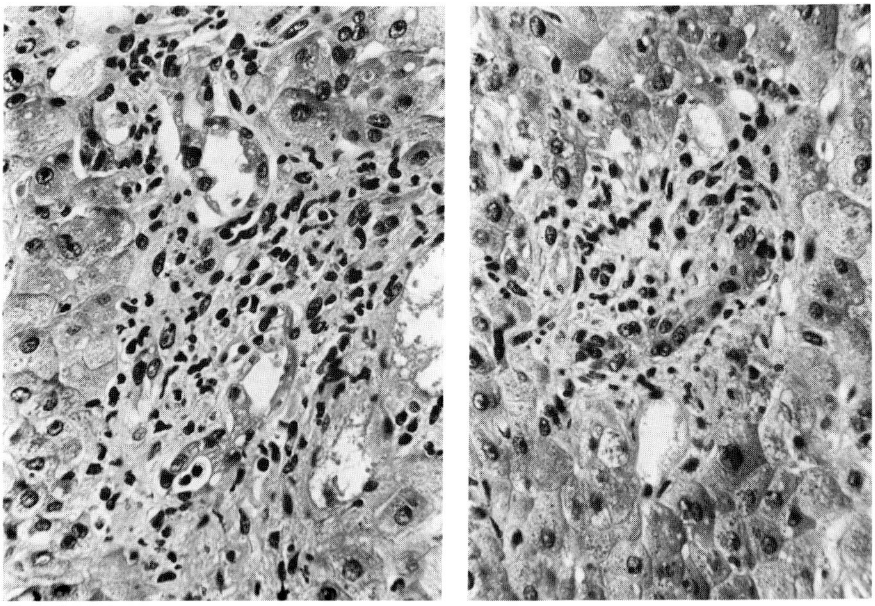

A *B*

Figure 9.14
Liver biopsy on day 40 after transplant and day 18 after clinical onset of multisystem GVHD associated with rise in LFTs. A. Dilated, irregular bile ducts show cytoplasmic vacuolization and flattening with loss of epithelium. B. Longitudinal section of the small bile duct shows nuclear abnormalities, cell dropout, and periductular edema. These are classic changes of acute GVHD. (From Sale GE, Shulman HM. The pathology of bone marrow transplantation. New York: Masson Publishing USA, 1984.)

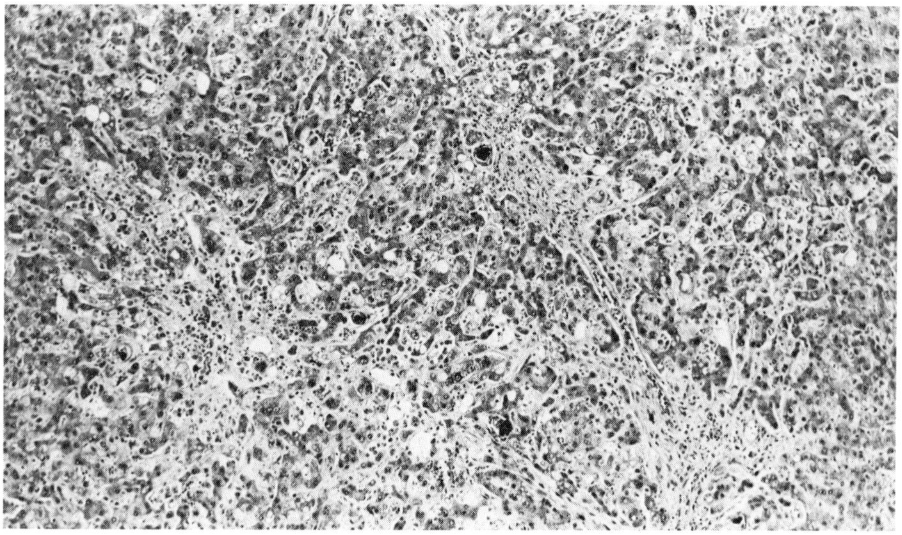

Figure 9.15
Characteristic picture of severe prolonged GVHD of the liver showing severe cholestasis with bile plugs within pericentral cholangioles, marked inflammation, and early fibrosis. (From Sale GE, Shulman HM. The pathology of bone marrow transplantation. New York: Masson Publishing USA, 1984.)

Summary of Pathologists' Role in Management of GVHD

For a more detailed essay on the pathologic diagnosis of GVHD in skin, liver, gut, and mouth, see Sale and Shulman [13]. For the pathologist's orientation we summarize our general guidelines.

Acute skin GVHD is diagnosed on or after day 21 if eosinophilic bodies and a lymphocytic infiltrate are present in epidermis. This frequently is noted at rete ridge bases or in hair follicles at the shoulder of the bulb or at the neck of a sebaceous duct. *Serial* skin biopsies in the period before day 21 are often necessary to evaluate whether there is progression to bulla formation or regression. Clinically, the latter is ignored, the former deemed GVHD and treated. This clinical situation is not quite as urgent as in heart or renal graft rejection: a few days' observation is usually affordable. The exception is "hyperacute" GVHD in the mismatched or undersuppressed recipient. Unfortunately, there are no good clinical or histologic criteria for a sharply defined diagnosis of hyperacute GVHD because of the competing causes of epidermal atypia and necrosis, so that clinical judgment decides on treatment.

Gut GVHD is usually not approached safely by endoscopy before day 21 to 30 due to thrombocytopenia or leukopenia. The rectal biopsy is quite useful thereafter, using the "exploding crypt" [18] as the criterion (in the absence of CMV, which clouds diagnostic criteria). Chronic nausea and

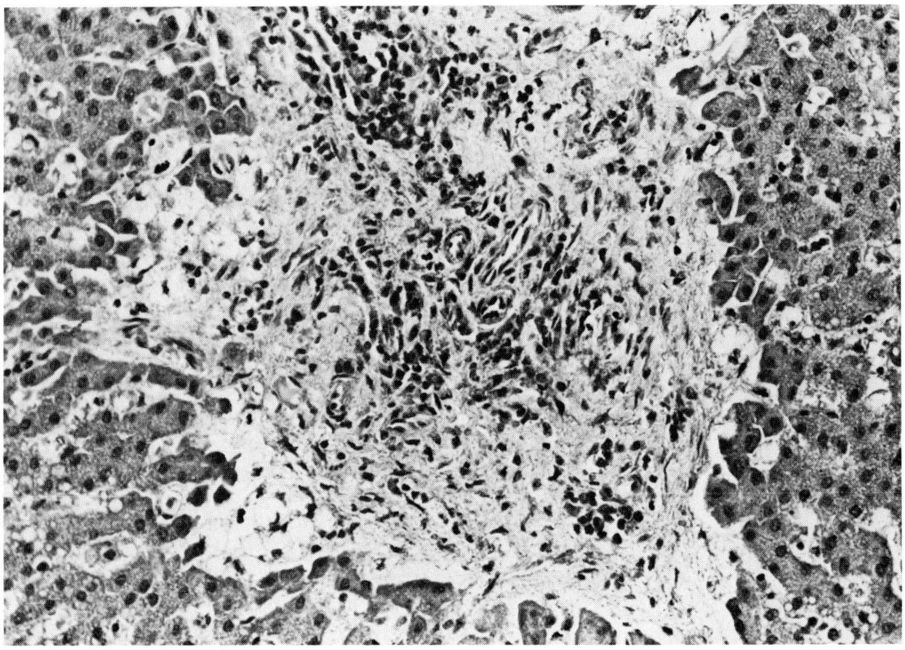

Figure 9.16
Medium-power view of severe chronic GVHD of the liver with pattern of a chronic septal fibrosis progressing toward early cirrhosis shows marked ductal reduction, day 350 after transplantation. (From Sale GE, Shulman HM. The pathology of bone marrow transplantation. New York: Masson Publishing USA, 1984.)

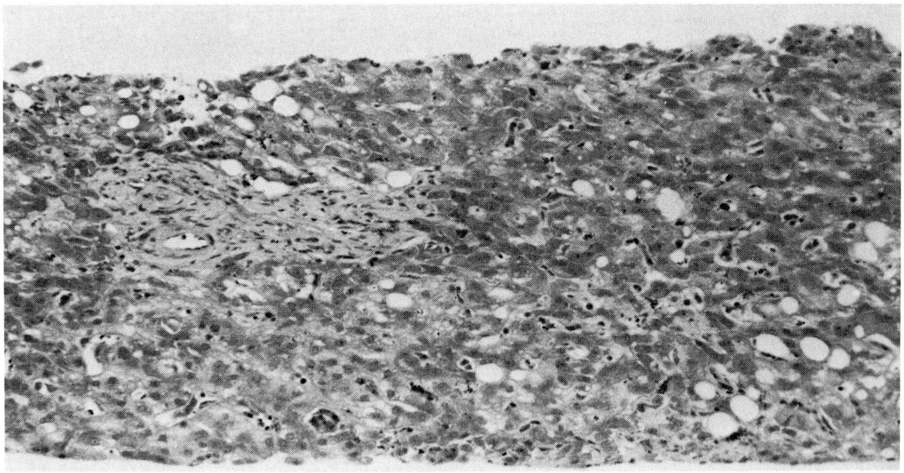

Figure 9.17
Liver biopsy obtained 324 days after allograft showing chronic GVHD of the liver with hepatocyte disarray, focal dropout, and absence of ducts within the triad marked by focal fibrosis and a small hepatic arterial branch. (From Sale GE, Shulman HM. The pathology of bone marrow transplantation. New York: Masson Publishing USA, 1984.)

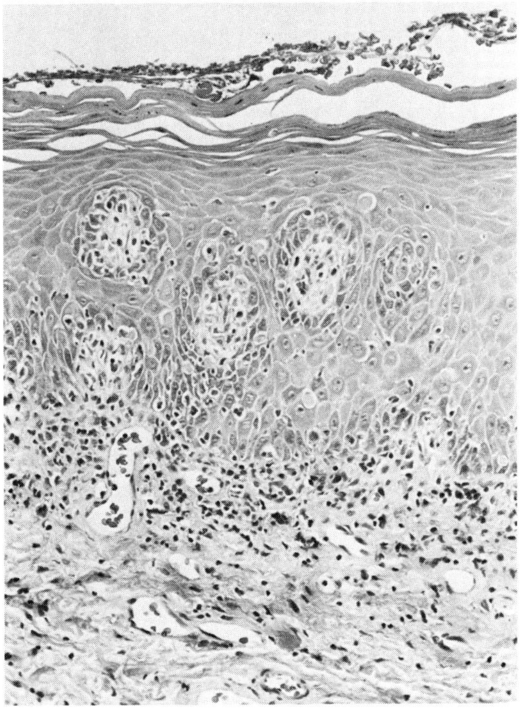

Figure 9.18
Medium-power view of lip biopsy showing grade II GVHD with characteristic lichenoid infiltrate, eosinophilic bodies, satellitosis, and the characteristically parakeratotic epithelium of the lip. Such findings are usually seen on biopsies obtained day 80 through 150 after transplantation in patients with chronic GVHD. Biopsies of the oral surfaces are usually avoided before day 50 because the patient is recovering from the mucositis caused by radiation and chemotherapy, and biopsies are not considered diagnostically useful during that period. (From Sale GE, Shulman HM. The pathology of bone marrow transplantation. New York: Masson Publishing USA, 1984.)

vomiting after about day 30 is approached by esophageal, gastric, and duodenal endoscopy and biopsy. CMV, herpes, and fungi can be reliably diagnosed in this manner and the patient treated. GVHD can be assessed well in the esophagus in the absence of severe acute inflammation and in stomach and duodenum in the absence of evidence of CMV infection. (CMV mimics the apoptotic lesion of GVHD and makes GVHD diagnosis impossible when it is present.)

Liver biopsy diagnosis of veno-occlusive disease rests on a good trichrome stain and the assessment of several central veins. Bile duct lesions during the first 100 days, with characteristic lymphoid infiltration, apoptosis, and atypical regeneration, are reliable criteria for GVHD. B or non-A, non-B hepatitis can produce difficult differential diagnostic problems, especially after about day 60 to 100, in separating GVHD. Protracted liver GVHD (2 to 4 weeks) produces bizarre cholangiolar structures with bile plugs.

Chronic GVHD of the skin and mouth is easily diagnosed by lichen planus–like lesions. The lip biopsy also usually shows concomitant interlobular duct damage in the minor salivary gland. Skin biopsy is the gold standard at this point (100 days) after transplantation. Skin findings are similar to those of acute GVHD but are often more exuberant and may involve sweat glands. Occasionally, minimal and focal GVHD involvement of rete ridges and hair follicles only may be present at this time. A full assessment

clude chronic lymphocytic leukemia with secondary immunodeficiency and chronic GVHD in marrow transplant recipients. No clear evidence of long-term benefit has been achieved in these groups. One successful case of thymic transplantation for chronic mucocutaneous candidiasis has also been reported. Recent attempts to transplant thymuses to acquired immunodeficiency syndrome (AIDS) patients were reported by Hong. Although the patients all died, one clearly showed evidence of residual thymic tissue in the transplant site at 3 months after transplantation, suggesting that such grafts may show success in other patients if support can be improved. This may be more likely to succeed in AIDS patients than in patients undergoing marrow transplantation due to the markedly smaller risk involved in the procedure itself.

Summary

Marrow transplantation is fundamentally a refinement of transfusion therapy using certain spectra of hematopoietic stem cells or their immunologic derivatives. The information derived from 30 years of experimental and clinical studies is encyclopedic. The potential refinements are many, especially when combined with gene transfer therapy. Thymic transplantation, still in its infancy, is bound to benefit from the new knowledge and techniques of marrow transplantation, adoptive immunotherapy, and in vitro manipulation of the cells to be transplanted. Circumvention or solution of many of the problems (rejection, GVHD, and toxicity) appears to be on the immediate horizon. Data and methods explored in this field will benefit solid organ transplantation, and vice versa. The concept of using isolated, cloned, and cultured cells has already profoundly affected pancreatic and skin transplantation and shows promise for thymic, neural, endocrine, and other tissues, particularly in inborn errors of metabolism.

References

1. Thomas ED, Storb R, Clift RA, et al. Bone marrow transplantation. N Engl J Med 1975;292:832–43, 895–902.
2. Hobbs JR. Bone marrow transplantation for inborn errors. Lancet 1981;2:735–9.
3. O'Reilly RJ. Allogeneic bone marrow transplantation: current status and future directions. Blood 1983;62:941–62.
4. Storb R, Prentice RL, Thomas ED. Marrow transplantation for treatment of aplastic anemia. An analysis of factors associated with graft rejection. N Engl J Med 1977;296:61–6.
5. Beatty P, Clift RA, Michelson E, et al. Marrow transplantation from related donors other than HLA identical siblings. N Engl J Med 1985;313:765–71.

6. Sale GE, Buckner CD. Pathology of bone marrow in transplant recipients. In: Yeager E, ed. Hyun B, guest ed. Bone marrow examination. Hematol Oncol Clin North Am 1988;4:735–56.
7. Thomas ED, Marmont AM, Sale GE. Aplastic anemia and hematopoiesis following marrow transplantation. In: Zucker-Franklin D, ed. Atlas of blood cell function and pathology. Philadelphia: Lea & Febiger, 1988.
8. Berk PD, Popper H, Krueger GRF, et al. Venocclusive disease of the liver after allogeneic bone marrow transplantation: possible association with graft-versus-host disease. Ann Intern Med 1979;90:158–64.
9. Shulman HM, McDonald GB, Matthews D, et al. An analysis of hepatic venocclusive disease and centrilobular hepatocyte degeneration following bone marrow transplantation. Gastroenterology 1980;79:1178–91.
10. McDonald GB, Sharma P, Matthews D, et al. Venocclusive disease of the liver after bone marrow transplantation: diagnosis, incidence, and predisposing factors. Hepatology 1984;4:116–22.
11. McDonald GB, Sharma P, Matthews D, et al. The clinical course of 53 patients with venocclusive disease of the liver after marrow transplantation. Transplantation 1985;39:603–8.
12. Shulman HM, Gown AM, Nugent DJ. Hepatic venocclusive disease after bone marrow transplantation: identification of the occlusive material within occluded central venules. Am J Pathol 1987;127:549–58.
13. Sale GE, Shulman HM. The pathology of bone marrow transplantation. New York: Masson Publishing USA, Inc., 1984.
14. Ralph DD, Springmeyer SC, Sullivan KM, et al. Rapidly progressive air-flow obstruction in marrow transplant recipients: possible association between obliterative bronchiolitis and chronic graft-versus-host disease. Am Rev Respir Dis 1984;129:641–4.
15. O'Brien KD, Hackman RC, Sale GE, et al. Lymphocytic bronchitis in canine marrow graft recipients. Transplantation 1984;37:234–8.
16. Billingham RE. The biology of graft-versus-host reactions. Lectures 1966-67;62:21–78.
17. Sale GE, Lerner KG, Barker EA, et al. The skin biopsy in the diagnosis of acute graft-versus-host disease in man. Am J Pathol 1977;89:621–35.
18. Sale GE, Shulman HM, McDonald GB, et al. Gastrointestinal graft-versus-host disease in man. A clinicopathological study of the rectal biopsy. Am J Surg Pathol 1979;3:291–9.
19. Shulman HM, Sale GE, Lerner KG, et al. Chronic cutaneous graft-versus-host disease in man. Am J Pathol 1978;91:545–70.
20. Shulman HM, Sullivan KM, Weiden PL, et al. Chronic graft-versus-host syndrome in man. A long term clinicopathologic study of 20 Seattle patients. Am J Med 1980;69:204–17.
21. Sullivan KM, Shulman HM, Storb R, et al. Chronic graft-versus-host disease in 52 patients. Adverse natural course and successful treatment with combination immunosuppression. Blood 1981;57:267–76.
22. Parkman R. Clonal analysis of murine graft-versus-host disease. I. Phenotypic and functional analysis of T lymphocyte clones. J Immunol 1986;136:3543–8.
23. Hamilton BL, Bevan MJ, Parkman R. Anti-recipient cytotoxic T-lymphocyte precursors are present in the spleens of mice with acute graft-versus-host disease due to minor histocompatibility antigens. J Immunol 1981;126:621.
24. Hamilton BL, Parkman R. Acute and chronic graft-versus-host disease induced by minor histocompatibility antigens in mice. Transplantation 1983;36:150.

25. Seemayer TA. The GVHR: a pathogenetic mechanism of experimental and human disease. Perspectives in pediatric pathology, vol. 5. H.S. Rosenberg and R.P. Bolande, eds. New York: Masson Publishing, 1979:93–136.
26. Steinmuller D, Tyler JD, David CS. Cell-mediated cytotoxicity to non-MHC alloantigens on mouse epidermal cells. I. H-2 restricted reactions. J Immunol 1981;126:1747–53.
27. Steinmuller D, Tyler JD, David CS. Cell-mediated cytotoxicity to non-MHC alloantigens on mouse epidermal cells. II. Genetic basis of the response of C3H mice. J Immunol 1981;126:1754–58.
28. Namnoum JD, Hess AD, Shinn CA, Santos GW. Cyclosporin A and the thymus: immunopathology. Am J Pathol 1987;126:487–96.
29. Sale GE, Shulman HM, Gallucci BB, et al. Young rete ridge keratinocytes are preferred targets in cutaneous graft-versus-host disease. Am J Pathol 1985;118:278–87.
30. Sloane JP, Thomas JA, Imrie SF, et al. Morphological and immunohistological changes in the skin in allogeneic bone marrow recipients. J Clin Pathol 1984;37:919–30.
31. Sale GE, Storb R, Kolb H. Histopathology of hepatic acute graft-versus-host disease in the dog. A double-blind study confirms the specificity of small bile duct lesions. Transplantation 1978;26:103–6.
32. Bernuau D, Gisselbrecht C, Devergie A, et al. Histological and ultrastructural appearance of the liver during graft-versus-host disease complicating bone marrow transplantation. Transplantation 1980;29:236–44.
33. Bernuau D, Feldman G, Degott C, et al. Ultrastructural lesion of bile ducts in primary biliary cirrhosis. A comparison with the lesions observed in graft-versus-host disease. Hum Pathol 1981;12:782–93.
34. Berman MD, Rabin L, O'Donnell J, et al. The liver in long term survivors of marrow transplant—chronic graft-versus-host disease. J Clin Gastroenterol 1980;2:53–63.
35. Sloane JP, Farthing MJ, Powles RL. Histopathological changes in the liver after allogeneic bone marrow transplantation. J Clin Pathol 1980;33:344–50.
36. Shulman HM, Sharma P, Amos D, et al. A coded histologic study of hepatic graft-versus-host disease after human bone marrow transplantation. Hepatology 1988;3:463–70.
37. Fennel RH Jr. Ductular damage in liver transplant rejection: its similarity to that of primary biliary cirrhosis and graft-versus-host disease. Pathol Annu 1981;16:289–94.
38. Snover D. Hepatic graft-versus-host disease: a study of the predictive value of the liver biopsy. Hepatology 1984;4:127–30.
39. Kolb H, Sale GE, Lerner KG, et al. Pathology of acute graft-versus-host disease in the dog. An autopsy study of 95 dogs. Am J Pathol 1979;96:581–94.
40. Izutsu KT, Truelove EL, Shulman HM, et al. The predictive value of elevated labial saliva sodium concentration. Its relation to labial gland pathology in bone marrow transplant recipients. Hum Pathol 1983;13:29–35.
41. Izutsu KT, Sullivan KM, Schubert MM, et al. Disordered salivary immunoglobulin secretions and sodium transport in human chronic graft-versus-host disease. Transplantation 1983;35:441–6.
42. Beschorner WE, Saral R, Hutchins GM, et al. Lymphocytic bronchitis associated with graft-versus-host disease in recipients of bone marrow transplants. N Engl J Med 1978;299:1030–6.

43. Hong R. Reconstitution of T cell deficiency by thymic hormone or thymic transplantation therapy. Clin Immunol Immunopathol 1986;40:136–41.
44. Borzy MS, Hong R, Horowitz S, et al. Fatal lymphoma after transplantation of cultured thymus. N Engl J Med 1979;301:565–8.
45. Reece ER, Gartner JG, Seemayer TA, et al. Epstein-Barr virus in a malignant lymphoproliferative disorder of B cells occurring after thymic epithelial transplantation for combined immunodeficiency. Cancer Res 1981;41:4243–7.

10

Corneal Transplantation

GEORGE E. SALE
JOHN CHANDLER

After ulcers of the cornea which have been large, the inequalities and opacity of the cicatrix obscure the sight: in this case could not a small piece of the cornea be cut out by a kind of trephine about the size of a thick bristle, or a small crow quill, and would it not heal with a transparent scar?

Erasmus Darwin, 1796 [1]

Corneal grafting is a 200-year-old procedure that became very successful in the mid-twentieth century, and newer immunologic research has fine tuned our knowledge. The general histopathologic findings of corneal graft rejection were described over 20 years ago and subsequently subcategorized into epithelial, stromal, and endothelial rejection. It is crucial to avoid vascularization of the graft for successful long-term tolerance, as noted empirically. Recently, the concept that the cornea is an immunologically privileged site has been strongly challenged by experimental work on the effect of major histocompatibility complex (MHC) differences on corneal rejection in animals. Epidemiologic studies of many human patients have also shown that rejection tends to be greater when the donor and the recipient have substan-

This work was supported in part by grants CA 15704 and CA 18029 from the National Cancer Institute and HL 36444 from the National Heart and Lung Institute, NIH.

tial MHC differences. In addition, Langerhans cells have been described by some authors as being present in corneal epithelium, so that graft tolerance can be successfully induced by removing or inactivating Langerhans cells experimentally with anti-class II antibodies or ultraviolet light. Thus, modern immunologic research continues to refine our knowledge of the several factors important in corneal graft rejection and seems likely to add to the substantial clinical success already achieved by the pioneers in this field.

The opening quote by Erasmus Darwin was stimulated by an epidemic of corneal inflammation occurring at the end of the eighteenth century. For a century thereafter, many attempts at corneal grafting failed. But by 1888, von Hippel reported the first successful human corneal grafts. His method was to insert full-thickness rabbit cornea into intralamellar pockets. The first full-thickness penetrating homograft in humans was performed by Zirm in 1906. Elschnig of Prague and Filatov of the Soviet Union began to refine the original techniques, which many workers developed through the 1950s, although the present techniques remain very similar. Microsurgery and materials science have considerably improved these techniques' precision and control. The success rate has risen from 22% in 1930 to over 90% today, with the major causes of failure now being biologic rather than technical [2].

Clinical Aspects of Corneal Transplantation

The general success of corneal engraftment has widened the range of indications while, at the same time, known contraindications have imposed new limitations. A number of safe optical, preparatory, structural, therapeutic, cosmetic, and refractive indications are currently accepted [10]. However, neuroparalytic keratitis, trichiasis, abnormal lid posture, severe sicca syndrome, and uncontrollable glaucoma are contraindications. Unfortunately, of the 30 million blind people in the world, the majority are blind from corneal opacification caused by diseases associated with eyelid and other external eye diseases, often disqualifying them from grafting.

Risk Factors for Graft Survival

Vascularization of the cornea is a dominating risk factor for graft survival. Another important factor is HLA matching. A number of studies have demonstrated such matching to be of relative value in vascularized recipients. Batchelor et al. reported prognostic variables in 200 cases [3]. In the group of patients with vascularized corneas, the proportion of grafts functioning was found to be proportional to the number of HLA antigens shared by donor and recipient. A similar preliminary retrospective report on a series of 222 cases was published by Ehlers and Kissmeyer-Nielsen [4]. The same year Volker-Dieben et al. reported similar results in 49 "high-risk" corneal graft recipients [5]. Perhaps the best designed of several subsequent studies was that of Sanfilippo and colleagues, who reported a masked study of 97 patients in 1986 [6]. This clearly showed, by Cox analysis, a lower rejection rate in matched combinations, agreeing in general with the other studies. However, rejection does occur even in well-matched situations, probably due to minor antigen mismatches between unrelated donor-recipient pairs.

Storage Techniques

Storage technology has improved markedly over the last 15 years. Before 1974, stored donor corneas were felt to be viable only for 48 hours. Refrigeration in a modified tissue culture medium allows up to 96 hours' storage [7]. New methods of storage of donor cornea with a 3 to 4 mm scleral rim in prepared synthetic media have improved this situation so that storage for up to a month is possible with excellent viability [8]. A recent study of short- (mean 14.3 days) and long- (mean 29.8 days) term "cultured" storage showed no significant differences in graft viability [9]. Cryopreservation methods allow up to 18 months' storage [7].

Surgical Method of Transplantation

The usual technique of grafting is penetrating keratoplasty, in which the full-thickness recipient cornea is excised and replaced by donor cornea. Some of the earlier methods and the experimental methods include intralamellar insertion, much as introduced by von Hippel. Modern lamellar corneal grafting is a variant used in some superficial lesions of the cornea and other special situations. It requires a functioning host endothelial layer. The complications of the full-thickness corneal graft include at least 16, of which one is the biologic complication of rejection. Most of the others are related to surgical technique or to complicated wound healing. Grossly, the earliest sign of an allograft reaction is localized conjunctival hyperemia or the appearance of one or more keratic precipitates on a donor cornea. This may be followed by vasodilatation of the limbus and abnormal edema, vascularization, and opacification of the graft [11]. The reaction may be roughly proportional to the size of the corneal graft, with the optimal size being 6 to 8 mm in diameter [10]. Larger grafts or eccentrically positioned grafts approach the corneoscleral junction and, like a vascularized host cornea, significantly increase the risk of allograft rejection.

Infection

If infection is absent before the graft, it is rare after grafting. However, keratitis of the graft may occur if the disease that caused the original corneal opacity becomes active soon after operation. Such conditions include bacterial and viral infections. Continued treatment may be required; if that fails, a second graft may eventually be considered. Herpetic infections may occur in a graft even though the entire recipient lesion was removed because reactivated virus may reach the reinnervated graft through neurons from the latently infected trigeminal ganglion.

Immunosuppression

At the first sign of corneal graft rejection, topical and systemic steroids are given. Prompt administration of steroids may save the graft if initiated within 24 to 48 hours, but if administration is delayed 4 or 5 days, the graft may be irreversibly rejected. Therapy with topical steroids and cycloplegics may need to be continued for several weeks. The steroids are usually discontinued in 10 to 14 days. In general, the longer a rejection episode is delayed, the better the overall prognosis [10].

The recent experimental literature shows that systemically administered cyclosporine and some forms of local instillation may be quite helpful in delaying graft rejection in animal models, particularly rabbits. There is some evidence that the same problem of dependence on cyclosporine for continued tolerance that occurs in other settings may be present in the corneal graft situation [12].

Immunopathology of Corneal Transplantation

Polack [13] described the pathologic anatomy of corneal graft rejection in human beings and in rabbit experimental models. In both species, rejection was accompanied by grossly visible changes of vascular congestion, aqueous flare, and edema of the deep layers of the graft stroma. This is accompanied by lymphoid hyperplasia in the limbus and conjunctiva (Fig. 10.1). The growth of host blood vessels toward and into the donor cornea seemed a prerequisite for opacification and irreversible rejection in both species. The vessels usually reach the scar, consisting of proliferating fibroblasts, through the anterior third of the host cornea (Fig. 10.2). The border of the scar is infiltrated by lymphocytes and plasma cells and, occasionally, by small numbers of polymorphonuclear leukocytes (Fig. 10.3). A line of leukocytic infiltration moves across the endothelial layer of the cornea beginning with lymphocytes. This is followed by cytolytic destruction of endothelial cells. Often stromal and epithelial rejection proceed in tandem. However, individual portions of the allograft may be rejected. Of particular interest was that expansion of adjacent conjunctival and limbic lymphoid tissue precedes corneal rejection in the heterografted animal studies. It is very likely that similar reactions precede the rejection of human cornea. At that point in the development of immunology, the dichotomy between the B and T cell systems was poorly understood, and there was some doubt about the precise immunologic nature of corneal graft sickness and the relative contributions of cellular and humoral immune systems to rejection. It was clear that the vigor of rejection could be enhanced, even to the degree expected of a second-set graft rejection, if skin grafts were exchanged between donor and host animals before grafting to sensitize the host. This hastened the onset and increased the frequency of rejection for the purposes of the experimental rejection model.

In 1969, Khodadoust and Silverstein [14] published classic studies of experimental corneal graft rejection in which they clearly elucidated the nature

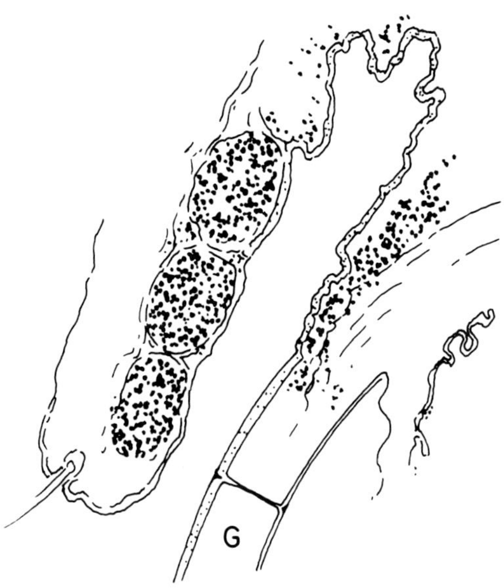

Figure 10.1
Lymphoid hyperplasia of the limbus and subconjunctival tissue early in graft rejection. G, *graft. (From Polack FM. The pathological anatomy of the corneal graft rejection. Excerpta Medica International Congress Series no. 146. Proceedings of the Twentieth International Congress of Ophthalmology, Munich, Aug. 14–19, 1966;885–90.)*

of the epithelial line, showing that this represents a wave of inflammation in which the host epithelium is replaced by donor epithelium. In some experimental rabbit studies using this model, the graft can remain clear despite a rejection line and a host epithelial replacement. Reactions of rejection in the epithelial, stromal, and endothelial layers often accompany each other. The stromal and endothelial reactions produce more lasting cloudiness of vision. A study of induced graft-vs-host reaction in the corneal endothelium was of particular interest [15]. Introduction of specifically sensitized lymphocytes into the anterior chamber caused a random distribution of "pocks" on the corneal endothelium. In the grafting of cornea, on the other hand, the rejec-

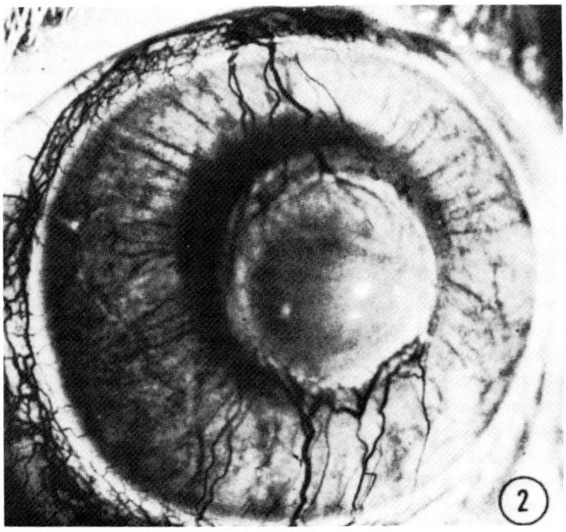

Figure 10.2
Corneal graft rejection in the eye of a rabbit. Opacification begins peripherally near the blood vessels and advances centripetally. (From Polack FM. The pathological anatomy of the corneal graft rejection. Excerpta Medica International Congress Series no. 146. Proceedings of the Twentieth International Congress of Ophthalmology, Munich, Aug. 14–19, 1966;885–90.)

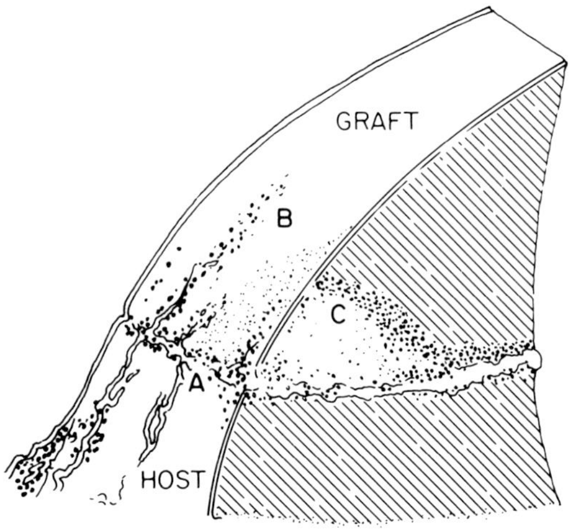

Figure 10.3
Schema showing alterations in different graft layers. A. Scar shows edema, a mononuclear cell infiltrate, and neovascularization. B. Vessels and lymphocytes invade the stroma, which also shows edema in the posterior layers. This edema may be secondary to alterations in the endothelium, C, which in the early stages shows mononuclear cell infiltrate, edema, and, posteriorly, destruction of cells. (From Polack FM. The pathological anatomy of the corneal graft rejection. Excerpta Medica International Congress Series no. 146. Proceedings of the Twentieth International Congress of Ophthalmology, Munich, Aug. 14–19, 1966;885–90.)

tion is a linear progression across the cornea, coming from the limbus. The latter pattern has been interpreted as far more consistent with vascular ingrowth as a prerequisite for rejection of the cornea. During this period, Polack [13], in transmission and scanning electron microscopic studies, showed that infiltration of lymphocytes into the graft endothelium preceded the endothelial blebbing and breakdown associated with the rejection process.

In 1969, Waltman et al. [16] showed that antilymphocyte globulin could completely prevent penetrating corneal graft rejection in animals. Additional studies of experimental animals in 1978 by Gronemeyer et al. with very careful analysis of sequential changes every two days generally confirmed prior work on the rejection process [17]. These studies involved lamellar implants rather than full-thickness corneal grafts. Generally, the scar heals 6 to 10 days after grafting in the syngeneic animal combinations. After day 10, the allograft reaction begins to occur in the others with characteristic inflammatory lesions not present in the syngeneic animals. From days 7 to 17, lymphocytes, many stimulated into blast transformation, infiltrate the graft and are associated with macrophages and plasma cells. Then between days 18 and 35, a phase of phagocytic and postrejection healing occurs. Here the predominating cell types are macrophages, fibroblasts, and mature fibrocytes.

The significance of the degree of tissue matching between donor and host was shown in other studies. Stark showed that mixed lymphocyte culture reaction screening (crossmatching) of donor-host corneas predicted graft success [18]. Data from others suggested that the Ia-like antigen (HLA-DR) was present in the cornea. In 1979. Streilein and others published data suggesting that Ia (class II)-bearing Langerhans cells (LHC) are absent from the central cornea but present in the limbus [19]. The same year, Klareskog et al. reported immunofluorescent evidence that LHC are present in the cornea [20]. In 1982, Gillette et al. [21] clarified this issue by publishing evidence that in several species, including humans, the central cornea does have some class II positive dendritic cells with adenosinetriphosphatase positivity, making them consistent with Langerhans cells, and that steroids may deplete these cells from the cornea. Furthermore, the concentrations of these cells may increase in infection and other inflammatory states. The dendritic cells, in contrast to those in other epithelia, are OKT6 negative [22]. They are presumably of bone marrow origin, but this has not been proved by experimental bone marrow transplantation, as has been demonstrated, for example, for pulmonary macrophages [23], Kupffer cells [24], epidermal Langerhans cells [25,26], and osteoclasts [27]. These studies suggest that matching, particularly at the DR locus, may improve success in grafting. In addition, class II expression on epithelial cells may be important in the pathogenesis of vaccinia or herpes viral infections of the cornea, as recently discussed by Streilein et al. [19] and Gillette et al. [21].

This recent research on corneal immunology may also shed light on the pathogenesis of graft-versus-host disease (GVHD). In marrow transplant recipients with chronic GVHD, the increased susceptibility to herpetic keratitis has been attributed to the sicca syndrome, producing dry cornea, due to lack of tear IgA [28]. A relative lack of host Langerhans cells, delayed repopulation by donor LHC, or the effects of systemic steroid therapy (possibly decreasing the concentration of central corneal Langerhans cells) in these patients may serve as alternative explanations for their marked susceptibility to herpetic keratitis.

Subsequent experimental studies by Ray-Keil and Chandler [29] have shown that treatment of cornea with appropriate wavelengths of ultraviolet light, which inactivates Langerhans cells, will decrease the rate of corneal graft rejection. Similar therapy has been reported by Atkinson and colleagues and by Honigsman and colleagues to ameliorate chronic GVHD of the skin even when the disease was refractory to immunosuppressive therapy with prednisone and cyclosporine [30,31].

References

1. Darwin E. Zoonomia or the laws of organic life, vol 2. London: J. Johnson, 1796, cited by Coster [2].
2. Coster DJ. Factors affecting the outcome of corneal transplantation. Ann R Coll Surg Engl 1981;63:91–7.
3. Batchelor JR, Casey TA, Werb A, et al. HLA matching and corneal grafting. Lancet 1976;1:551–4.
4. Ehlers H, Kissmeyer-Nielsen F. Corneal transplantation and HLA histocompatibility. A preliminary communication. Acta Ophthalmol (Copenh) 1979; 57:738–41.

5. Volker-Dieben HJ, Kok-von Alphen CC, Kruitt PJ. Advances and disappointments, indications and restrictions regarding HLA matched corneal grafts in high risk cases. Doc Ophthalmol 1979;46:219–26.
6. Sanfilippo F, MacQueen JM, Vaughn WK, et al. Reduced graft rejection with good HLA-A and B matching in high risk corneal transplantation. N Engl J Med 1986;315:29–35.
7. Smith RS. Corneal transplantation. In: Cerilli GJ, ed. Organ transplantation and replacement. Philadelphia: Lippincott, 1988;625–9.
8. Harbour RC, Stern GA. Variables in McCarey-Kaufman corneal storage. Their effect on corneal graft success. Ophthalmology 1983;90:668–72.
9. Andersen J, Ehlers N. Corneal transplantation using long-term cultured donor material. Acta Ophthalmol (Copenh) 1986;64:93–6.
10. Roper-Hall MJ. Stallard's eye surgery, ed. 6. Philadelphia: Lippincott, 1980;392–442.
11. Chandler JW. Immune reactions and corneal graft rejection. Trans Pac Coast Oto-Ophthalmol Soc 1974;2:209–16.
12. Hunter PA, Wilhelmus KR, Rice NS, Jones BR. Cyclosporine A applied topically to the recipient eye inhibits corneal graft rejection. Clin Exp Immunol 1981;45:173–7.
13. Polack FM. The pathologic anatomy of corneal graft rejection. Surv Ophthalmol 1966;11:391–404.
14. Khodadoust NA, Silverstein AM. The survival and rejection of epithelium in experimental corneal transplantation. Invest Ophthalmol 1969;8:169–89.
15. Khodadoust NA, Silverstein AM. Induction of corneal graft rejection by passive cell transfer. Invest Ophthalmol 1976;15:89–95.
16. Waltman SR, Faulkner HW, Burde RM. Modification of the ocular immune response. I. Use of antilymphocytic serum to prevent immune rejection of penetrating corneal homografts. Invest Ophthalmol 1969;8:196–200.
17. Gronemeyer U, Pulhorn G, Muller-Ruchholtz W. Allogeneic corneal grafting in inbred strains of rats. Graefes Arch Ophthalmol 1978;208:247–62.
18. Stark WJ. Transplantation immunology of penetrating keratoplasty. Trans Am Ophthalmol Soc 1980;78:1079–1117.
19. Streilein JW, Toews GB, Bergstresser PR. Corneal allografts fail to express Ia antigens. Nature 1979;282:326–7.
20. Klareskog L, Forsum U, Tjernlund UM, et al. Expression of Ia antigen-like molecules on cells in the corneal epithelium. Invest Ophthalmol Vis Sci 1979;18:310–3.
21. Gillette TE, Chandler JW, Greiner JV. Langerhans cells of the ocular surface. Ophthalmology 1982;89:700–11.
22. Seto SK, Gillette TE, Chandler JW. HLA-DR+/T6-Langerhans cells of the human cornea. Invest Ophthalmol 1987;28:1719–22.
23. Thomas ED, Ramberg R, Sale GE, et al. Direct evidence for a bone marrow origin of the alveolar macrophage in man. Science 1976;192:1016–8.
24. Gale RP, Sparkes RS, Golde DW. Bone marrow origin of hepatic macrophages (Kupffer cells) in humans. Science 1978;201:937–8.
25. Katz SI, Tamaki K, Sachs DH. Epidermal Langerhans cells are derived from cells originating in bone marrow. Nature 1979;282:324–6.
26. Pelletier M, Perreault C, Landry D, et al. Ontogeny of human epidermal Langerhans cells. Transplantation 1984;38:544–6.
27. Loutit JF, Nisbet NW. The origin of osteoclasts. Immunobiology 1982; 161:193–203.

28. Sale GE. The sicca syndrome of graft-versus-host disease. In: Sale GE, Shulman HM, eds. The pathology of bone marrow transplantation. New York: Masson Publishing USA, 1984.
29. Ray-Keil L, Chandler JW. Reduction in the incidence of rejection of heterotopic murine corneal transplants by pretreatment with ultraviolet radiation. Transplantation 1986;42:403–6.
30. Atkinson K, Weller P, Ryman W, Biggs J. PUVA therapy for drug-resistant graft-versus-host disease. Bone Marrow Transplant 1986;1:227–36.
31. Volc-Platzer B, Honigsmann H, Hinterberger W, Wolff K. Chronic cutaneous graft-versus-host reaction: treatment with photochemotherapy. J Invest Dermatol 1987;89:444.

survivors. Infection associated with engraftment of individual organs such as kidney, pancreas, and cornea is covered in the individual chapters on those organs. This chapter focuses on special differences and unique problems for the settings of solid organ versus marrow transplantation. It will also discuss the fascinating new problem of neolymphoma associated with infection by the Epstein-Barr (EBV) and human immunodeficiency (HIV) viruses.

An important difficulty is diagnosing some lesions that are not clearly infectious. Examples include bronchiolitis obliterans in the heart-lung and marrow transplant recipient, the acute interstitial pneumonia of the marrow recipient, and the difficulty in the gut and marrow transplant recipient of distinguishing lesions of gut rejection or GVHD from those of gram-negative or viral infection. Precise answers to many of these dilemmas remain unavailable. Most pathologists are well aware of the imprecision of terminology in some of these areas and of the limited range of responses to injury mounted by a given organ, but other medical personnel tend to use syndromic or descriptive terms loosely in a type of slang, as if they represented well-understood pathogenetic entities (e.g., "adult respiratory distress syndrome," "hyaline membrane disease"). Part of the pathologist's job may be to separate jargon from objective evidence and rational argument.

Perhaps the most important role of a chapter on this subject, however, is to stimulate sympathy in pathologists for the sense of urgency appropriately felt by clinicians caring for such patients. The request for a rapid, even immediate work-up in such a patient is reasonable and necessary. Almost any infection in such a patient is an emergency.

Summary of Problems in Organ Transplantation

The general problem of infections in solid organ transplant recipients is well reviewed by Tolkoff-Rubin and Rubin [4]. Figure 11.1 diagrams the time course of infectious problems for renal and other solid transplant recipients in general.

Skin Transplantation Serious infections in the skin transplant patient are basically those associated with burns and their treatment. Infections have always been the major cause of death in burn patients. Success in treatment of infections in this population has been good, but not complete. Survival rates of patients with three degrees of burn severity increased between the 1960s and 1970s (Fig. 11.2). The predominant organisms have changed from streptococci to staphylococci, then *Pseudomonas* sp., and gram-negative bacteria since 1935 (Fig. 11.3). Two of the advances making this possible have been the team-oriented burn center and the *Pseudomonas* vaccine (Fig. 11.4).

Burn wound infections are classified as noninvasive or invasive depending on the viability of the eschar and the concentration of organisms; over 10^5 organisms per gram of tissue and an eschar with areas of dry necrosis characterize an invasive infection.

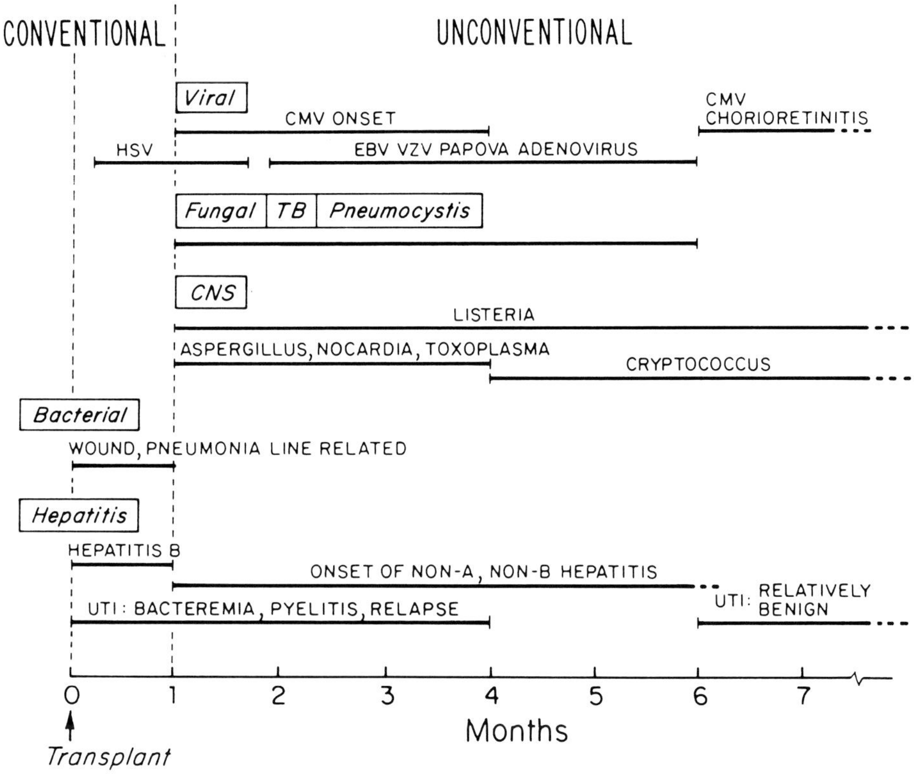

Figure 11.1
Timetable of the occurrence of infection in solid organ transplant recipients. (From Rubin RH, Wolfson JS, Casini AB, et al. Am J Med 1981;70:405–11.)

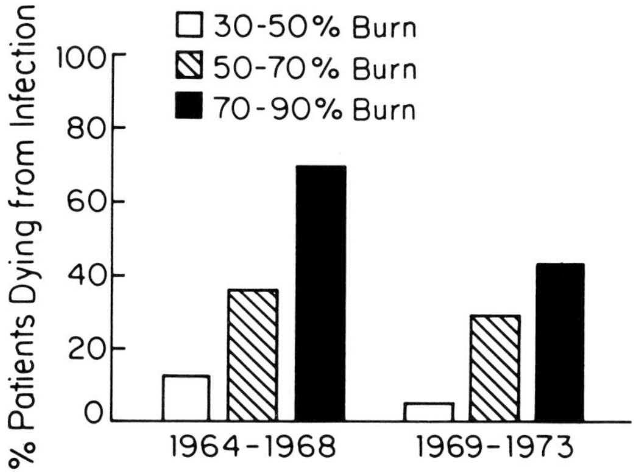

Figure 11.2
Percentage of burned body surface area associated with a 50% mortality for the years 1964 to 1968 vs 1969 to 1973. (From Alexander JW. Infectious problems in the burn patient. In: Artz CP, Moncrief JA, Pruitt BA, eds. Burns: a team effort. Philadelphia: Saunders, 1979.)

Figure 11.5
Predisposing risk factors and common infections by time after marrow transplantation. (From Meyers JD. In: Mandell G, et al., eds. Principles and practice of infectious diseases, 2nd ed. New York: John Wiley & Sons, 1985.)

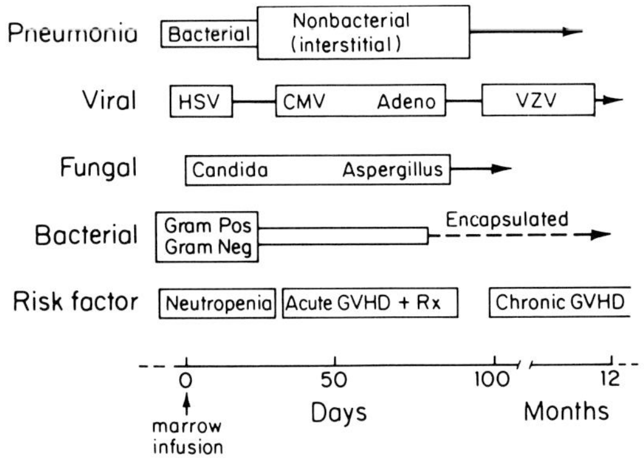

chronic GVHD. The use of trimethoprim sulfa has rendered *P. carinii* infection unusual in the early period and decreased it in the late. Coagulase-negative staphylococci, *Candida* sp., and *Aspergillus* sp. are now the major pathogens of the early period. Systemic antibiotic administration and laminar air flow room isolation have been effective methods of decreasing the frequency of septicemia in the early period. They may also reduce the severity of GVHD, as has been demonstrated now for aplastic but not leukemic patients [5].

The course of infectious disease within the marrow transplant population cannot necessarily be expected to take the classic path. One example of this is that *Staphylococcus epidermidis* can be a pathogen in these patients and has caused significant septicemias. The second point is that *P. carinii* does not behave in this population as it does either in other populations that are immunosuppressed by drugs or in the AIDS population. For example, the frequency of *Pneumocystis* organisms per gram tissue seems smaller in our population and the number of interstitial organisms is higher, compared with alveolar organisms, than that in other populations. The AIDS population tends to have the capacity for a chronic *Pneumocystis* infection with high numbers of organisms in the alveoli and alveolar ducts which does not progress as rapidly as the usual case reported outside that population.

The third example of importance is aspergillosis, which in the marrow transplant population can take several forms. One of the more common is a blood-borne dissemination with embolization to various organs. It is perhaps not as widely recognized that a rapidly progressive form of bronchopulmonary aspergillosis is also seen in this patient population. Rampant examples in our earlier experiences included cases in which large and medium-sized airways were totally plugged with huge masses of *Aspergillus*. A milder form of this may be difficult to distinguish clinically in the early post-transplant period from bronchiolitis obliterans or evidence of the controversial acute GVHD of the lung. A recent example is a 32-year-old Hawaiian male with myelodysplastic syndrome dying 102 days after bone marrow transplantation who, after developing some early skin GVHD and liver disease associated with veno-occlusive disease, developed an obstructive pulmonary picture on day 35 with markedly reduced forced expiratory volume (FEV) reminiscent of the clinical course of bronchiolitis obliterans. Over the period of 2 weeks, a cavity developed in this patient's left upper lobe during worsening pneumonitis. At autopsy on day 102, the patient showed evidence of diffuse intrapulmonary bronchopulmonary aspergillosis with many plugs within small bronchioles, which could easily have explained the FEV.

The second period's major pathogen is CMV infection, which had been an extremely refractory problem for over a decade. Recent important advances have occurred in this area, particularly in the lethal interstitial pneumonia that has plagued these patients. That infection is a diffuse interstitial process of relatively rapid onset associated with miliary lesions of CMV-infected lung [6,7] and progressing in more than 80% of cases to death. Recent advances have taken three forms: (1) use of seronegative donor blood products, (2) gancyclovir (DHPG) therapy, and (3) CMV immune globulin. Meyers [3] showed some years ago that some CMV may be transmitted by blood products. A protective effect could be demonstrated when only seronegative blood products were given to seronegative recipients. No other combination (e.g., seronegative blood products into seropositive patients) appeared protective. The practical effect of this is somewhat limited because many people are seropositive. But the acyclovir derivative, DHPG, has recently been shown, when used alone, to decrease markedly the titer of virus in lung tissue of infected patients when levels are measured in serial biopsy and some autopsy samples [8]. This, among other data, has led to the interpretation that the "autoimmune" response to CMV is an important pathogenetic mechanism. Recent trials of DHPG combined with CMV immune globulin have had very promising preliminary results in at least two centers, suggesting a significant decrease in mortality from CMV pneumonia.

Diagnostic efforts have also markedly improved in that CMV pneumonia can now clearly be diagnosed using bronchoalveolar lavage combined with "shell vial" culture and immunocytologic detection with monoclonal antibody [9,10]. This has markedly decreased the use of open lung biopsy.

Corneal Transplantation Herpetic keratitis and other problems are discussed in Chapter 10.

AIDS in the Transplant Recipient

AIDS is already a problem in the field of transplantation. Transfusions, a form of transplant, are a major risk factor for AIDS patients. Transplants of marrow or other organs from HIV-infected patients obviously should be avoided. Marrow transplantation has even been proposed and carried out as a treatment for AIDS patients with what would appear to be little real hope for success, since transplantation itself is quite immunosuppressive and may aggravate AIDS infection. It is a serious problem in the field of marrow grafting that many patients now presenting with leukemia in remission were given transfusions between 1980 and 1984, when blood banks were unable to screen for HIV. Some of these patients are found to be HIV-antibody positive when evaluated for transplantation. It is uncertain how successful marrow transplantation will be in such patients; but our first such patient showed rapid growth and dissemination of virus during the first weeks after transplantation and died soon after of other infections.*

Diagnostic Pathologic Findings of Infections

Biopsy Diagnosis of Infections

Skin Immunosuppressed patients frequently exhibit skin lesions in which biopsy is tried for diagnosis. Disseminated embolic fungal infection can often be so diagnosed using silver or periodic acid–Schiff (PAS) stain. In hematologic malignancies, bacterial infections may require separation from chloromas and Sweet's syndrome, in which nodular collections of mature, presumably nonmalignant polymorphonuclear leukocytes collect without evidence of infection. Infrequently parasitic (*Demodex* sp.) or superficial dermatophyte infections are found. Viral infections, such as herpes zoster, can be confirmed by immunohistology, but Tzanck preparations (direct smears of vesicles) are extremely useful, being rapid and noninvasive.

Lung Differential diagnosis of bronchopulmonary infections has evolved with developments in antibiotics and methodology. Focal (especially cavitary) lesions located by computed tomography (CT) scans are now approached with fine needle aspiration whose yield is high in cavitary fungal or bacterial infections. Many transplant recipients, especially those receiving marrow, develop diffuse pneumonitis. Within a few days of grafting, this often represents edema, hemorrhage, or transient radiation or endotoxic damage. Days to weeks later, true interstitial pneumonia may develop, with or without an infectious etiology. *P. carinii* pneumonia can be studied at biopsy or lavage using a rapid silver stain [11]. The most frequent infectious pneumonia is CMV. The danger of rapid progression had for many years prompted aggressive early open lung biopsy because other methods had low yields. Direct smear imprint cytologic study, monoclonal antibody immunofluorescence on frozen section and smear, immunoenzyme techniques on paraffin section, and in situ hybridization using viral DNA segments as probes have rendered diagnostic histology extremely sensitive and specific since then. Furthermore, bronchoalveolar lavage [9], when combined with the "shell vial" accelerated centrifugation culture technique and monoclonal antibody diagnosis, has rendered lung biopsy necessary in markedly fewer cases. Furthermore, antibodies to adenovirus, respiratory syncytial virus, herpes simplex 1 and 2, and herpes zoster have markedly sped the diagnosis

*Bowden R, personal communication, 1988.

of these viruses on many fixed, frozen, or freshly smeared tissue samples [10,12,13].

In situ hybridization methods, which identify specific viral DNA genomic sequences even in paraffin-embedded tissues, may not only help in diagnosis of active infection but also in latent infection [12]. Blot technology may soon allow rapid identification of virus in circulating lymphocytes, and a new polymerase chain reaction may geometrically increase the sensitivity of such methods.

Gastrointestinal Tract Lessons learned from the study of lung biopsies were applied to the gastrointestinal tract by Spencer et al. [14]. Marrow transplant recipients often develop chronic anorexia, nausea, and vomiting. Distinguishing GVHD, reflux, fungus, or virus is difficult. Fiberoptic endoscopy was employed in a study of these patients, and the results proved informative (half the patients had viral infections; a smaller fraction had fungus or GVHD) and very useful for guiding therapy. Furthermore, unexpectedly, many patients with CMV esophagitis or gastroenteritis failed to progress to CMV pneumonia.

Liver Fine needle aspiration is useful for cavitary lesions, although hemorrhagic complications may be more frequent than in other patient groups (especially after marrow transplantation). Needle biopsies are a distinctly low-yield procedure for viral infection other than hepatitis A or B. Open biopsy can often assist in distinguishing infection from veno-occlusive disease or GVHD. Pretransplant biopsies may be needed in patients with elevated LFTs to assess tumor status and to evaluate the risk of veno-occlusive disease.

Mouth *Candida* infection and chronic GVHD are the major diagnoses separated by biopsy. Viral lesions are occasionally mistaken clinically for GVHD and noted on biopsy with cytologic or immunohistologic study.

Genitourinary Tract Infrequently outside the renal transplant setting, renal biopsy or renal pelvic cytologic study through ureterostomy may be undertaken to address the differential diagnosis of obstruction or hemorrhagic cystitis. Adenovirus infection of the kidney or bladder may present in this way [15]. BK virus, an RNA virus occasionally infecting humans, may infect the bladder or the renal pelvis and mimic hemorrhagic cystitis. Frequently, asymptomatic CMV infection of the kidney will be detected by urine culture or cytologic study, procedures that are used with serology to assess the status of marrow graft recipients, for example.

Bone Marrow Only occasionally will a marrow biopsy yield histologic evidence of viral or fungal infection. CMV is also difficult to culture from bone marrow aspirates, although the association of CMV infection with marrow depression in transplant recipients is highly suspicious for direct infectious damage to the marrow [16].

Autopsy Diagnosis of Infections

Unfortunately, some infections in transplant recipients are not diagnosed until autopsy. Two important explanations are as follows: (1) biopsy of a suspected organ may be too risky at certain post-transplant intervals because of problems such as thrombocytopenia and (2) some fungal infections never reveal positive cultures of blood or other specimens before death and may produce no distinct radiographic findings. In transplant recipients, therefore, autopsy data are extremely important, because without such data many epidemiologic patterns would never be suspected. Viral cultures of autopsy specimens are important in all immunosuppressed transplant recipients because viral infection is very frequent and is often undiagnosed or unsuspected during life.

Heart Toxoplasmosis, fungal emboli, Chagas' disease, and cardiomyopathy due to chemotherapy with adriamycin, for instance, may surface only at necropsy. Cardiac biopsy is unusual in transplantation outside the cardiac transplantation group.

Brain and Spinal Cord Unsuspected infections and undiagnosed focal lesions are often clarified at autopsy. Unsuspected toxoplasmosis, herpetic, and even bacterial infections may occasionally be discovered only at brain autopsy. Recently, brain biopsy has been used successfully to diagnose focal lesions in AIDS patients (and recently in one of our bone marrow transplant patients) if toxoplasmosis is suspected. Wright-Giemsa stains of brain tissue smears seem to be the most effective approach.

New Neoplasia in Transplant Patients

Introducing an article on the incidence of tumors in cyclosporine-treated transplant recipients, Israel Penn stated that "any form of immunosuppression, if of sufficient duration and intensity, will lead to the development of certain forms of cancer" [17,18]. He then reported that lymphoproliferative lesions were more frequent than skin tumors in cyclosporine-treated patients, whereas the reverse is true in transplant recipients with other types of immunosuppression (as he had reported 8 years earlier) [19]. It is clear that his bold statement about the incidence of cancer is correct based on these data. Most fascinating from a conceptual point of view was the reaction to these earlier tumor statistics by Streilein [20].

Matching bold statements with Penn, Streilein proposed that Penn's data on skin tumors permitted the postulation of a SALT (skin-associated lymphoid tissue) similar to the previously proposed GALT (gut-) and BALT (bronchus-) associated lymphoid tissues. (Not to be outdone, Chandler and Axelrod subsequently proposed a CALT, or conjunctiva-associated lymphoid tissue [21].) Streilein suggests that indeed the strongest data supporting an immunosurveillance mechanism in humans have come from this early experience with human skin tumors in transplant recipients. What antigenic determinants are involved or what relative growth advantages might be conferred on subpopulations of epidermal cells remain unknown. However, clues can be seen in the fact that basal cell carcinomas were much less frequent than were squamous cell carcinomas in Penn's studies. Relevant is the fact that we have seen one, and others have seen six, cases of porokeratosis of Mibelli [22] in transplant recipients, which represents a local proliferative lesion of an epidermal cell subset. Further understanding of these cutaneous tumors will be one important test for the theory of immunosurveillance.

Fisher and Kripke [23] have clearly shown that ultraviolet light systemically immunosuppresses and is associated with an increased incidence of skin tumors even in nonexposed areas. The mechanism is apparently complex and involves both T-suppressor and dendritic cells. Recent data by Cruz et al. [24] show that ultraviolet light may induce tolerance in dendritic cells to delayed-type hypersensitivity. Theoretically this may be extended to the tolerance of tumors.

Lymphoproliferative disorders were reported as frequent in the renal transplant population, along with nonmelanotic skin and lip cancers. Congenitally immunodeficient patients showed a high incidence of lymphoma. Some of the unusual features reported include a 40- to 350-fold relative risk of developing malignant lymphomas in renal transplant recipients and a high frequency of CNS involvement (49%), a presumably privileged site. The leading hypothesis is EBV-induced lymphomagenesis for this population. Renal and cardiac transplants are said to carry between 2% and 20% incidence of EBV-associated lymphoma. In the case of marrow transplant recipients, radiation and carcinogenic alkylating agents such as cyclophosphamide are also probable causes of post-transplant cancer [25–27].

Recently, Nalesnik and colleagues from Pittsburgh summarized 43 patients with post-transplant immunoproliferative disorders derived from the Denver-Pittsburgh experience in solid organ transplantation between 1980 and 1987 [28]. They found a spectrum of lesions from monomorphic to polymorphic and some impressive evidence of reversibility in the nonclonal and half the clonal cases. Some of the patients had a mononucleosislike syndrome. All the patients had received cyclosporine. Four patients with multiple tumors could be studied in more detail. Clonality by gene rearrangement did not always correlate with a "monoclonal" light chain ratio. Different gut tumors often represented either different clonal tumors or polyclonal tumors.

Thymic transplantation has also been associated with EBV-associated immunoblastic lymphoma as reported by Reece et al. [29] and Borzy et al. [30]. As late as 1978, EBV infection was regarded as an insignificant problem in recipients of marrow and other transplants [7]. That consensus has radically changed. We recently analyzed 15 cases of EBV-associated lymphoma in Seattle [31] occurring among 2192 allogeneic marrow transplant recipients. Fourteen of the 15 were large cell noncleaved immunoblastic lymphomas, and one was an angioimmunoblastic lymphadenopathy. Thirteen of the 15 cases occurred in donor cell types as determined by cytogenetic and molecular analysis. Studies of surface light chain expression and immunoglobulin heavy chain gene rearrangement analysis indicated that most of these lesions seem to begin as polyclonal populations, giving rise to oligoclonal or monoclonal subpopulations. The risk factor analysis implicated T-cell monoclonal antibody directed against the T-cell receptor (CD3) used in marrow depletion or GVHD therapy. Mismatched marrow recipients with GVHD were also at higher risk. It is of interest that these patients seem to have disease in abdominal sites rather than putatively privileged (CNS) sites more frequently than do recipients of solid organ grafts. This may imply that abnormal B-cell proliferation is more frequent in the peripheral lymphoid tissues of marrow recipients who are attempting to regenerate totally ablated lymphoid systems and that such sites are also particularly predisposed to EBV-induced proliferation.

Three more recent cases have been particularly fascinating. One of these is a polyclonal diffuse T-cell proliferation with no evidence of HTLV-I.* Two others were T-cell neoplasms 1 and 2 years after transplantation arising in patients with B-cell lymphoma and acute myelogenous leukemia, respectively, as original diagnoses. The cases were negative by DNA hybridization studies for EBV or HTLV-I, II, or III in preliminary studies [32].

References

1. Sale GE, Shulman HM, Hackman RC. Pathology in bone marrow transplant recipients. In: Said J, Nash G, eds. The pathology of acquired immune deficiency. Major problems in pathology series. Philadelphia: Saunders, in press.
2. Rubin RH, Wolfson JS, Cosini AB, et al. Infection in the renal transplant recipient. Am J Med 1981;70:405–11.
3. Meyers JD. Infection in marrow transplant recipients. Am J Med 1986;81:27–38.
4. Tolkoff-Rubin NE, Rubin RH. Infection in the organ transplant recipient. In: Cerelli CJ, ed. Organ transplantation and replacement. Philadelphia: Lippincott, 1988;445–61.
5. Storb R, Prentice RL, Buckner CD, et al. Graft-versus-host disease and survival in patients with aplastic anemia treated by marrow grafts from HLA-identical siblings. Beneficial effect of a protected environment. N Engl J Med 1983;308:302–7.
6. Beschorner WE, Hutchins GM, Burns WH, et al. Cytomegalovirus pneumonia in bone marrow transplant recipients: miliary and diffuse patterns. Am Rev Respir Dis 1980;122:107–14.
7. Sale GE, Hackman RC. Pathology of infections after bone marrow transplantation. In: Sale GE, Shulman HM, eds. The pathology of bone marrow transplantation. New York: Masson, 1984.
8. Shepp DH, Dandliker PS, de Miranda P, et al. Activity of 9-[2-hydroxy-1-(hydroxymethyl) ethoxymethyl] guanine in the treatment of cytomegalovirus pneumonia. Ann Intern Med 1985;103:368–73.
9. Crawford SW, Bowden RA, Hackman RC, et al. Rapid detection of cytomegalovirus pulmonary lavage and centrifugation culture. Ann Intern Med, 1988;108:180–5.
10. Hackman RC. Immunohistology for the rapid diagnosis of viral infections. West J Med 1986;145:373.

*Hackman RC, unpublished data.

11. Mahan CT, Sale GE. Rapid methenamine silver stain for *Pneumocystis* and fungi. Arch Pathol Lab Med 1978;102:351–2.
12. Myerson D, Hackman RC, Nelson JA, et al. Widespread presence of histologically occult cytomegalovirus. Hum Pathol 1984;15:430–9.
13. Springmeyer SC, Hackman RC, Holle R, et al. Diagnosis of acute diffuse pneumonia in the immunocompromised host: use of bronchoalveolar lavage. J Infect Dis 1986;154:604–10.
14. Spencer GD, Hackman RC, McDonald GB, et al. A prospective study of unexplained nausea and vomiting after marrow transplantation. Transplantation 1986;6:602–7.
15. Shields AF, Hackman RC, Fife KH, et al. Adenovirus infections in patients undergoing bone marrow transplantation. N Engl J Med 1985;312:529–33.
16. Sale GE. Pathology of bone marrow with marrow transplantation. In: Sale GE, Shulman HM, eds. The pathology of bone marrow transplantation. New York: Masson, 1984.
17. Penn I. Cancers following cyclosporine therapy. Transplantation 1987;43:32–5.
18. Penn I. The development of new tumors after transplantation. In: Cerilli GJ, ed. Organ transplantation and replacement. Philadelphia: Lippincott, 1988;439–44.
19. Penn I. Tumor incidence in human allograft recipients. Transplant Proc 1979;11:1047–52.
20. Streilein W. Skin associated lymphoid tissue (SALT): origins and functions. J Invest Dermatol 1983;80:12–6s.
21. Chandler JW, Axelrod AJ. Conjunctiva associated lymphoid tisssue: a probable component of the mucosa associated lymphoid system. In: O'Connor GR, ed. Immunologic diseases of the mucous membranes. Pathology, diagnosis, and treatment. New York: Masson, 1980;63–70.
22. Komorowski RA, Clowry LJ. Porokeratosis of Mibelli in transplant recipients. Am J Clin Pathol 1989;91:71–4.
23. Fisher M, Kripke N. Suppressor T cells mediate resistance to ultraviolet induced tumors in mice. Science 1982;216:1133–4.
24. Cruz PD, Nixon-Fulton J, Tigelaar RE, Bergstresser PR. Disparate effects of in vitro low dose UVB irradiation on intravenous immunization with purified epidermal cell subpopulations for the induction of contact hypersensitivity. J Invest Dermatol 1989;92:160–5.
25. Deeg HJ, Prentice R, Fritz TE, et al. Increased incidence of malignant tumors in dogs after total body irradiation and marrow transplantation. Int J Radiat Oncol Biol Phys 1983;9:1505–11.
26. Witherspoon R, Fisher LD, Schoch G. Secondary cancers after marrow transplantation for leukemia or aplastic anemia. New Engl J Med, 1989;321:784–9.
27. Hanto DW, Frizzera G, Gajl-Peczalsca KJ, et al. Epstein-Barr virus, immunodeficiency, and B cell lymphoproliferation. Transplantation 1985;39:461–72.
28. Nalesnik MA, Jaffe R, Starzl TE, et al. The pathology of posttransplant lymphoproliferative disorders occurring in the setting of cyclosporine A–prednisone immunosuppression. Am J Pathol 1988;133:173–92.
29. Reece ER, Gartner JG, Seemayer TA, et al. Epstein-Barr virus in a malignant lymphoproliferative disorder of B cells occurring after thymic epithelial transplantation for combined immunodeficiency. Cancer Res 1981;41:4243–7.
30. Borzy MS, Hong R, Horowitz SD, et al. Fatal lymphoma after transplantation of cultured thymus in children with combined immunodeficiency disease. N Engl J Med 1979;301:565.
31. Zutter MM, Martin PJ, Sale GE, et al. Epstein-Barr virus lymphoproliferation after bone marrow transplantation. Blood 1988;72:520–9.

32. Zutter MM, Loughran T, Martin PJ, et al. T-cell lymphoproliferation after marrow transplantation. Blood 1987;70:317a.
33. Alexander JW. Infectious problems in the burn patient. In: Artz CP, Moncrief JA, Pruitt BA, eds. Burns: a team effort. Philadelphia: Saunders, 1979.
34. Martin PJ, Shulman HM, Schubach WH, et al. Fatal EBV associated proliferation of donor B cells after treatment of acute GVHD with a murine anti T cell antibody. Ann Intern Med 1984;101:310–5.

12

Fine Needle Aspiration in Transplantation Pathology

PEKKA HÄYRY
EEVA VON WILLEBRAND
JUHANI AHONEN

Numerous attempts have been made to monitor rejection episodes from blood specimens [1]. However, needle biopsy is still the only reliable method to assess the graft and serves as a "gold standard" in clinical trials [1].

Excluding hyperacute rejection, histologic analysis of the allograft has demonstrated two major venues of rejection: cellular and vascular [2]. *Cellular rejection* indicates accumulation of "round" inflammatory cells, predominantly lymphocytes, blast cells, and mononuclear phagocytes, into the transplant. This infiltrate is seen initially in the vicinity of the blood vessels particularly around arterioli, but later diffusely throughout the graft. Cellular rejections usually occur relatively soon after the transplantation. Most can be readily reversed with drugs. Hallmarks of *vascular rejection* are vasculitis, fibrointimal thickening of the graft arteriolar endothelium leading to "onion skinning," and obliteration of the arteries and, in renal grafts, destruction of glomeruli. Most of these changes are irreversible. Vascular rejections are usually assigned to humoral immunity [3,4]. However, on most

This study was supported in part by grants IRO1AM26882 and IRO1AM31730 from the NIH, Bethesda, MD, and in part by the Association of Finnish Life Insurance Companies, the Sigrid Juselius Foundation, and the Academy of Finland, Helsinki, Finland.

Table 12.1
FNA reporting form for use with the "increment" method of interpreting inflammation

Inflammatory cells	*FNAB (%)*	*Blood (%)*	*Increment*	*Correction factor*	*Corrected increment (%)*
Lymphoblasts	2		2	1.0	2.0
Plasmablasts and plasma cells	4		4	1.0	4.0
Activated lymphocytes	4		4	0.5	2.0
Large granular lymphocytes				0.2	
Lymphocytes (others)	20	5	15	0.1	1.5
Polymorphonucleaar leukocytes					
Juvenile forms				0.1	
Neutrophils	61	87		0.1	
Basophils		1		0.1	
Eosinophils	3	2	1	0.1	0.1
Monoblasts				1.0	

Monocytes	6	5	1	0.2	0.2
Macrophages				1.0	
Total score (sum of corrected increments)					9.8

	Grade			
Parenchymal Cells	*1 (no change)*	*2 (swelling)*	*3 (swelling & vacuolization)*	*4 (necrosis)*
Endothelial cells		x		
Tubular cells		x		
Parenchymal cells: 10 per 100 inflammatory cells				
Conclusion: Acute cellular rejection; moderate				

FNAB, fine needle aspiration biopsy.

Table 12.2
International quality control workshop, 1984: rate of agreement with Helsinki diagnosis according to diagnosis

		Helsinki diagnosis		*Center diagnosis*[a] *(No. of centers)*					
					Disagree				
Group no.	*Slide no.*	*Primary*	*Secondary*	*Agree*	*x*	*xx*	*xxx*	*Total*	*Centers agree (%)*
1	1	Normal (no inflammation)		16				16	100
	11	Normal (no inflammation)		15	1			16	94
	15	Normal (no inflammation)	CsA toxicity	12	2		2	16	75
2	7	Normal (no inflammation)		1	1	1	2	5	20
	16	Normal (no inflammation)		1	2		1	4	25
1	2	Blastogenic inflammation		16				16	100
	12	Blastogenic inflammation		13		2	1	16	81
	13	Blastogenic inflammation		16				16	100
2	6	Blastogenic inflammation		5				5	100
	8	Blastogenic inflammation		5				5	100
	17	Blastogenic inflammation	ATN	2		2		4	50
	19	Blastogenic inflammation		4				4	100
	20	Blastogenic inflammation	ATN	4				4	100
1	3	CsA toxicity		12	2		2	16	75
2	9	CsA toxicity	ATN	2		1	2	5	40
1	4	Necrosis	ATN	12	2	2		16	75
1	5	Nonblastogenic inflammation		10	2	4		16	63
	14	Nonblastogenic inflammation		9	1	4	2	16	56
2	10	Nonblastogenic inflammation		2	2		1	5	40
	18	Nonblastogenic inflammation		4			4		100

[a]Designated "agree" if compatible with the primary diagnosis of Helsinki; x, minor disagreement; xx, marked disagreement; xxx, complete disagreement.
Source: Häyry P. Transplant aspiration cytology. A quality control analysis in 1984. Transplant Proc 1985;17:2100–5. With permission of the author and Grune & Stratton.

In acute cellular rejection, without cyclosporine toxicity or acute tubular necrosis, the graft parenchymal cells appear usually normal in the beginning. With prolonged rejection, their morphology gradually deteriorates. In late and irreversible rejection, necrotic cells are frequently seen in FNAB specimens [7,46]. All these parenchymal cell changes are nonspecific, except perhaps for isometric vacuolization in cyclosporine toxicity. Thus the interpretation of these changes requires concomitant assessment of inflammation, sometimes staining of cyclosporine in cellular cytoplasm, and knowledge of the recipient's clinical background [45]. Some of the characteristic parenchymal cell changes are shown in Figure 12.1.

Components of Inflammation

Lymphoblasts representing primarily T blast cells, plasmablasts representing primarily B blast cells, plasma cells, "activated lymphocytes," "large

Figure 12.1
Parenchymal cells in fine needle aspirates. A. A group of normal tubular cells. B. Endothelial cells with normal morphology. C. Swelling of tubular cells during acute tubular necrosis. D. Tubular cells with swelling and strong isometric vacuolation in the cytoplasm in cyclosporine nephrotoxicity.

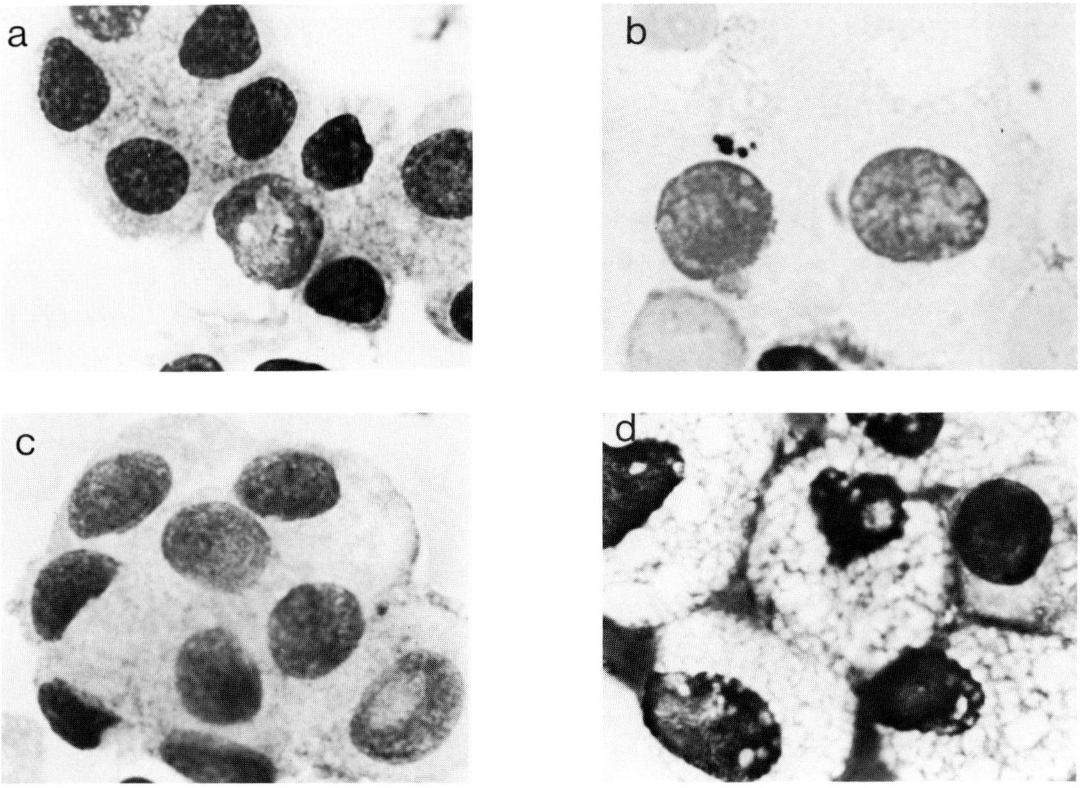

granular lymphocytes" (GL) representing primarily the graft-infiltrating natural killer (NK) cells [47], small lymphocytes and early monoblasts, monocytes, and tissue macrophages at different stages of maturation [7,46] are easily identified in MGG-stained cytosmears. Granulocytes appear later along with necrotic changes [7,8]. According to our experience [48], eosinophils are not recorded in excess over the blood background; however, this might be a visual artifact related to the increment method [48], or the eosinophils may exist in degranulated forms. Some of the inflammatory cell types present in renal FNAB are shown in Figure 12.2.

Figure 12.2
Inflammatory cells in fine needle aspirates during rejection. A. A blast cell with intense cytoplasmic basophilia and a perinuclear halo and an activated lymphocyte. B. A blast cell with a less prominent perinuclear halo. C. A large granular lymphocyte with azurophilic granulation in the cytoplasm (to the left) and a lymphocyte. D. A basophil and an eosinophil. E. A monocyte with normal morphology. F. Macrophages with vacuolation and inclusions in the cytoplasm surrounding a tubular cell.

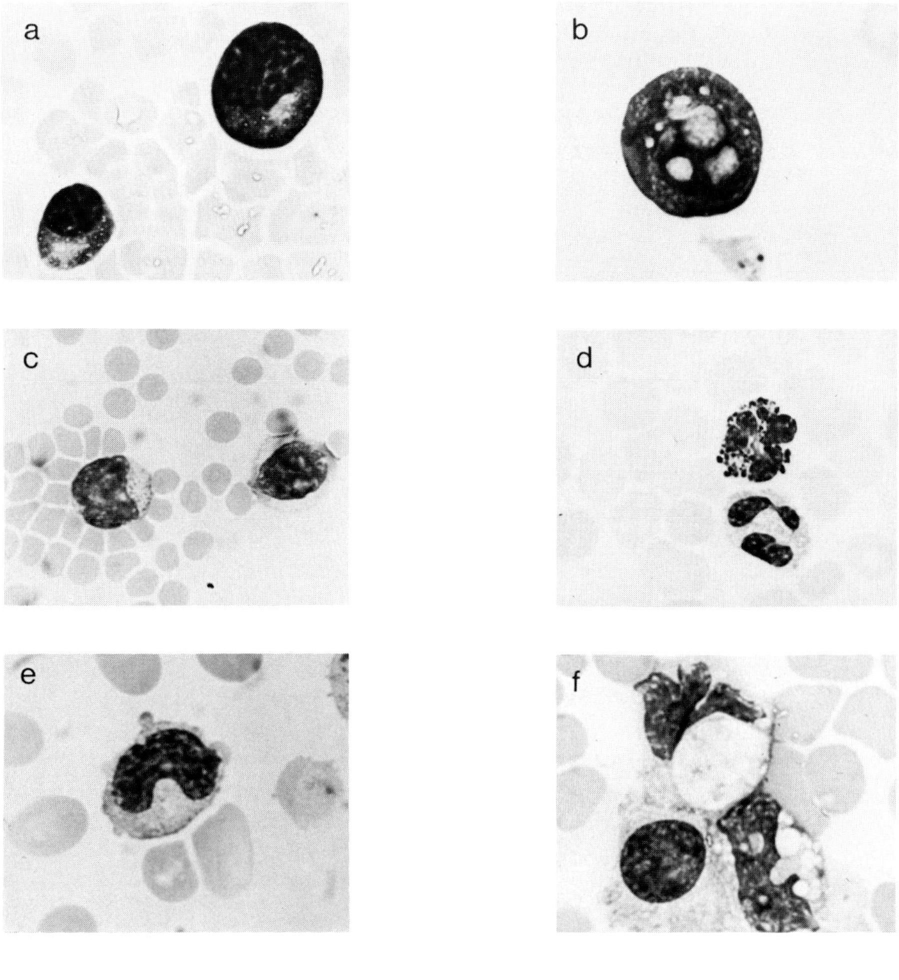

Thrombocytes are slightly difficult to visualize in ordinary MGG staining, but they can be analyzed adequately by proper monoclonal antibodies to the thrombocyte lineage [22]. Indium-labeled thrombocytes [49,50] have been demonstrated in the allograft during rejection. This has been confirmed by the FNAB [22]. Moreover, the FNAB analysis indicates that entrapment of the thrombocytes is a two-stage process, where "loose" aggregates are invariably seen, approximately two times the blood background level in all acute episodes of rejection. Agglutination of thrombocytes onto the graft endothelium is limited primarily to prolonged and irreversible rejections.

A "Common" Pattern of Inflammation

Lymphocytes and monocytes are the first inflammatory cells to appear in the transplant during rejection. Concomitantly, blast cells appear and the transplant function begins to deteriorate. Some inflammation is present in most allografts even without evidence of clinical rejection, and some low-grade blast cell–dominated episodes may pass clinically unnoticed [1]. Intensified anti-inflammatory treatment clears the inflammatory cells from the graft, and the graft resumes normal function. Maturation of blood-borne monocytes into tissue macrophages is the most prominent cytologic hallmark of acute irreversible rejection [6–8].

Most early inflammatory episodes follow this pattern, with some deviation [51]. The inflammatory episode may persist for several days or even weeks, or multiple peaks of inflammation may be encountered with frequent exacerbations and remissions. Sometimes the FNAB shows inflammation 2 or 3 days before deterioration in graft function begins, whereas in some cases a high peak of inflammation may mount within hours (Fig. 12.3).

Effect of Immunosuppression on the Pattern of Inflammation

Prophylactic immunosuppression may influence the cytologic pattern of inflammation. One example is the higher (background) inflammation observed under cyclosporine compared with azathioprine plus steroids [52,53]. In the azathioprine and low-dose steroid regimen, the first episodes of inflammation occur early; most of them are blast cell dominated and intense [54]. Under azathioprine and high-dose steroids, the onset of inflammation is delayed, the intensity is reduced, and fewer blast cells and macrophages are seen in the aspirates during the first episode of rejection [54]. Immunosuppression with cyclosporine A alone, without steroids, is usually accompanied by prominent inflammation the first days after transplantation. Lymphocytes and mononuclear phagocytes dominate; high numbers of mature macrophages are characteristic. A persistent low-grade inflammation is also more common in cyclosporine-treated patients than in patients receiving azathioprine plus steroids. The incidence of intense inflammatory episodes is higher under cyclosporine compared with regimens containing azathioprine plus steroids or cyclosporine plus steroids [52,53]. If cyclo-

tion may be visualized in aspiration cytology as lymphocyte- and mononuclear phagocyte–dominated inflammation without any clear blastogenic component. A close correlation between isometric vacuolation of the tubular and endothelial cells in the FNAB and similar changes in the graft tubular cells in histologic specimens in the context of cyclosporine toxicity is also reported [25,72,73]. Cyclosporine deposits may be visualized concomitantly in the FNAB with proper antibodies, although demonstration of these deposits is obviously more difficult from tissue sections.

However, only cellular rejections can be visualized accurately in the FNAB; it is far more difficult to visualize vascular rejections, and quantitation of the extent of vascular damage is definitely not possible. The FNAB and the needle biopsy are by no means alternative methods of transplant monitoring but should be used concomitantly (Table 12.3).

Table 12.3
Differences between needle biopsy and fine needle aspiration biopsy

	Needle biopsy	*Fine needle aspiration biopsy*
Glomeruli	Transplant glomerulopathy, (recurrent) glomerulonephritis	
Tubuli	Atrophy, vacuolization, necrosis, calcification	Swelling, vacuolization, inclusions, necrosis of single tubular cells
Blood vessels	Transplant vasculopathy, vasculitis	Number of endothelial cells, activated endothelial cells
Interstitium	Edema, fibrosis	
Inflammation	Density, expansion, distribution of cellular infiltrate, immunohistochemistry	Quantification, state of activation, phenotypic differentiation of infiltrating cells, course of inflammation

Source: Hammer C. Personal communication, 1987.

Fine Needle Aspiration Biopsy as a Differential Diagnostic Tool

The following intragraft disorders can be adequately diagnosed by FNAB: acute tubular necrosis, cyclosporine nephrotoxicity, and inflammation (cellular rejection) (Table 12.4).

If in an initially nonfunctioning transplant, tubular cell changes compatible with acute tubular necrosis are observed, this diagnosis is likely. Improvement of tubular cell morphology in the absence of inflammation is usually associated with the onset of urine production. In the context of more severe acute tubular necrosis, monocytes and macrophages can be seen in the aspirate, this probably being a scavenger phenomenon unrelated to any irreversible rejection process. These cells also disappear with the onset of graft function. A rapid deterioration of parenchymal cell morphology and appearance of necrotic parenchymal cells in the cytologic specimens indicate discontinuation of the vascular supply. If during acute tubular necrosis blastogenic inflammation is observed, rejection has been superimposed. It is safest to treat, regardless of minimal or nonexisting clinical signs of rejection, in the absence of urine production. Persistent inflammation with gradually deteriorating parenchymal cell morphology indicates nonresponsiveness to therapy and suggests a change in the treatment protocol. Demonstration of tissue macrophages and necrotic parenchymal cells in the FNAB specimen, in the context of a late inflammatory episode, indicates prolonged and irreversible rejection. Disappearance of inflammatory cells

Table 12.4
Differential diagnosis of early renal transplant failure by fine needle aspiration biopsy

	FNAB cytology			
Serum creatinine	*Inflammation*	*Tubular cell*	*Isometric vacuolization and (possibly) CyA deposits in the graft*	*Explanation*
Normal	—	—	—	Well functioning graft
Elevated	—	+ +	—	ATN
Elevated	±[a]	+ + +	+ + +	CyA toxicity
Elevated	+ + +	+	—	Rejection
Elevated	+ + +	+ + +	+ + +	Rejection and CyA toxicity

Source: Häyry P, von Willebrand E. Transplant aspiration cytology in the evaluation of a renal allograft. In: Touraine JL, ed. Transplantation and clinical immunology, vol. XV. Immunosuppression. Amsterdam: Excerpta Medica, 1983;124–37.

concomitantly with treatment, and improvement in graft parenchymal cell morphology, indicate a good response to treatment or a spontaneous resolution of the episode. Distinct tubular cell changes with isometric vacuolation (and concomitant deposits of cyclosporine) are compatible with cyclosporine nephrotoxicity. If such alterations are seen together with blastogenic inflammation, this indicates rejection regardless of maximal cyclosporine treatment. Thus no therapeutic margin is left, and a change in immunosuppressive protocol is indicated. Persistent inflammation with lymphocytes and mononuclear phagocytes and the presence of activated vascular endothelial cells indicate that vascular alterations are present; to confirm vascular rejection, a needle biopsy must be performed. At present no universal agreement exists on the changes associated with viral infections in FNAB.

In other words, the possibility of performing *repeated* biopsies with FNAB gives a dynamic picture of the process. As Claus Hammer states: "A needle biopsy gives a pathologist a comprehensive although spot-lit picture of the phenomenon: the situation may be visualized within seconds, but whether the bicycle rider is moving forward or backward cannot be stated."

Fine Needle Aspiration Biopsy as an Investigative Tool

Expression of Histocompatibility Antigens

The expression of MHC antigens in a renal transplant is regulated by extraneous factors, such as the type of immunosuppression or presence of rejection [23]. We have earlier shown that both sets of MHC antigens are prominently visualized on the surface of normal renal microvascular endothelial cells. However, they (and, in particular, class II) are usually undetectable in well-functioning transplants. On the other hand, in most transplants undergoing rejection, these antigens are again prominently expressed. This has been confirmed both in experimental conditions [74] and in humans [24]. In addition, we know now that upregulation of class II antigens is primarily due to gamma-interferon and other lymphokines released in situ by inflammatory blast cells [75] and that a major downregulating mechanism is administration of steroids and other concomitant immunosuppression [75,76]. These observations have in many ways aided the understanding of the "vicious cycles" of rejection and induction of rejection episodes in the context of virus infection [77].

Isolation and Experimental Analysis of the Functions of the Inflammatory Cells

Several investigators [78,79] have isolated allograft-infiltrating lymphoid cells during rejection by FNAB and expanded them in situ. Buurman et al. [79] and Doveren et al. [80] have used the same procedure and limited dilution assays to quantitate the frequency of cytotoxic T lymphocytes and their precursors in dog renal transplants and Manca et al. the frequency of T helper lymphocytes in rat renal allografts [81,82]. These clones may be immortalized by hybridization to appropriate T-cell lines and their functions analyzed further [81]. Using exogenous interleukin-2 (IL-2) [78,79], this experimental setup favors the cloning efficacy of CD8 cytotoxic and NK cells. If IL-2 is excluded and high stimulator-responder ratios employed [82], the cloning efficacy of CD4 helper cells is favored. As an extension of FNAB to tumor immunology, an assay has been devised to monitor splenic white blood cell populations in experimental animals with transplanted tumors, with subcutaneous transposition of the spleen and frequent aspiration biopsies [83].

Clinical Trials

In many recent clinical trials the gold standard of needle biopsy has been partially replaced by a "silver standard" of FNAB [84–86]. Our own experience deals mostly with the impact of various immunosuppressive protocols on the frequency, type, and duration of the inflammatory episodes of rejection. As this experience has been reported in detail elsewhere [52,54,82,87,88], it will not be discussed here.

Fine Needle Aspiration Biopsy and Other Organs

Liver Transplants

FNAB has been successfully used to monitor liver transplants in both Europe and the United States [18,89]. Our experience is based on experimental work in the pig [90]. Using immunosuppressed and nonimmunosuppressed piglets we demonstrated that the inflammatory components of rejection were similar in liver transplants when compared with kidney transplants in humans. We also identified in cytologic specimens the various parenchymal components of the liver (i.e., hepatocytes and bile duct and vascular endothelial cells), correlated the cytologic findings to graft histology, and subsequently employed this in human liver transplantation. At present there is a good reason to believe that aspiration cytology will become a major method for monitoring liver allografts in humans.

Pancreatic Transplants

Two Middle-European groups [91,92] have performed duct-obliterated pancreatic transplants in the dog and attempted to analyze these by FNAB. Both report difficulty in obtaining FNABs from the fibrotic pancreas. Reading of the biopsies has been laborious because of the high level of background inflammation due to the obliteration procedure.

Heart Transplants

There have been no attempts to monitor heart transplants with classic aspiration cytology.

Lung Transplants

Bronchoalveolar lavage provides easy access to the lung, and the lavage fluid faithfully describes the inflammatory changes in alveolar interstitium [93]. Bronchoalveolar lavage has been used to monitor inflammatory processes mimicking rejection in the lung [94]. Krombach et al. [95] have demonstrated that if lavages are repeatedly performed into the same segment, nonspecific changes are frequently associated with subsequent aspirates.

FNAB has been used to monitor lung transplants under experiment conditions as demonstrated by Hoyer et al. [96] in the dog. The biopsies were performed through a window of partial pleurectomy and confirmed by open biopsy. The group reports similar inflammatory changes in both types of specimens and no complications due to pneumothorax.

Monitoring of Graft-vs-Host Disease in Bone Marrow Recipients

Liver FNAB and lung bronchoalveolar lavage provide a means to analyze these organs during a GVHD episode in bone marrow transplant recipients. Our mostly unpublished experience with more than 100 liver FNABs [97] has demonstrated that the appearance of lymphoid and monocytoid blasts together with activated lymphocytes in the FNAB correlate with clinical GVHD. In bronchoalveolar lavage, relative and absolute lymphocytosis are seen during acute pulmonary complications.

Summary

Transplant aspiration cytology is a new diagnostic and investigative method that has been developed for continuous monitoring of intragraft events in clinical organ transplantation. Worldwide experience has demonstrated that repeated aspiration biopsies of, e.g., human renal allografts make it possible to evaluate the onset, type, size, and duration of the inflammatory episodes of rejection; to monitor concomitant changes in the graft tubular and vascular endothelial components; and to evaluate the impact of immunosuppressive and anti-inflammatory treatment on these parameters. Application of monoclonal marker antibodies may be used to dissect the inflammatory episodes further and to quantitate, e.g., the regulation of MHC antigen expression in the graft or the presence of cyclosporine deposits in the transplant. The technology of FNAB and related cytologic methods have not been developed to replace the needle biopsy: only needle biopsy makes it possible to evaluate the graft comprehensively. FNAB makes it possible to monitor intragraft parameters daily or even more frequently. Thus the two procedures, which yield largely different types of information, should be used together.

References

1. Häyry P, von Willebrand E. Transplant aspiration cytology. Transplantation 1984;38:7–12.
2. Porter KA. Rejection in treated renal allografts. J Clin Pathol 1967;20:518–25.
3. Porter KA, Andres GA, Colder MW, et al. Human renal transplants. II. Immunofluorescent and immunoferritin studies. Lab Invest 1968;18:159–62.
4. Andres GA, Accinni L, Hsu KC, et al. Human renal transplants. III. Immunopathologic studies. Lab Invest 1970;2:558–62.
5. von Willebrand E. Fine needle aspiration cytology of human renal transplant. Clin Immunol Immunopathol 1980;17:309–22.
6. Häyry P, von Willebrand E. Monitoring of human renal allograft rejection with fine-needle aspiration cytology. Scand J Immunol 1981;13:87–97.
7. Häyry P, von Willebrand E. Practical guidelines for fine needle aspiration biopsy of human renal allografts. Ann Clin Res 1981;13:288–306.
8. Häyry P, von Willebrand E, Ahonen J, et al. Monitoring of organ allograft rejection by transplant aspiration cytology. Ann Clin Res 1981;13:264–87.
9. Kreis HA. Use of fine needle aspiration cytology to diagnose rejection. Transplant Proc 1984;16:1569–72.
10. Belitsky P. Transplant fine needle aspiration cytology. Transplant Immunol Lett 1986;3:8–9.
11. Kirby JA, Reader JS, Pepper JR. Lung transplantation: effect of cyclosporine A on the frequency of cytolytic lymphocytes recovered from blood and the bronchoalveolar space. J Heart Transplant 1986;5:33–8.
12. Leskinen R, Tukiainen P, Taskinen E, et al. Bronchoalveolar lavage in the diagnosis of pulmonary complications in bone marrow transplant recipients. Exp Hematol 1984;12(Suppl 15):24–5.
13. Klima G, Spielberger M, Konig P, Margreiter R. Fine needle aspiration biopsy and urinary sediment cytology in renal allograft recipients. Transplant Proc 1985;17:2083–4.
14. Gupta R, Campbell J, Om A, Belitsky P. Serial monitoring of cellular rejection by simultaneous histology and fine needle aspiration cytology. Transplant Proc 1985;17:2123–4.
15. von Willebrand E, Soots A, Häyry P. In situ effector mechanisms in rat kidney allograft rejection. I. Characterization of host cellular infiltrate in rejecting allograft parenchyma. Cell Immunol 1979;46:309–26.
16. Häyry P, von Willebrand E, Soots A. In situ effector mechanisms in rat kidney allograft rejection. III. Kinetics of the inflammatory response and generation of donor-directed killer cells. Scand J Immunol 1979;10:95–108.
17. Hancock WW, Thomson NM, Atkins AF. Composition of interstitial cellular infiltrate identified by monoclonal antibodies in renal biopsies of rejecting human renal allografts. Transplantation 1983;35:458–63.
18. Lautenschlager I, Hockerstedt K, von Willebrand E, et al. Aspiration cytology of a human liver allograft. Transplant Proc 1984;16:1243–6.
19. Wood RFM, Bolton EM, Thompson JF, Morris PJ. Monoclonal antibodies and

fine needle aspiration cytology in detecting renal allograft rejection. Lancet 1982;II:278–80.
20. Bolton EM, Thompson JF, Wood RFM, Morris PJ. Lymphocyte subpopulations in fine needle aspiration biopsies determined by immunoperoxidase staining. In: Kreis H, Droz D, eds. Renal transplant cytology. Milan: Wichtig Editore, 1984;204–9.
21. von Willebrand E. OKT4/8 ratio in the blood and in the graft during episodes of human allograft rejection. Cell Immunol 1983;77:196–201.
22. von Willebrand E, Zola H, Häyry P. Thrombocyte aggregates in renal allografts. Analysis with fine needle aspiration biopsy and monoclonal antithrombocyte antibodies. Transplantation 1985;39:258–62.
23. Häyry P, von Willebrand E, Ahonen J, Eklund B. Do well-to-do and repeatedly rejecting renal allografts express the transplantation antigens similarly on their surface? Scand J Urol Nephrol Suppl 1981;64:52–5.
24. Hall BM, Dugging GG, Philips J, et al. Increased expression of HLA-DR antigens on renal tubular cells in renal transplants: relevance to the rejection response. Lancet 1984;2:247–51.
25. von Willebrand E, Häyry P. Cyclosporine A deposits in renal allografts. Lancet 1983;2:189–92.
26. Carter NP, Bewick ALT, Bolton EM, et al. Flow cytometric analysis of fine needle aspiration biopsies of human renal allografts. In: Kreis H, Droz D, eds. Renal transplant cytology. Milan: Wichtig Editore, 1984:45–55.
27. Koller C, Stadler J, Hammer C, et al. Evaluation of FNAB and TAC by coulter counting. In: Kries H, Droz D, eds. Renal transplant cytology. Milan: Wichtig Editore, 1984:39–44.
28. Wilson RG, Shenton BK, Taylor RM, Proud G. Aspirate cellularity as a rapid indicator of renal allograft rejection. Br J Surg 1986;73:116–7.
29. Pasternack A, Helin H, Tornroth T, et al. Aspiration biopsy of the kidney with a new fine needle: a way to obtain glomeruli for morphological study. Clin Nephrol 1978;10:78–81.
30. Rowden G, Dean S, Campbell J, Belitsky P. Electronmicroscopic analysis of kidney glomeruli obtained by fine needle aspiration. J Electron Microsc Tech 1985;2:547–55.
31. Waugh J, Bishop A, Hall BM, et al. Assessment of fine needle aspiration biopsies from renal transplants using monoclonal antibodies as lymphocyte markers. Transplant Proc 1986;18:267–9.
32. Koller C, Stadler J, Hammer C, et al. Evaluation of FNAB and TAC by coulter counting. In: Kreis H, Droz D, eds. Renal transplant cytology. Milan: Wichtig Editore, 1984:39–44.
33. Kormendi F, Perner F, Beregi E, et al. New corrective calculation to compensate the error of blood contamination in aspiration cytology specimens of human renal allografts. Transplant Proc 1985;17:2075–6.
34. von Willebrand E, Häyry P. Reproducibility of the fine needle aspiration biopsy. Analysis of 93 double biopsies. Transplantation 1984;38:314–6.
35. Belitsky P, Campbell J, Gupta R. Serial biopsy controlled evaluation of fine needle aspiration in renal allograft rejection. Lab Invest 1985;53:580–5.
36. Vereerstraeten P, Romasco F, Monsieur R, et al. Representativeness and reproducibility of WBC counts in fine needle aspiration specimens from kidney transplants. Transplant Proc 1985;17:2106–7.
37. Morris PJ. T cells in the blood and kidney after transplantation. In: Kreis H, Droz D, eds. Renal transplant cytology. Milan: Wichtig Editore, 1984:113–9.
38. Swobodnik W, Spohn B, Schusdziarra V, et al. Ultrasonically targeted fine

needle aspiration cytology in the immediate postoperative followup of transplanted kidneys. Ultraschall Med 1985;6:147–51.
39. Reitamo S, Konttinen YT, Ranki A, Häyry P. The relation of different inflammatory cell types to the various parenchymal components of rejecting kidney allografts. Histopathology 1980;4:517–32.
40. Leskinen R, Häyry P. Topographical distribution of inflammatory leukocyte subsets in acute cellular rejection of a kidney allograft. Acta Pathol Microbiol Scand Sect C 1985;94:69–76.
41. Kolbeck PC, Tatum AH, Sanfilippo F. Relationships among the histologic pattern, intensity, and phenotypes of T cells infiltrating renal allografts. Transplantation 1984;38:709–13.
42. Häyry P. Transplant aspiration cytology. A quality control analysis in 1984. Transplant Proc 1985;17:2100–5.
43. Belitsky P, Gupta R, Campbell J. Diagnosis of acute cellular rejection in kidney allografts by fine needle aspiration cytology. Transplant Proc 1984;16:1076–9.
44. Wahlberg J, Backman U, Frodin L, et al. Fine needle biopsies of renal transplants in clinical rejection monitoring. Uppsala J Med Sci 1985;90:163–8.
45. Ahonen J. Clinical use of FNAB in renal transplantation. In: Kreis H, Droz D, eds. Renal transplant cytology. Milan: Wichtig Editore, 1984:31–5.
46. Häyry P, von Willebrand E. Aspiration cytology in monitoring of human allografts. In: Williams GM, Burdick JF, Solez K, eds. Kidney transplant rejection: diagnosis and treatment. New York: Marcel Dekker, 1986;247–62.
47. Saksela E, Timonen T, Ranki A, Häyry P. Morphological and functional characterization of isolated effector cells responsible for human natural killer cell activity to fetal fibroblasts and to cultured cell line targets. Immunol Rev 1979;44:71–123.
48. Lautenschlager I, von Willebrand E, Häyry P. Blood eosinophilia, steroid and rejection. Transplantation 1985;40:354–7.
49. Smith N, Chandler S, Hawker RJ, et al. Indium-labeled platelets as diagnostic aid after renal transplantation. Lancet 1979;2:1241–2.
50. Leithner OH, Sinzinger H, Angelberger P, Syre P. Indium-111 labeled platelets in chronic kidney transplant rejection. Lancet 1980;2:213–4.
51. Häyry P, von Willebrand E. Transplant aspiration cytology in the evaluation of a renal allograft. In: Touraine JL, ed. Transplantation and clinical immunology, vol XV. Immunosuppression. Amsterdam: Excerpta Medica, 1983;124–37.
52. Häyry P, Ahonen J, von Willebrand E, et al. Effect of cyclosporine A on the in situ inflammatory response of human renal allograft rejection: a preliminary report. Scand J Immunol 1983;16:135–49.
53. Egidi F, Tarantino A, De Vecchi A, Zubani R, Ponticelli C. Patterns of inflammation in fine needle aspiration biopsies in renal transplant patients treated with different immunosuppressive agents. Transplant Proc 1985;17:2091–3.
54. Häyry P, von Willebrand E, Ahonen J, Eklund B. Glucocortisteroids in renal transplantation. I. Impact of high vs. low dose postoperative methyl-prednisolone administration on the first episode(s) of rejection. Scand J Immunol 1982;16:39–49.
55. Vereerstraeten P, Romasco F, Kinnaert P, et al. T cell subset patterns in peripheral blood and in fine needle aspiration lymphocytes after kidney transplantation. Transplant Proc 1985;17:2115–6.
56. Waugh J, Bishop GA, Hall BM, et al. T cell subsets in fine needle aspiration biopsies from renal transplant recipients. Transplant Proc 1985;17:1701–3.
57. Lautenschlager I, von Willebrand E, Häyry P. Does T4 predominance in the graft signify severe rejection? Transplant Proc 1986;18:1311–3.

58. Taube D, Welsh K, Hobby P, Williams DG. Human renal allograft and peripheral blood T lymphocyte subpopulations during the onset and treatment of rejection. Clin Nephrol 1984;22:127–32.
59. Tufveson G, Backman U, Claesson K, et al. Renal transplant cytology: impact of different immunosuppressive protocols and biopsy techniques. Transplant Proc 1985;17:2087–8.
60. Nguyen L, Hammer C, Dendorfer U, et al. Changes in large granular lymphocyte size and number in kidney-transplant patients during rejection and viral infection. Transplant Proc 1985;17:2110–1.
61. von Willebrand E, Pettersson E, Ahonen J, Häyry P. CMV infection, class II antigen expression and human kidney allograft rejection. Transplantation 1986;42:364–7.
62. Ouziala M, Santelli G, Charpentier B, Fries D. Diagnostic value of fine needle aspiration biopsy during viral infections in renal transplant recipients. Transplant Proc 1985;17:2098–9.
63. Surachno S, van Oers MH, Wilmink JM. Early diagnosis of bacterial infection of renal allografts by fine needle aspiration biopsy (letter). Lancet 1986;1:686–7.
64. Wernecke K, Heckemann R, Jakubowski HD. Perirenal masses following kidney transplantation. Ultrasonically guided punctures and aspirate analyses. ROFO 1982;137:403–9.
65. Hildell J, Aspelin P, Nyman U, et al. Ultrasonography in complications of renal transplantation. Acta Radiol (Diagn) (Stockholm) 1984;25:299–304.
66. Droz D, Campos H, Noel LH, et al. Renal transplant fine needle aspiration cytology: correlations to renal histology. In: Kreis H, Droz D, eds. Renal transplant cytology. Milan: Wichtig Editore, 1984;59–65.
67. De Vecchi A, Egidi F, Banfi G, et al. Comparison of fine needle aspiration biopsy and needle biopsy in renal transplantation. In: Kreis H, Droz D, eds. Renal transplant cytology. Milan: Wichtig Editore, 1984;67–72.
68. Koeller C, Hammer C, Gokel JM, et al. Correlation between core biopsy and aspiration cytology. Transplant Proc 1984;16:1298–1300.
69. Bolton EM, Thompson JF, Wood RF, Morris PJ. Immunoperoxidase staining of fine needle aspiration biopsies and needle core biopsies from renal allografts. Transplantation 1983;36:728–31.
70. Cooksey G, Reeve RS, Paterson AD, et al. Lymphocyte subpopulations in cytologic aspirates from human renal allografts. Transplant Proc 1985;17:630–2.
71. Reeve RS, Cooksey G, Wenham PW, et al. A comparison of fine needle aspiration cytology and tru-cut tissue biopsy in the diagnosis of acute renal allograft rejection. Nephron 1986;42:68–71.
72. Egidi F, De Vecchi A, Pagliari B, et al. Lack of relationship between blood cyclosporine levels and nephrotoxicity as assessed by fine needle aspiration biopsy of renal allografts. Transplant Proc 1985;17:2096–7.
73. Santelli G, Ouziala M, Charpentier B, Fries D. Predictive value of fine needle aspiration biopsy for cyclosporine nephrotoxicity. Transplant Proc 1985;17: 2094–5.
74. de Wall RMW, Bogman MJJ, Maass CN, et al. Variable expression of Ia antigens on the vascular endothelium of mouse skin allografts. Nature 1983;303:426–9.
75. Häyry P, von Willebrand E. The influence of the pattern of inflammation and administration of steroids on class II MHC antigen expression in renal transplants. Transplantation 1986;42:358–63.
76. Leszczynski D, Ferry B, Schellekens H, et al. Antagonistic effects of gamma-interferon and steroids on tissue antigenicity. J Exp Med 1986;164:1470–7.

77. Häyry P, Ferry B, Leszczynski D, et al. Generation and breakdown of a vicious cycle in context of acute allograft rejection. Transplant Proc 1986;18(Suppl 4):52–62.
78. Wolff JL, Beaurain G, Campos H, et al. Characterization of T cells cultured from fine needle aspirates of human renal allografts during rejection. Kidney Int 1985;27:469–71.
79. Buurman WA, Doveren RFC, Vanderlinden CJ, Kootstra G. Limiting dilution analysis permits accurate measurement of CTL response in rejection. Transplant Proc 1986;18:745–7.
80. Doveren RFC, Buurman WA, Vanderlinden CJ, et al. Analysis of cytotoxic lymphocyte T response in rejecting allografted canine kidneys. Transplantation 1986;41:33–8.
81. Manca F, Halttunen J, Ferry B, et al. Allospecific rat-mouse hybridoma clones generated from kidney graft infiltrating cells. Transplantation 1987;44:440–2.
82. Manca F, Ferry B, Jaakkola MM, et al. Frequency and functional characterization of specific T helper cells infiltrating rat kidney allografts during acute rejection. Scand J Immunol 1987;25:255–64.
83. Lersch C, Thiel M, Hammer C, et al. Splenic fine needle aspiration cytology in small animals with transplanted tumors. Transplant Proc 1985;17:2132–3.
84. Fill H, Spielberger M, Leidlkair K, Klima G. Nephrography with radioactive hippuran in transplanted kidneys—interpretation, limitations, and usefulness. Eur J Nucl Med 1985;11:171–8.
85. Baillet G, Ballarin J, Urdaneta N, et al. Evaluation of allograft perfusion by radionuclide first-pass study in renal failure following renal transplantation. Eur J Nucl Med 1986;11:463–9.
86. Maury CP, Teppo AM, Ahonen J, von Willebrand E. Measurement of serum amyloid A protein concentrations as test of renal allograft rejection in patients with initially non-functioning grafts. Br Med J 1984;288:360–1.
87. Häyry P, Ahonen J, Kock B, et al. Glucocorticosteroids in renal transplantation. II. Impact of high versus low dose postoperative methyl-prednisolone administration on graft survival and on the frequency and type of complications. Scand J Immunol 1985;19:211–8.
88. Häyry P, von Willebrand E, Ahonen J, et al. Effects of cyclosporine, azathioprine and steroids on the renal transplant, on the cytological patterns of intragraft inflammation and on concomitant rejection-associated changes in the recipient blood. Transplant Proc 1988;20:153–62.
89. Vogel W, Margreiter R, Schalzl F, Judmaier G. Preliminary results with fine needle aspiration biopsy in liver grafts. Transplant Proc 1984;16:1240–2.
90. Lautenschlager I, Hockerstedt K, Taskinen E, et al. Fine needle aspiration cytology of liver allografts in the pig. Transplantation 1984;38:330–4.
91. Baumgartner D, Buerger H, Rubelli M, Mona D. Changes in pancreatic aspiration cytology induced by duct obliteration. In: Kreis H, Droz D, eds. Renal transplant cytology. Milan: Wichtig Editore, 1984:167–71.
92. Steiner E, Hammer C, Land W, et al. Fine needle biopsy of canine pancreas graft—an attempt at cytologic diagnosis in graft rejection. Transplant Proc 1984:16:789–90.
93. Hunninghake GW, Gadek JE, Kawanami O, et al. Inflammatory and immune processes in the human lung in health and disease: evaluation by bronchoalveolar lavage. Am J Pathol 1979;97:149–52.
94. Schorer C, Konig G, Hammer C, et al. Monitoring of pulmonary inflammation by bronchoalveolar lavage. Transplant Proc 1985;17:2137–9.

95. Krombach F, Konig G, Wanders A, et al. Effect of repeated bronchoalveolar lavage on free lung cells and peripheral leukocytes. Transplant Proc 1985; 17:2134–6.
96. Hoyer J, Sellin D, Keck H, Kotschau H. Value of fine needle aspiration biopsy in allogeneic lung transplantation in dogs. Transplant Proc 1986;17:2130–1.
97. Leskinen R, Volin L, Taskinen E, et al. Monitoring of bone marrow transplant recipient liver by fine needle aspiration biopsy. Transplant Proc 1986;18:115–6.

Index